ACSM's
Certification
Review

FIFTH EDITION

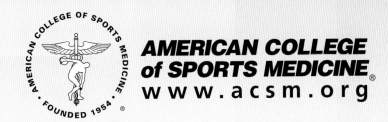

AMERICAN COLLEGE
of SPORTS MEDICINE®
w w w . a c s m . o r g ®

ACSM's
Certification
Review

FIFTH EDITION

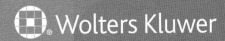 Wolters Kluwer

Philadelphia • Baltimore • New York • London
Buenos Aires • Hong Kong • Sydney • Tokyo

Executive Editor: Michael Nobel
Senior Product Development Editor: Amy Millholen
Marketing Manager: Shauna Kelley
Designer: Stephen Druding
Production Project Manager: David Saltzberg
Manufacturing Coordinator: Margie Orzech
Compositor: Absolute Service, Inc.

ACSM Committee on Certification and Registry Boards Chair: William Simpson, PhD, FACSM
ACSM Publications Committee Chair: Jeffrey A. Potteiger, PhD, FACSM
ACSM Group Publisher: Katie Feltman

Fifth Edition

9 8 7 6 5 4 3 2 1

Printed in China

Library of Congress Cataloging-in-Publication Data

Names: Churilla, James R., editor. | Bosak, Andrew, editor. | Montes,
  Brittany, editor. | Sorace, Paul, editor. | American College of Sports
  Medicine.
Title: ACSM's certification review / senior editor, James R. Churilla ;
  associate editors, Andrew Bosak, Brittany Montes, Paul Sorace.
Description: Fifth edition. | Philadelphia : Wolters Kluwer Health, [2018] |
  Includes bibliographical references and index.
Identifiers: LCCN 2016052001 | ISBN 9781496338778
Subjects: | MESH: Sports Medicine | Certification | Exercise | Physical
  Fitness | Examination Questions | Case Reports
Classification: LCC RC1210 | NLM QT 18.2 | DDC 617.1/027076—dc23 LC record
available at https://lccn.loc.gov/2016052001

DISCLAIMER

Care has been taken to confirm the accuracy of the information present and to describe generally accepted practices. However, the authors, editors, and publisher are not responsible for errors or omissions or for any consequences from application of the information in this publication and make no warranty, expressed or implied, with respect to the currency, completeness, or accuracy of the contents of the publication. Application of this information in a particular situation remains the professional responsibility of the practitioner; the clinical treatments described and recommended may not be considered absolute and universal recommendations.

The authors, editors, and publisher have exerted every effort to ensure that drug selection and dosage set forth in this text are in accordance with the current recommendations and practice at the time of publication. However, in view of ongoing research, changes in government regulations, and the constant flow of information relating to drug therapy and drug reactions, the reader is urged to check the package insert for each drug for any change in indications and dosage and for added warnings and precautions. This is particularly important when the recommended agent is a new or infrequently employed drug.

Some drugs and medical devices presented in this publication have Food and Drug Administration (FDA) clearance for limited use in restricted research settings. It is the responsibility of the health care provider to ascertain the FDA status of each drug or device planned for use in their clinical practice.

As an undergraduate student at Wake Forest University, I took my first American College of Sports Medicine (ACSM) certification examination in 1978 — which I had to retake in 1979! The experience of being certified by ACSM was one of the great accomplishments of my young career and helped me get my first job with Dr. Noel Nequin at Swedish Covenant Hospital in Chicago. Under Noel's guidance and urging, I became certified as an ACSM program director for Preventive and Rehabilitative Exercise Programs (which is no longer an ACSM certification) in 1983. At about that same time (1981), I was invited to sit on the ACSM Certification and Education Committee (now known as the Committee on Certification and Registry Boards [CCRB]), and I have held various positions on that committee for more than 30 years. For six of those years, I served as the chair. During those 30 years, there has been an exponential growth in the number of certification candidates and in the resources being provided to certification candidates.

This fifth edition of *ACSM's Certification Review* follows the comprehensive update from the fourth edition. Senior Editor James R. Churilla and his talented team of associate editors (Andrew Bosak, Brittany Montes, and Paul Sorace) and writers have updated the quintessential review for ACSM Certified Personal Trainer (CPT), ACSM Exercise Physiologist-Certified (EP-C), and ACSM Certified Clinical Exercise Physiologist (CEP). Although the scope of this fifth edition targets these three certifications, the ACSM Certified Group Exercise Instructor, ACSM Registered Clinical Exercise Physiologist, and those preparing for the Exercise is Medicine® Credential will also find this book to be very useful.

The fifth edition maintains the strategic organization of three parts for each certification — cases for each certification, a detailed breakdown of the knowledge and skills for each certification, and sample questions that are similar to those found on each certification examination. One of the more unique features of this edition is the cases, which are organized within the text according to the domains, a result of the recent job task analysis. The four domains include health and fitness assessment (initial client consultation and assessment for CPT, health and fitness assessment for EP-C, and patient/client assessment for CEP); exercise programming (exercise programming and implementation for CPT, exercise prescription and implementation for EP-C, and exercise prescription for CEP); exercise counseling and behavioral strategies (exercise leadership and client education for CPT, exercise counseling and behavioral strategies for EP-C, and program implementation for CEP); program administration (legal/professional/business/marketing for CPT, management for EP-C, and leadership and counseling for CEP); and legal and professional considerations for all three certifications.

JC, Andy, Brittany, and Paul will receive much praise for the contents of this book and their professional approach to providing for certification candidates the very best resource to prepare for their examinations. For me, it is a simple "thank you" to them for their dedication and their friendship. To present and future certification candidates — this book will be your guide to success.

Walter R. Thompson, PhD, FACSM
Regents Professor
Department of Kinesiology and Health
(College of Education) and
Division of Nutrition
(Byrdine F. Lewis School of Nursing and
Health Professions)
Georgia State University
Atlanta, Georgia

Preface

This fifth edition of the *ACSM's Certification Review* has been extensively revised from previous editions of this text. This edition covers all the current knowledge and skills (KSs) for the certifications of the Certified Personal Trainer (CPT), the Certified Exercise Physiologist (EP-C), and the Certified Clinical Exercise Physiologist (CEP).

TEXT ORGANIZATION

This text is organized into parts by certification level and is further subdivided into three main sections in each part as follows:

- **Case studies** that involve both multiple-choice questions as well as open-ended discussion questions are divided by certification level and domain. There are 21 case studies (and 13 accompanying electrocardiograms [ECGs]) in the book.
- **Job task analysis (JTA) tables** that contain a detailed breakdown of all the KSs by certification level and domain. In this section, there is a further breakdown of what each KSs statement refers to as well as helpful study resources for each KSs. The KSs section was extensively impacted by the recent ACSM JTA that was performed on all certification levels.
- **Practice examinations**, one for each certification, contain 100 multiple-choice practice questions with answers and explanations. At the end of each exam, a table indicates which questions in that practice test correspond to which domain(s).

STUDYING FOR A CERTIFICATION EXAM

The many individuals involved in the preparation of this text intend that it be used as a review aid for the certification exams and assume that the reader is actively preparing to sit for one of the three ACSM certifications covered. This text represents one of many study tools available and should not be viewed as the sole source of information to use in preparing to take one of these three certification exams.

As a study or review tool, this text may help you clarify areas of strengths and weaknesses. Your individual weaknesses should be eliminated by further study. This text should be viewed as part of a study kit that each of you needs to identify for yourself. Certainly, *ACSM's Guidelines for Exercise Testing and Prescription*, Tenth Edition (*GETP10*) must be considered as part of that package.

ACSM certification levels build upon one another. For instance, the CEP certification encompasses all EP-C and CPT KSs. Thus, individuals who intend to use this book to review for the CEP certification are responsible for all KSs covered in the EP-C and CPT sections as well as all KSs covered in the CEP section. Similarly, individuals preparing for the EP-C certification are responsible for all KSs covered in the CPT section.

We are aware that facts, standards, and guidelines change on a regular basis in this ever growing field of knowledge. Hence, in the event that conflict may be noted between this book and the *GETP10*, the latter text should be used as the **definitive and final resource**. In such cases, where an update is needed or where a conflict or error is identified, we will make every effort to provide further explanations or corrections online. The web address for any corrections is http://certification.acsm.org/updates

If I can play a small role in your ACSM certification success, I would feel truly happy that all the hard work put into this project has paid off.

**James R. Churilla, PhD, MPH, MS, FACSM, ACSM-PD,
ACSM-RCEP, ACSM-CEP, ACSM EP-C**
Senior Editor

ADDITIONAL RESOURCES

ACSM's Certification Review, Fifth Edition, includes additional resources for instructors that are available on the book's companion Web site at http://thepoint.lww.com/ACSMCR5e. In previous editions, there was an appendix featuring images and other supporting content from related ACSM titles. We are now providing that as a digital resource that can be found on the book's page on thePoint®.

Instructors

Approved adopting instructors will be given access to the following additional resource:

- Image bank

Acknowledgments

I owe a great deal of gratitude to a number of people who have helped me throughout my life. I have been privileged to work as a fitness professional and academician during my 28-year professional career. To all my friends and colleagues who have believed in me, supported me, and help guide me along the way, I say thank you. There are two special individuals that I need to personally thank, Dr. Anthony Abbott and Dr. Ed Howley. Dr. Abbott's no nonsense approach to fitness education and training is unequivocally the best. Dr. Howley's approach to teaching, research, and developing people should be modeled by all academia. Thank you both for your mentorship and friendship, I would never have enjoyed the level of success I have as a fitness professional and academic professional without these two great people. I would like to thank my three associate editors for their willingness to be part of this book and their expertise. Brittany, Andy, and Paul, I chose you three because of my experiences with you, and I knew you would exceed my expectations, and you did. To all my chapter contributors, both new and returning, you all stepped up and delivered an excellent, relevant work that will help people in preparing for ACSM certifications for years to come. To everyone who contributed new practice examination questions, this is not an easy task, but each of you submitted excellent case studies and questions. Thank you to Katie and everyone on her team at ACSM and Wolters Kluwer Health/Lippincott Williams & Wilkins for their support on this project.

This project would not have been possible without the support of my family. I would like to thank my wife Mirtha and my two boys Cameron and Tyler for their love and support every day.

—James R. Churilla

First, I want to thank Dr. James Churilla, ACSM, and the textbook publishers for giving me the chance to be a part of this exceptional project and process. Working with Dr. Churilla has been a blessing and his attention to detail and hardworking mentality is second to none! Second, a massive thank you goes to the case study authors and the self-test question writers as their efforts contributed a great deal. My participation in this project would not have been possible without my family and former professors. Many thanks to my professors and mentors who contributed to my academic training and career. Finally, I owe a lifetime of gratitude to my wife (Betsy), children (Katherine, Evan, Dylan, Megan, and Robyn), parents (Walter and Laramie), and the Lord, who constantly provide love and support while giving me the inspiration and opportunity to work in this extraordinary field.

—Andrew Bosak

A special thank you to all the individuals who stewarded their time and gifts to such an important project. To my graduate mentor, Dr. James Churilla, I am exceptionally grateful for the incredible and humbling opportunity you provided me to be a part of this project. You have a very special gift of infusing fervor into your students through your teaching, thank you. To my mentor, sounding-board, and dearest friend Dr. Barbara Bushman, thank you for your guidance and encouragement over the years. Finally, to my very best friend and husband Jonathan, thank you for your love, steadfast encouragement, and support in all I pursue.

—Brittany Montes

I want to give a special thanks to the contributing authors and the self-test question writers. Their contributions helped make this book such an asset for ACSM certification candidates. I want to say thank you to Tom LaFontaine, PhD, FACSM. Tom took me under his wing when I was just starting my career as an exercise professional. His mentoring as an exercise professional, author and editor played a signifcant role in my professional development. I also want to thank Dr. James Churilla for leading the development of this new edition of *ACSM's Certification Review*. I value our professional relationship and more importantly our friendship.

—Paul Sorace

Contributing Authors to the Fifth Edition*

Clinton A. Brawner, PhD, MS, FACSM, ACSM-RCEP, ACSM-CEP

Henry Ford Hospital
Detroit, Michigan
Cases: Domain of Patient/Client Assessment for CEP
(Electrocardiograms)

Melissa Conway-Hartman, MEd, LAT, ATC, ACSM EP-C

Brooks College of Health
University of North Florida
Jacksonville, Florida
Cases: Domain on Exercise Leadership and Client Education of
CPT, Domain on Legal, Professional, Business, and Marketing
of CPT, Domain on Exercise Counseling and Behavioral
Strategies of EP-C

Donald M. Cummings, PhD

East Stroudsburg University
East Stroudsburg, Pennsylvania
Cases: Domain of Exercise Prescription for CEP

Shala E. Davis, PhD, FACSM

East Stroudsburg University
East Stroudsburg, Pennsylvania
Cases: Domain of Leadership and Counseling for CEP

Shawn Drake, PT, PhD, ACSM-RCEP, ACSM-PD, ACSM-CEP

Arkansas State University
Jonesboro, Arkansas
Cases: Domain of Exercise Prescription and Implementation
for EP-C

Trent A. Hargens, PhD, FACSM, ACSM-CEP

James Madison University
Harrisonburg, Virginia
Cases: Domain of Patient/Client Assessment for CEP

Shenelle E. Higbee, MS, ACSM-RCEP, ACSM-CEP, ACSM EP-C

PeaceHealth St. Joseph Medical Center
Bellingham, Washington
Cases: Domain of Legal and Professional Considerations of CEP

Dennis Kerrigan, PhD, ACSM-CEP

Henry Ford Hospital
Detroit, Michigan
Cases: Domain of Patient/Client Assessment for CEP
(Electrocardiograms)

Frederick Klinge, MBA, ACSM EP-C

Ochsner Health System/Varsity Sports
New Orleans, Louisiana
Cases: Domain of Management for EP-C

Angela Kvies, BS, ACSM-CEP

Cardiac/Pulmonary Rehabilitation
Baptist Medical Center Beaches
Jacksonville, Florida
Cases: Domain on Exercise Leadership and Client Education of CPT

Brittany C. Montes, MSH, ACSM-CEP, ACSM EP-C

Brooks College of Health
University of North Florida
Jacksonville, Florida
Cases: Domain on Exercise Programming and Implementation
of CPT

Matthew W. Parrott, PhD, ACSM EP-C

H-P Fitness, LLC
Kansas City, Missouri
Cases: Domain of Legal and Professional for EP-C

Will Peveler, PhD

Northern Kentucky University
Highland Heights, Kentucky
Cases: Domain on Health and Fitness Assessment of EP-C

M. Ryan Richardson, MSH, ACSM EP-C

Brooks College of Health
University of North Florida
Jacksonville, Florida
Cases: Domain of Initial Client Consultation and Assessment of CPT

Joselyn M. Rodriguez, MSH, ACSM EP-C

Cardiopulmonary Rehabilitation and H.E.A.R.T. Fitness
Memorial Hospital
Jacksonville, Florida
Cases: Domain on Exercise Prescription of CEP

Peter Ronai, MS, FACSM, ACSM-RCEP, ACSM-CEP

Sacred Heart University
Fairfield, Connecticut
Cases: Domain on Exercise Programming and Implementation
of CPT

Mandy J. Van Hofwegen, BS, ACSM-RCEP, ACSM-CEP

PeaceHealth St. Joseph Medical Center
Bellingham, Washington
Cases: Domain of Legal and Professional Considerations of CEP

David E. Verrill, MS, FAACVPR

University of North Carolina at Charlotte
Charlotte, North Carolina
Cases: Domain of Program Implementation and Ongoing
Support for CEP, Domain on Exercise Prescription of CEP

*See Appendix B for a list of contributors to the previous two editions.

Reviewers for the Fifth Edition

Mindy Caplan, ACSM EP-C
Yoga by Julie
Albuquerque, New Mexico

Ashley Haave, BS
Medtronic
Tacoma, Washington

Aimee Katona, ACSM-CEP, ACSM EP-C
University of Michigan Health System
Canton, Michigan

Jessica Keudell, BS
Epic Fitness
Silverton, Oregon

Carrie Oestreich, ACSM-CEP
Veterans Health Administration
Ann Arbor, Michigan

Holly Winchel, BS, ACSM-CEP
Mayo Clinic Health System
Sparta, Wisconsin

Review Question Contributors to the Fifth Edition

Travis Armstrong, BS, ACSM-CEP, ACSM EP-C, ACSM EIM II

HealthLink Fitness & Wellness Center
Baptist Health System
San Antonio, Texas

Robert Berry MS, ACSM-CEP, ACSM-RCEP

Henry Ford Health System
Detroit, Michigan

Melissa Conway-Hartman, MEd, LAT, ATC, ACSM EP-C

Brooks College of Health
University of North Florida
Jacksonville, Florida

Gregory B. Dwyer, PhD, ACSM-CEP, RCEP, ETT, PD, EIMIII, FACSM

East Stroudsburg University
East Stroudsburg, Pennsylvania

Michael A. Figueroa, EdD

William Paterson University
Wayne, New Jersey

Amanda K. Hovey, BS, ACSM-CEP, ACSM EP-C

Olmsted Medical Center
Rochester, Minnesota

Kevin Huet, MS, EP-C, CSCS

Kennesaw State University
Kennesaw, Georgia

Dana Killefer, MS, ACSM-RCEP

Touro Infirmary Cardiac and Pulmonary Rehabilitation and
    Wellness Center
New Orleans, Louisiana

Thomas P. Mahady, MS, CSCS

Center for Cardiac Prevention and Rehabilitation
Hackensack University Medical Center
Hackensack, New Jersey

Joseph A. Mychalczuk, MS, ACSM-RCEP

Sacred Heart University
Fairfield, Connecticut

Matthew Owens, MS, ACSM-CEP

East Stroudsburg University
East Stroudsburg, Pennsylvania

Will Peveler, PhD

Northern Kentucky University
Highland Heights, Kentucky

Greg Ryan, PhD, CSCS

Georgia Southern University
Statesboro, Georgia

Natalie Santillo, BS, MS

Precision Sports Performance
East Hanover, New Jersey

Brianna Trump, MS, ACSM-CEP

East Stroudsburg University
East Stroudsburg, Pennsylvania

David E. Verrill, MS, FAACVPR

University of North Carolina at Charlotte
Charlotte, North Carolina

Brianna Wells, MS, CSCS

Henry Mayo Fitness and Health
Valencia, California

Contents

Foreword / v
Preface / vi
Acknowledgments / vii
Contributing Authors to the Fifth Edition / viii
Reviewers for the Fifth Edition / ix
Review Question Contributors to the Fifth Edition / x

PART 1 ACSM CERTIFIED PERSONAL TRAINER (CPT) / 1

Associate Editor: Brittany Montes, MSH, ACSM-CEP, ACSM EP-C

Section 1   CPT Case Studies / 3

Case Study CPT.I / 3
Case Study CPT.II(1) / 4
Case Study CPT.II(2) / 6
Case Study CPT.III(1) / 8
Case Study CPT.III(2) / 9
Case Study CPT.IV / 11
CPT Case Studies Answers and Explanations / 12

Section 2   CPT Job Task Analysis / 21

Domain I: Initial Client Consultation and Assessment / 21
Domain II: Exercise Programming and Implementation / 29
Domain III: Exercise Leadership and Client Education / 41
Domain IV: Legal, Professional, Business, and Marketing / 46

Section 3   CPT Examination / 59

CPT Examination Answers and Explanations / 67
CPT Examination Questions by Domain / 77

PART 2 ACSM CERTIFIED EXERCISE PHYSIOLOGIST (EP-C) / 79

Associate Editor: Andrew Bosak, PhD, ACSM EP-C

Section 4   EP-C Case Studies / 81

Case Study EP-C.I / 81
Case Study EP-C.II / 83
Case Study EP-C.III / 84
Case Study EP-C.IV / 85
Case Study EP-C.V / 87
EP-C Case Studies Answers and Explanations / 90

Section 5   EP-C Job Task Analysis / 97

Domain I: Health and Fitness Assessment / 97
Domain II: Exercise Prescription, Implementation, and Ongoing Support / 106
Domain III: Exercise Counseling and Behavioral Strategies / 121
Domain IV: Legal and Professional / 126
Domain V: Management / 130

Section 6   EP-C Examination / 135

EP-C Examination Answers and Explanations / 143
EP-C Examination Questions by Domain / 153

PART 3 ACSM CERTIFIED CLINICAL EXERCISE PHYSIOLOGIST (CEP) / 155

Associate Editor: Paul Sorace, MS, FACSM, ACSM-RCEP

Section 7   CEP Case Studies / 157

Case Study CEP.I / 157
Case Study CEP.II(1) / 158
Case Study CEP.II(2) / 161
Case Study CEP.II(3) / 163
Case Study CEP.II(4) / 165
Case Study CEP.II(5) / 167
Case Study CEP.III / 169
Case Study CEP.IV / 172
Case Study CEP.V(1) / 173
Case Study CEP.V(2) / 174

ECG Case Studies / 175

CEP.ECG(1) / 175
CEP.ECG(2) / 176
CEP.ECG(3) / 177
CEP.ECG(4) / 178
CEP.ECG(5) / 178
CEP.ECG(6) / 179
CEP.ECG(7) / 180
CEP.ECG(8) / 180
CEP.ECG(9) / 181
CEP.ECG(10) / 182
CEP.ECG(11) / 182
CEP.ECG(12) / 183
CEP.ECG(13) / 184
CEP Case Studies Answers and Explanations / 185
ECG Case Studies Answers and Explanations / 202

Section 8   CEP Job Task Analysis / 207
Domain I: Patient/Client Assessment / 207
Domain II: Exercise Prescription / 214
Domain III: Program Implementation and Ongoing Support / 219
Domain IV: Leadership and Counseling / 226
Domain V: Legal and Professional Considerations / 231

Section 9   CEP Examination / 235
CEP Examination Answers and Explanations / 244
CEP Examination Questions by Domain / 253

Appendix A Editors for the Previous Two Editions / 255

Appendix B Contributors to the Previous Two Editions / 257

Index / 261

PART

1

ACSM Certified Personal Trainer (CPT)

BRITTANY MONTES, MSH, ACSM-CEP, ACSM EP-C
Associate Editor

CPT Case Studies

DOMAIN I: INITIAL CLIENT CONSULTATION AND ASSESSMENT

CASE STUDY
CPT.I

Author: **M. Ryan Richardson, MSH**
Author's Certifications: **ACSM EP-C**

You have been assigned a new client, Bill (62 yr old), by your health club manager. Bill would like to begin a guided exercise program focused on his goals of weight loss and becoming more active. During your initial appointment with Bill, you perform routine health assessment revealing the following information:

Height	6 ft 2 in
Weight	255 lb
Body mass index (BMI)	32.7 kg $\cdot$ m^{-2}
Resting blood pressure (BP)	136/86 mm Hg
Resting heart rate (HR$_{rest}$)	82 bpm
Lipids	High-density lipoprotein (HDL): 47; low-density lipoprotein (LDL): 128; triglycerides: 132 (all mg $\cdot$ dL^{-1})
Fasting blood glucose	114 mg $\cdot$ dL^{-1}
Family history	Bill informs you that his father had a coronary revascularization procedure at the age of 58 yr; this procedure is referred to as a coronary artery bypass graft, often referred to as a CABG. His mother died from cancer at 76 yr of age and his younger brother had a myocardial infarction (heart attack) at age 56 yr.
Smoking status	Never smoked
Current medications	Lipitor, a statin drug used to treat high cholesterol Zestril, an angiotensin-converting enzyme (ACE) inhibitor used to treat high BP and heart failure Prilosec, an antacid drug used to treat heartburn, stomach ulcers, and gastroesophageal reflux disease Advil, a nonsteroidal anti-inflammatory drug Bill occasionally takes to treat back and joint pain
Exercise history and/or sedentary lifestyle	Played golf, using a powered golf cart, two times per week until a back injury 5 yr ago; played baseball and football in high school
Surgeries	Bill had his gallbladder removed 2 yr ago. He also had an endoscopic outpatient procedure to treat his stomach ulcer 1 yr ago. He reports no orthopedic surgeries or active injuries other than occasional low back pain following activities like yard work.

Bill is interested in lower intensity exercise due to his concerns regarding joint pain in his lower back and extremities. His stated goal is to lose a minimum of 30 lb. At the conclusion of the initial appointment, you decide on a combination of resistance training using machines and body weight exercises and aerobic exercise on the treadmill and recumbent bicycle. He will also begin a stretching program with a focus on the lower back and extremities.

MULTIPLE-CHOICE QUESTIONS FOR CASE STUDY CPT.I

1. Bill should be characterized as meeting all defining criteria for American College of Sports Medicine (ACSM) risk factors for atherosclerotic cardiovascular disease, *except*
   A) Hypertension
   B) Obesity
   C) Sedentary lifestyle
   D) Family history

2. According to his history and goals, your next session would occur when?
   A) Immediately, including high-intensity exercise
   B) Immediately, only for resistance training
   C) After meeting with the dietician
   D) After medical clearance has been obtained

3. Based on Bill's fasting glucose level, he would be classified as
   A) Normal
   B) Prediabetic
   C) Hypoglycemic
   D) Diabetic

4. What would be Bill's estimated maximum HR (using the formula 220 − age)?
   A) 145 bpm
   B) 158 bpm
   C) 186 bpm
   D) Cannot be determined

5. Based on Bill's lipid profile, he would be classified as
   A) Normal
   B) Hyperlipidemic
   C) Dyslipidemic
   D) At risk for atherosclerosis

DISCUSSION QUESTIONS FOR CASE STUDY CPT.I

You have reviewed Bill's history and received his informed consent, and the medical clearance has been obtained for the possible inclusion of vigorous intensity exercise. You now decide to perform a fitness assessment.

1. Identify appropriate fitness assessments and explain why these are appropriate protocols.

2. Use the Karvonen heart rate reserve (HRR) formula to calculate the training HR range for Bill during his initial training phase for aerobic exercise. Discuss the reasoning for choosing this training range.

DOMAIN II: EXERCISE PROGRAMMING AND IMPLEMENTATION

CASE STUDY CPT.II(1)

Author: **Brittany C. Montes, MSH**
Author's Certifications: **ACSM-CEP, ACSM EP-C**

You are a CPT at a local fitness center and have acquired a new client, Marie, a fit young woman and expectant mother currently in her first trimester. She has recently joined your facility and feels that exercising in an environment with other people around would give her peace of mind. She informs you that she was a collegiate cross-country runner and prefers outdoor activity but would like an exercise prescription that includes aerobic, resistance, and balance activities modified for pregnancy. Marie expresses to you that although she hopes to maintain as much of her fitness as possible throughout her pregnancy, her main goals are to maintain her health and the health of her baby. She enjoys running in the morning with her husband for anywhere between 30 and 45 min (approximately 150–225 min · wk^{-1}) 5 d · wk^{-1} and performs additional full-body resistance training at 40%–60% of her one repetition maximum (1-RM); this has been her exercise routine for the previous 3 yr. She hands you the bottom portion of the *PARmed-X for Pregnancy Health Evaluation Form* with her obstetrician's signature and comment reading, "No contraindications." You have the following information:

Age	27
Height	5 ft 7 in (67 in)
Weight	130 lb (59.1 kg)
BMI	$20.4 \text{ kg} \cdot \text{m}^{-2}$
Resting BP	110/60 mm Hg
HR_{rest}	62 bpm
LDL cholesterol (LDL-C)	$86 \text{ mg} \cdot \text{dL}^{-1}$
HDL cholesterol (HDL-C)	$89 \text{ mg} \cdot \text{dL}^{-1}$
Total cholesterol	$175 \text{ mg} \cdot \text{dL}^{-1}$
Fasting glucose	$90 \text{ mg} \cdot \text{dL}^{-1}$
Current medication use	None; daily vitamin supplements

MULTIPLE-CHOICE QUESTIONS FOR CASE STUDY CPT.II(1)

1. Which of the following is an appropriate frequency, intensity, time, and type (FITT) exercise prescription for Marie?
   A) Continue with current aerobic program of moderate intensity running for $150–225 \text{ min} \cdot \text{wk}^{-1}$. Use resistance bands, machines, and body weight exercises in place of free weights and perform high repetition sets (12–15 repetitions) to moderate fatigue at 40%–60% of estimated 1-RM. Include at least 10 min $2–3 \text{ d} \cdot \text{wk}^{-1}$ of flexibility exercise.
   B) Decrease current aerobic program to a maximum of $150 \text{ min} \cdot \text{wk}^{-1}$. Include resistance exercises targeting large muscle groups at a frequency of $3 \text{ d} \cdot \text{wk}^{-1}$ and intensity of 50%–80% of estimated 1-RM; three sets of 8–10 repetitions using free weights should be performed. Include at least 10 min $2–3 \text{ d} \cdot \text{wk}^{-1}$ of flexibility exercise.
   C) Continue with current aerobic program of moderate intensity running for $150–225 \text{ min} \cdot \text{wk}^{-1}$. Include resistance exercises targeting large muscle groups at a frequency of $3 \text{ d} \cdot \text{wk}^{-1}$ and intensity of 50%–80% of estimated 1-RM; three sets of 8–10 repetitions using free weights should be performed. Include at least 10 min $2–3 \text{ d} \cdot \text{wk}^{-1}$ of flexibility exercise.
   D) Decrease current aerobic program to a maximum of $150 \text{ min} \cdot \text{wk}^{-1}$. Use resistance bands, machines, and body weight exercises in place of free weights and perform high repetition sets (12–15 repetitions) to moderate fatigue at 40%–60% of estimated 1-RM. Include at least 10 min $2–3 \text{ d} \cdot \text{wk}^{-1}$ of flexibility exercise.

2. Which of the following would be a safe exercise testing assessment for Marie if she has an uncomplicated pregnancy?
   A) Submaximal cycle ergometer testing; YMCA cycle ergometer protocol
   B) Maximal treadmill test using a Bruce protocol
   C) Submaximal treadmill test using a modified Balke protocol
   D) Both A and C

3. All of the following are appropriate exercise modifications during pregnancy for Marie *except*
   A) Swim, cycle, or elliptical trainer if low back pain or joint pain occur
   B) Transition from using free weights to weight machines and resistance bands
   C) Decrease aerobic activity from moderate-vigorous to light activity only
   D) Run on a treadmill or track instead of a sidewalk

4. Which of the following is an appropriate method of monitoring exercise intensity for Marie?
   A) %HRR or %HR max (*i.e.*, target HR)
   B) The talk test
   C) $\%\dot{V}O_2R$ (*i.e.*, target $\dot{V}O_2$)
   D) Rating of perceived exertion (RPE)
   E) Both B and D

5. All of the following are warning signs to terminate exercise during pregnancy *except*
   A) Severe dizziness or headache
   B) Chest pain
   C) Calf pain or swelling
   D) Increased fetal movement

DISCUSSION QUESTIONS FOR CASE STUDY CPT.II(1)

1. What changes can Marie expect in her fitness level over the duration of her pregnancy?

2. Why is it important that women not perform any exercises in the supine position after the first trimester?

DOMAIN II: EXERCISE PROGRAMMING AND IMPLEMENTATION

CASE STUDY CPT.II(2)

Author: **Peter Ronai, MS, FACSM**
Author's Certifications: **ACSM-RCEP, ACSM-CEP**

You are a CPT at a corporate fitness center, and Roger, a 50-yr-old architect, is a new client who has recently joined your facility. He is seeking his initial fitness evaluation and first workout session. He is 5 ft 7 in and weighs 220 lb (100 kg). His waist circumference is 40.5 in, and his hip circumference is 37 in. Roger is a nonsmoker with an HR_{rest} of 74 bpm, BP of 132/82 mm Hg, total cholesterol of 200 mg $\cdot$ dL^{-1}, HDL-C of 45 mg $\cdot$ dL^{-1}, LDL-C of 121 mg $\cdot$ dL^{-1}, triglycerides of 170 mg $\cdot$ dL^{-1}, and fasting glucose of 90 mg $\cdot$ dL^{-1}. His father and mother are in their 70s and are apparently healthy.

These are the results of his initial screening and fitness assessment with you.

Predicted $\dot{V}O_{2max}$ YMCA bike test	31.5 mL $\cdot$ kg $\cdot$ min^{-1} or 9 metabolic equivalents (METs) Some low back and leg pain at the end of test which he alleviated by standing and gently leaning backward
Flexibility/sit and reach with a ruler	15 in; he experienced some low back and leg pain after the test, which he alleviated by standing and gently leaning backward (above average)
1-RM bench/chest press (selectorized machine)	150 lb; 40th percentile (fair)
1-RM leg press (selectorized machine)	300 lb; 35th percentile (below average)
Pull-ups/chin-ups	2 repetitions (poor)
Push-ups	9 repetitions (fair)
ACSM Abdominal Crunch Test	23 repetitions He experienced some low back and leg pain after the test, alleviated by standing and gently leaning backward (above average).
Surgeries	None Occasional low back pain that his physician has defined as chronic and has cleared him to participate in a comprehensive exercise program
Contraindications to exercise	None

During additional preactivity screening, Roger had difficulty holding his extended arms directly overhead without arching his back, pushing his head and neck forward, and flexing at his waist when performing a series of overhead squats. He also seemed to become very knock kneed (genu valgus) during the descent phase of the overhead squat. He also stands with a forward head, rounded shoulders, and an anteriorly tilted pelvis. Roger does not currently have back pain; however, he did have some low back and leg pain after the bike test, sit-and-reach test, and the abdominal crunch test, which was alleviated by standing and gently leaning backward.

Upon discussing his medical history, Roger reports occasionally taking Advil for low back pain. His physician told him that he has slight degeneration of a disc in his low back and metabolic syndrome. He wants him to get in shape and lose weight before he considers placing Roger on medications.

His current activity includes walking his energetic 5-mo-old black Labrador retriever, Midas, for about 2 miles (approximately 40 min) daily, a 3-MET activity. Additionally, he plays seasonal golf and softball, and he used to play three-on-three basketball 2 yr ago, an activity he would like to be able to participate in again. He often feels "tired all over" after walking Midas and hopes that a structured exercise routine that combines endurance training and full-body strength training will help him lose weight and stay healthy, making walking Midas easier, improving his golf game, and enabling him to start playing basketball again.

MULTIPLE-CHOICE QUESTIONS FOR CASE STUDY CPT.II(2)

1. Based on Roger's profile, the initial phase of his resistance training program should include (all RPE values refer to a 10-point scale):
   A) Training each muscle group for 3–6 sets with 3–5 repetitions at a high intensity of ≥85% of 1-RM per set, with a rest interval of 5 min between sets at an RPE of 8–9.
   B) Training each muscle group for 2 sets with 15–25 repetitions at a low intensity of ≤50% of 1-RM per set, with a rest interval of 1 min between sets at an RPE of 3–4.
   C) Training each muscle group for 2–4 sets with 8–12 repetitions at a moderate to high intensity of >60%–80% of 1-RM per set, with a rest interval of 3–5 min between sets at an RPE of 7–8.
   D) Training each muscle group for ≥1 set with 10–15 repetitions at a moderate intensity of 60%–70% of 1-RM per set, with a rest interval of 2–3 min between sets at an RPE of 5–6.

2. During the first 4 wk, Roger's aerobic exercise program should include everything below *except*
   A) ≥5 d · wk⁻¹ at an intensity of 40%–75% of $\dot{V}O_2R$ or HRR
   B) Exercises performed primarily in an upright or standing position
   C) An initial exercise HR and MET range of approximately 146–170 bpm and 7–7.8 METs, respectively (using the HRR and $\dot{V}O_2R$ methods)
   D) A gradual weekly increase in exercise volume

3. Roger wants to achieve an exercise volume of 1,000 MET-min · wk⁻¹. How long must each of his aerobic exercise sessions last if he is working at an exercise intensity of 5 METs five times per week? How many kilocalories would he expend at the end of a week if he did this?
   A) 20 min per session; equivalent to 831 kcal · wk⁻¹
   B) 40 min per session; equivalent to 1,670 kcal · wk⁻¹
   C) 60 min per session; equivalent to 2,494 kcal · wk⁻¹
   D) 80 min per session; equivalent to 3,325 kcal · wk⁻¹

4. Which initial resistance training workout will best enable Roger to safely enhance his muscle function and perform better during his follow-up fitness assessments?
   A) Bicep curls, triceps pushdowns, knee extensions, chest flys, sit-ups, lateral shoulder raises, front shoulder raises, straight-leg raises and reverse sit-ups, weighted side bends, accompanied by posterior shoulder and standing floor touch stretches
   B) Straight-leg deadlifts, barbell rows, barbell squats, roman chair sit-ups, barbell bench press, bent-over rear shoulder dumbbell raises, standing barbell bicep curls, overhead dumbbell triceps extensions, Russian twists, accompanied by posterior shoulder and standing toe touch stretches
   C) Machine hack squats, prone hamstring curls, seated machine trunk rotation, seated machine back extensions, seated machine scapular rows (cable), standing barbell shoulder press, barbell lunges, lying barbell triceps press, decline barbell press, preacher barbell biceps curl, accompanied by prone trunk rotation and knee hug and supine double knee hug stretches
   D) Wall squats, body weight lunges, supine stability ball hamstring curls, standing cable chest press, cable scapular row in standing, machine shoulder press, latissimus dorsi pull-downs, opposite arm-leg raises (bird-dogs) in quadruped position, modified side bridges (side plank) with knees flexed, prone planks from the knees, accompanied by hip flexor and pectoral stretches

5. Roger wants to begin playing competitive three-on-three basketball (approximately an 8-MET activity) as an enjoyable means of attaining some of his goals. His maximal aerobic capacity is approximately 9 METs and his initial training intensity range will be between 60% and 80% of $\dot{V}O_2$ reserve ($\dot{V}O_2R$) or HRR. What is the corresponding MET range for him as he begins his exercise program over the first 4 wk? Is basketball within this range?
   A) Between 2.8 and 4.4 METs; no, basketball exceeds his current prescribed intensity range
   B) Between 3.8 and 5.4 METs; yes, basketball is within his prescribed intensity range
   C) Between 4.8 and 6.4 METs; yes, basketball is within his prescribed intensity range
   D) Between 5.8 and 7.4 METs; no, basketball exceeds his current prescribed intensity range

DISCUSSION QUESTIONS FOR CASE STUDY CPT.II(2)

1. In order to avoid dropping out due to business, boredom, burnout, and injury, Roger has requested a list of outdoor activities he can do occasionally to substitute and supplement his fitness center exercises. Where can he find a resource to help him locate appropriate physical activities based on effort levels and their corresponding MET levels and kilocalorie expenditure rates?

2. What seems to be Roger's exercise "directional preference" or "movement bias" and how should this guide the development of his comprehensive exercise program?

DOMAIN III: EXERCISE LEADERSHIP AND CLIENT EDUCATION

CASE STUDY CPT.III(1)

Author: **Angela Kvies, BS**
Author's Certifications: **ACSM-CEP**

Barbara is a 65-yr-old female and a new client. At her last appointment, Barbara's primary care physician reported that she needs to improve her lifestyle choices and recommended that she find a personal trainer to help her get started. You are eager to help her modify her cardiovascular disease risk factors and immediately set up an interview and evaluation.

Barbara lives alone, near her son and grandson. She used to be very active in her community but has recently stopped attending church and many other activities. She has a history of depression but denies any current symptoms. You ask her about coping techniques when she feels stressed, and she explains that she prays and talks to her friends and family. Over the course of the interview, Barbara shares that she enjoys social activities. Barbara's father died of a myocardial infarction when he was 62 yr old, but no other family members have had heart problems.

Barbara reports being inactive for the last few years. She would like to increase her endurance and strength so that she can keep up with her grandson. She has trouble walking long distances due to knee pain but does not report any other orthopedic limitations. She would like to lose some weight but expresses that she becomes very discouraged when she doesn't see immediate results. Barbara is very resistant to discuss her current nutritional habits and states that she tries to eat low-fat, low-sodium, and low-carbohydrate meals.

Barbara brought a copy of her most recent blood test with her for your review. She is currently taking medication for high BP and a statin for abnormal cholesterol levels. Her lipid profile reads as follows:

Total cholesterol	143 mg $\cdot$ dL^{-1}
Triglycerides	63 mg $\cdot$ dL^{-1}
HDL-C	46 mg $\cdot$ dL^{-1}
LDL cholesterol (LDL-C)	84 mg $\cdot$ dL^{-1}

Over the course of several visits, her resting BP has ranged between 130/88 and 138/90 mm Hg. She is a nonsmoker, reports not having diabetes, weighs 203 lb, and is 5 ft 2 in tall. Barbara has never had a stress test and denies any symptoms of angina or dyspnea with exertion. You have all the necessary clearance to begin an exercise regime with Barbara.

MULTIPLE-CHOICE QUESTIONS FOR CASE STUDY CPT.III(1)

1. What is her weight classification based on her calculated BMI?
   A) Overweight
   B) Class I obesity
   C) Class II obesity
   D) Class III obesity

2. Barbara would like to lose the minimal amount of weight to achieve a BMI that puts her in the "normal weight" category. How much weight will she need to lose to achieve this goal? Choose the closest answer.
   A) 42 lb
   B) 68 lb
   C) 75 lb
   D) 86 lb

3. Barbara calculated that she has reduced her caloric intake by 200 kcal $\cdot$ d^{-1}. At this rate, with no additional energy expenditure, how many pounds will she lose in 1 wk?
   A) 0.4 lb
   B) 0.6 lb
   C) 0.8 lb
   D) 1.0 lb

4. What would Barbara's recommended caloric deficit (by combination of diet and exercise) each day need to be in order to meet ACSM's guidelines for weight loss?
   A) 150–300 kcal
   B) 250–500 kcal
   C) 500–1,000 kcal
   D) 750–1,250 kcal

5. Weight loss would be an example of what type of motivation for Barbara? Keeping up with her grandson would be what type of motivation?
   A) Extrinsic motivation and intrinsic motivation, respectively
   B) Extrinsic motivation and extrinsic motivation, respectively
   C) Intrinsic motivation and intrinsic motivation, respectively
   D) Intrinsic motivation and extrinsic motivation, respectively

DISCUSSION QUESTIONS FOR CASE STUDY CPT.III(1)

1. Barbara looks at her long-term goals. She expresses to you that she is discouraged by the amount of time it will take her to reach her desired weight loss. She is still resistant to discussing her diet in detail. Describe the motivational strategies you would use to encourage Barbara and keep her interested in the program.

2. Barbara is willing enough to exercise at the gym with your guidance two times per week for 1 h. When you discuss additional activity, Barbara expresses that she tries to exercise at home but often lacks motivation. What alternatives can you give Barbara for additional physical activity to keep her engaged in the exercise program? What specific guidelines for cardiovascular exercise will you give her?

DOMAIN III: EXERCISE LEADERSHIP AND CLIENT EDUCATION

CASE STUDY CPT.III(2)

Author: **Melissa Conway-Hartman, MEd, LAT, ATC**
Author's Certifications: **ACSM EP-C**

Carl is a sedentary 45-yr-old African American male. He ran track in high school and ran recreationally in college, routinely competing in 5K races. He now works at a desk job 40 h a week. He is the father of three boys and has discovered he can no longer keep up with them. He gets winded playing touch football in the park with his friends and family. He wants to run 5K races with his boys who are at the age where they are playing organized sports. He has come to you, his personal trainer, seeking guidance to help him get back in shape.

He shares the following results of his recent physical examination with you:

Height	6 ft 2 in (187.9 cm)
Weight	250 lb (113.6 kg)
Percentage body fat	30%
Resting BP	138/86 mm Hg
Blood glucose	111 mg · dL^{-1}
Total cholesterol	209 mg · dL^{-1}
LDL-C	160 mg · dL^{-1}
HDL-C	45 mg · dL^{-1}
Triglycerides	150 mg · dL^{-1}
Three-day dietary recall results	Daily caloric intake: 2,600 cal Simple or refined carbohydrates: 60% Complex carbohydrates: 40% Protein: 115 g Carbohydrates: 400 g Fat: 60 g He drinks two cups of coffee a day and consumes no alcohol.

MULTIPLE-CHOICE QUESTIONS FOR CASE STUDY CPT.III(2)

1. What is Carl's BMI?
   A) 35.4 kg · m^{-2}
   B) 28.1 kg · m^{-2}
   C) 31.8 kg · m^{-2}
   D) 22.2 kg · m^{-2}

2. What is his BMI classification?
   A) Normal
   B) Underweight
   C) Overweight
   D) Class I obesity

3. You evaluate Carl's readiness to change and according to the transtheoretical model of behavior change, what stage of readiness is Carl currently experiencing?
   A) Action
   B) Preparation
   C) Contemplation
   D) Maintenance

4. In order to help Carl become successful at his behavioral change, what strategy can you use to move Carl to the next stage of readiness?
   A) Make a list of activities Carl likes so he won't get bored with his exercise
   B) Teach Carl about the benefits of regular exercise
   C) Emphasize self-liberation by helping Carl make a firm commitment to a goal and a start date
   D) Have Carl list the places around his home where he can be active (*i.e.*, the park)

5. What is Carl's daily energy intake of carbohydrates, fats, and proteins?
   A) 460 protein, 1,600 carbohydrate, 540 fat
   B) 1,600 protein, 460 carbohydrate, 540 fat
   C) 1,560 carbohydrate, 520 protein, 520 fat
   D) 1,040 carbohydrate, 780 protein, 780 fat

6. According to the socioecological model, the park close to Carl's house is an example of a
   A) Microsystem
   B) Mesosystem
   C) Exosystem
   D) Macrosystem

7. Carl sets a long-term goal of losing 20 lb at a rate of 1 lb · wk^{-1}. Assuming he will burn 2,000 cal through exercise each week and assuming all his weight loss is fat mass, what is his target for daily caloric intake?
   A) 2,386 cal
   B) 1,572 cal
   C) 984 cal
   D) 2,466 cal

DISCUSSION QUESTIONS FOR CASE STUDY CPT.III(2)

1. When examining the information provided by Carl, what barriers might he encounter to achieving his goal? How will you help him overcome those barriers?

2. Setting goals can help clients stay motivated. How will you help Carl set appropriate goals to ensure his success? List specific steps you will take and provide examples of goals you may set.

DOMAIN IV: LEGAL, PROFESSIONAL, BUSINESS, AND MARKETING

CASE STUDY CPT.IV

Author: **Melissa Conway-Hartman, MEd, LAT, ATC**
Author's Certifications: **ACSM EP-C**

You have just been hired as a fitness professional at the new fitness facility in your town. Most of your day is spent as a floor trainer. You orient new members to the facility while assisting current members with workouts, offering fitness advice, and keeping the fitness floor clean and safe. Part of your duty is to recruit new and current members to augment personal training clientele.

MULTIPLE-CHOICE QUESTIONS FOR CASE STUDY CPT.IV

1. During consultation with a new personal training client, you are recording her health history and she tells you she has high BP and high cholesterol. Her doctor wants her to start exercising and that is why she joined the gym. She states her BP is 138/86 mm Hg and her total cholesterol is 220 mg · dL^{-1}. You would like to start her out walking or using the stationary bike and doing light resistance exercises; however, before this can begin, she needs to
   A) Have a medically supervised maximal graded exercise test (GXT)
   B) Have a submaximal test with a physician present
   C) Have a maximal GXT without a physician present
   D) Have physician consent formed signed

2. While you are working the floor, you notice a member performing a push-up with his feet on the stability ball and his hands grasping the handles of a machine. What is the best course of action for you?
   A) Watch and cheer him on
   B) Explain to him the risks do not outweigh the benefits and how he can get hurt from this exercise
   C) Hold the stability ball so it will not roll away
   D) Stand close to him in case he loses control of the cable handles

3. The facility manager has asked for help in promoting the gym to the neighboring communities. You suggest she
   A) Use social media exclusively
   B) Put flyers up in the group fitness room
   C) Have the front desk staff greeters hand flyers out to each member
   D) Use direct mail and host a fitness activity in the neighborhood park

4. A member comes to you and states he has a superior labral tear from anterior to posterior lesion in his right shoulder from years ago that he never had repaired. He wants you to show him exercises to help treat his shoulder. What should you do?
   A) Try to convert him to a client
   B) Show him the close grip dumbbell bench press exercise but stay away from other free weights
   C) Refer him to his physician or physical therapist
   D) Teach him to work his biceps and triceps and not address the glenohumeral joint

5. While walking on the treadmill, one of the members attempted to remove her sweatshirt without stopping the treadmill. She fell while the belt was still moving and was thrown off the treadmill. As you help her, you discover that she has a few abrasions but nothing serious. She wants to finish her workout. What should you do?
   A) Make her go home and rest for the day
   B) Write an incident report describing what happened and have her sign it
   C) Give her a few adhesive bandages and leave her alone
   D) Try to convert her to be your client

6. During an initial interview with a client, you review the informed consent form. The purpose of this form is to
   A) Protect you from any legal action on the part of the client
   B) Provide information to the client regarding participation options and risks
   C) Prove you are not negligent
   D) Open a discussion about assessments

7. One of the members would like to attend a circuit class you are teaching. He asks if you think he can handle it because he suffered a second-degree hamstring strain 3 wk ago. What are the signs of a second-degree hamstring strain?
   A) Inability to contract the muscle
   B) Loss of sensation
   C) Painful active contraction with limited range of motion
   D) Point tenderness

DISCUSSION QUESTIONS FOR CASE STUDY CPT.IV

1. While working with your personal training client, she trips over a weight that was left on the floor. She says she felt a pop in her ankle. On observation, you notice swelling on the lateral aspect. What do you think her injury could be and how would you handle this situation?

2. The facility manager wishes to establish an hourly safety checklist of the fitness floor; this includes the cardio and flexibility areas, group fitness room, and locker rooms. She requests your assistance in completing the checklist. What tasks should be included on this list?

CPT CASE STUDIES ANSWERS AND EXPLANATIONS

CASE STUDY CPT.I

Multiple-Choice Answers for Case Study CPT.I

1—D. Family history

2—D. After medical clearance has been obtained

3—B. Prediabetic

4—B. 158 bpm

5—C. Dyslipidemic

> *Resource*: Riebe D, senior editor. *ACSM's Guidelines for Exercise Testing and Prescription*. 10th ed. Philadelphia (PA): Wolters Kluwer; 2018.

> *Notes for Risk Factors*

> *Risk Factors*

> **Age:** Yes, he is male $\geq$45 yr of age.

> **Family history:** No, father and brother were older than 55yr of age when they suffer their respective cardiovascular events.

> **Cigarette smoking:** No, he reports never smoking.

> **Sedentary lifestyle:** Yes, he is not meeting the minimum criteria of 30 min of moderate intensity physical activity on at least 3 d of the week during the past 3 mo.

Obesity: Yes, based on his current height and weight, his BMI exceeds 30 kg · m^{-2}.

Hypertension: Yes, he currently takes an ACE inhibitor which is an antihypertensive medication.

Dyslipidemia: Yes, he currently takes a statin medication for his cholesterol.

Prediabetes: Yes, his current fasting glucose meets the criteria for impaired (100–125 mg · dL^{-1}).

Negative Risk Factors

High HDL: No, his HDL concentration does not meet this criterion ($\geq$60 mg · dL^{-1}).

Bill is asymptomatic but has $\geq$2 cardiovascular disease risk factors including a history of hypertension that he currently takes an ACE inhibitor to treat. He will require a medical exam prior to vigorous exercise.

Resources: Battista R, senior editor. *ACSM's Resources for the Personal Trainer*. 5th ed. Philadelphia (PA): Wolters Kluwer; 2018.

Riebe D, senior editor. *ACSM's Guidelines for Exercise Testing and Prescription*. 10th ed. Philadelphia (PA): Wolters Kluwer; 2018.

Discussion Question Answers for Case Study CPT.I

1. Following physician clearance, Bill can begin an exercise program. Submaximal tests are appropriate. For estimation of cardiorespiratory fitness, tests may include submaximal cycle ergometer tests (*e.g.*, Åstrand-Ryhming bike test for unconditioned men, YMCA bike test), step tests (*e.g.*, Queens College, 3-min YMCA, Åstrand-Ryhming), submaximal treadmill protocols (shown to produce the highest $\dot{V}O_{2peak}$ in individuals with low back pain), and track tests (*e.g.*, 6-min walk, Rockport). For muscular strength assessment, a 10- to 15-RM is recommended for those considered higher risk. Muscular endurance tests may include the push-up or YMCA bench press test, and partial curl-up depending on Bill's back pain. Maximal testing would not be appropriate in a gym setting due to his moderate risk classification.

> ***Resources***: Battista R, senior editor. *ACSM's Resources for the Personal Trainer*. 5th ed. Philadelphia (PA): Wolters Kluwer; 2018.
>
> Riebe D, senior editor. *ACSM's Guidelines for Exercise Testing and Prescription*. 10th ed. Philadelphia (PA): Wolters Kluwer; 2018.

2. Because Bill is deconditioned with a moderate risk classification, a light to moderate range of 30%–40% is appropriate during the initial phase of aerobic training. This range can be beneficial in those who are deconditioned while also addressing the stated long-term goal of weight loss through a lower intensity exercise program.

Calculation
$HR_{max} = 220 - age$
Target HR (lower end of range) $= [(0.30) \times (HR_{max} - HR_{rest})] + HR_{rest}$
Target HR (higher end of range) $= [(0.40) \times (HR_{max} - HR_{rest})] + HR_{rest}$
$HR_{max} = 220 - 62$
Target HR (lower end of range) $= [(0.30) \times (158 - 82)] + 82$
Target HR (higher end of range) $= [(0.40) \times (158 - 82)] + 82$

The initial HR training range for Bill is 105–112 bpm.

> ***Resources***: Battista R, senior editor. *ACSM's Resources for the Personal Trainer*. 5th ed. Philadelphia (PA): Wolters Kluwer; 2018.
>
> Riebe D, senior editor. *ACSM's Guidelines for Exercise Testing and Prescription*. 10th ed. Philadelphia (PA): Wolters Kluwer; 2018.

CASE STUDY CPT.II(1)

Multiple-Choice Answers for Case Study CPT.II(1)

1—A. Continue with current aerobic program of moderate intensity running for 150–225 min · wk^{-1}. Use resistance bands, machines, and body weight exercises in place of free weights and perform high repetition sets (12–15 repetitions) to moderate fatigue at 40%–60% of estimated 1-RM. Include at least 10 min 2–3 d · wk^{-1} of flexibility exercise.

> ***Resources***: Bushman BA, senior editor. *ACSM's Complete Guide to Fitness & Health*. Champaign (IL): Human Kinetics; 2011.
>
> Riebe D, senior editor. *ACSM's Guidelines for Exercise Testing and Prescription*. 10th ed. Philadelphia (PA): Wolters Kluwer; 2018.

2—D. Both A and C

> ***Resources***: Mottola MF, Davenport MH, Brun CR, Inglis SD, Charlesworth S, Sopper MM. $\dot{V}O_{2peak}$ prediction and exercise prescription for pregnant women. *Med Sci Sports Exerc*. 2006;38(8):1389–95.
>
> Riebe D, senior editor. *ACSM's Guidelines for Exercise Testing and Prescription*. 10th ed. Philadelphia (PA): Wolters Kluwer; 2018.

3—C. Decrease aerobic activity from moderate-vigorous to light activity only

> ***Resource***: Bushman BA, senior editor. *ACSM's Complete Guide to Fitness & Health*. Champaign (IL): Human Kinetics; 2017.

4—E. Both B and D

> ***Resource***: Battista R, senior editor. *ACSM's Resources for the Personal Trainer*. 5th ed. Philadelphia (PA): Wolters Kluwer; 2018.

5—D. Increased fetal movement

> ***Resources***: Battista R, senior editor. *ACSM's Resources for the Personal Trainer*. 5th ed. Philadelphia (PA): Wolters Kluwer; 2018.
>
> Bushman BA, senior editor. *ACSM's Complete Guide to Fitness & Health*. Champaign (IL): Human Kinetics; 2017.

CPT

Discussion Question Answers for Case Study CPT.II(1)

1. Because Marie is already a very active and healthy young woman and plans to continue her activity throughout her pregnancy, she will preserve much of her aerobic fitness (although it will decrease slightly) and muscle mass and will gain less fat mass. Marie will notice an increase in her HR (due to increased gestational hormones during her first trimester and to maintain BP during second and third trimesters) and that her BP should remain relatively unchanged. Additionally, pregnant women experience a decrease in thermoregulatory control, so you will need to counsel Marie on wearing appropriate attire, maintaining adequate hydration, and refraining from exercising in hot and humid environments. As Marie progresses in her pregnancy, you should address modifications to her exercise prescription regarding her personal discomforts and abilities. You should also discuss the increased caloric need (approximately 300 kcal $\cdot$ d^{-1}) she will experience due to her pregnancy and determine the amount that will cover both this increased caloric need as well as cover the amount of kilocalories expended during her exercise sessions.

   Resources: Battista R, senior editor. *ACSM's Resources for the Personal Trainer*. 5th ed. Philadelphia (PA): Wolters Kluwer; 2018.

   Bushman BA, senior editor. *ACSM's Complete Guide to Fitness & Health*. Champaign (IL): Human Kinetics; 2017.

2. Blood flow to the heart is reduced during exercise performed in the supine position due to the weight of the fetus lying compressing the inferior vena cava. In order to ensure that orthostatic hypotension and obstruction of venous return do not occur, exercises performed in the supine position are discouraged.

   Resources: ACOG Committee on Obstetric Practice. ACOG Committee Opinion No. 650. Physical activity and exercise during pregnancy and the postpartum period. *Obstet Gynecol*. 2015;126:e135–e142.

   Battista R, senior editor. *ACSM's Resources for the Personal Trainer*. 5th ed. Philadelphia (PA): Wolters Kluwer; 2018.

   Bushman BA, senior editor. *ACSM's Complete Guide to Fitness & Health*. Champaign (IL): Human Kinetics; 2017.

CASE STUDY CPT.II(2)

Multiple-Choice Answers for Case Study CPT.II(2)

1—D. Training each muscle group for ≥1 set with 10–15 repetitions at a moderate intensity of 60%–70% of 1-RM per set, with a rest interval of 2–3 min between sets at an RPE of 5–6.

   Resources: Battista R, senior editor. *ACSM's Resources for the Personal Trainer*. 5th ed. Philadelphia (PA): Wolters Kluwer; 2018.

   Riebe D, senior editor. *ACSM's Guidelines for Exercise Testing and Prescription*. 10th ed. Philadelphia (PA): Wolters Kluwer; 2018.

   Roger is middle-aged, deconditioned, and unaccustomed to resistance training. A gradual progression using ≥1 set of 10–15 repetitions of moderate intensity (*i.e.*, 60%–70% 1-RM) resistance is recommended.

2—C. An initial exercise HR range and MET range of approximately 146–170 bpm and 7–7.8 METs, respectively (using the HRR and $\dot{V}O_2R$ methods)

   Resources: Battista R, senior editor. *ACSM's Resources for the Personal Trainer*. 5th ed. Philadelphia (PA): Wolters Kluwer; 2018.

   Riebe D, senior editor. *ACSM's Guidelines for Exercise Testing and Prescription*. 10th ed. Philadelphia (PA): Wolters Kluwer; 2018.

   Roger has the metabolic syndrome. The 40%–75% of $\dot{V}O_2R$ or HRR is recommended to help manage his dyslipidemia. This would equate to an intensity of 4.2–7 METs or an HR range of 112–146 bpm. Roger's directional preference is slight extension, so an upright posture will be most comfortable. Lastly, a progressively increasing exercise volume of ≥300 min $\cdot$ wk^{-1} will help him accomplish his weight loss and BP and blood lipid management goals.

3—B. 40 min per session; equivalent to 1,670 kcal $\cdot$ wk^{-1}

   Resources: Battista R, senior editor. *ACSM's Resources for the Personal Trainer*. 5th ed. Philadelphia (PA): Wolters Kluwer; 2018.

   Riebe D, senior editor. *ACSM's Guidelines for Exercise Testing and Prescription*. 10th ed. Philadelphia (PA): Wolters Kluwer; 2018.

   Roger must perform 200 MET-min of exercise per session. He must do that for 40 min if he wishes to achieve 200 MET-min.

The formula in Box 6.3 entitled "Calculation of METs, MET-min^{-1}, and kcal · min^{-1}" on page 166 of the *ACSM Guidelines* is as follows:

To convert METs to kcal · min^{-1}, use the formula: kcal · min^{-1} = METs × 3.5 mL · kg^{-1} · min^{-1} × body weight (in kg) ÷ 1,000 × 5. Roger would expend approximately 8.35 kcal and 334 kcal per session.

4—D. Wall squats, body weight lunges, supine stability ball hamstring curls, standing cable chest press, cable scapular row in standing, machine shoulder press, latissimus dorsi pull-downs, opposite arm-leg raises (bird-dogs) in quadruped position, modified side bridges (side plank) with knees flexed, prone planks from the knees, accompanied by hip flexor and pectoral stretches.

Resources: Battista R, senior editor. *ACSM's Resources for the Personal Trainer*. 5th ed. Philadelphia (PA): Wolters Kluwer; 2018.

Haney W, Pabian P, Smith M, Patel C. Low back pain: movement considerations for exercise and training. *Strength Cond J*. 2013;35:99–106.

Huynh L, Chimes GP. Get the lowdown on low back pain in athletes. *ACSM's Health & Fitness Journal*. 2014;18:15–22.

Lee BC, McGill SM. Effect of long-term isometric training on core/torso stiffness. *J Strength Cond Res*. 2014;29:1515–26.

Riebe D, senior editor. *ACSM's Guidelines for Exercise Testing and Prescription*. 10th ed. Philadelphia (PA): Wolters Kluwer; 2018.

All of the other answer choices include workouts which overemphasize activation of anterior chain muscles; use a preponderance of single-joint, isolation exercises; require extensive trunk flexion; or are too advanced for Roger's fitness level, training experience, and history of back pain and trunk flexion intolerance. Answer D includes exercises that promote muscle balance and adequate activation of posterior chain muscles, employ primarily multijoint exercises, elongate his overactive or shorter muscles, and avoid postures and motions which cause him discomfort.

5—D. Between 5.8 and 7.4 METs; no, basketball exceeds his current prescribed intensity range

Resources: Battista R, senior editor. *ACSM's Resources for the Personal Trainer*. 5th ed. Philadelphia (PA): Wolters Kluwer; 2018.

Riebe D, senior editor. *ACSM's Guidelines for Exercise Testing and Prescription*. 10th ed. Philadelphia (PA): Wolters Kluwer; 2018.

Roger would be engaging in "vigorous" activity for someone of his age, health, and fitness level and be above 80% of his V̇O$_2$R and HRR.

Discussion Question Answers for Case Study CPT.II(2)

1. The Compendium of Physical Activities is an alphabetized directory of physical activities that are indexed by activity type, MET level, and kilocalorie expenditure rate. Activities can be selected within a client's desired or prescribed intensity levels to help the client accomplish him or her exercise volume goals for health improvement, weight loss, or rehabilitation.

   Resource: Ainsworth BE, Haskell WL, Hermann, et al. 2011 Compendium of Physical Activities: a second update of codes and MET values. *Med Sci Sports Exerc*. 2011;43(8):1575–81.

2. It is apparent from Roger's fitness assessments and medical history that he is somewhat intolerant of trunk flexion, experiences relief from performing gentle extension exercises, and is doing his exercises in general with his spine in a neutral to slightly extended position. Exercise program design for persons with chronic low back pain should resemble those of apparently healthy individuals without low back pain. Exercise positions and postures (trunk flexion in Roger's case) which cause pain should be avoided, and exercises should be modified to accommodate client's exercise movement directional preferences. Roger will probably find it more comfortable to perform many of his exercises in a standing position or, if he must sit, with either a back support or chest pad.

   Resources: Haney W, Pabian P, Smith M, Patel C. Low back pain: movement considerations for exercise and training. *Strength Cond J*. 2013;35:99–106.

   Hislop H, Avers D, Brown M. *Daniels and Worthingham's Muscle Testing: Techniques of Manual Examination and Performance Testing*. 9th ed. St. Louis (MO): Elsevier Saunders; 2014. 528 p.

   Huynh L, Chimes GP. Get the lowdown on low back pain in athletes. *ACSM's Health Fitness J*. 2014;18:15–22.

   Lee BC, McGill SM. Effect of long-term isometric training on core/torso stiffness. *J Strength Cond Res*. 2014;29:1515–26.

   Long A, Donelson R, Fung T. Does it matter which exercise? A randomized control trial of exercise for low back pain. *Spine (Phila Pa 1976)*. 2004;29:2593–602.

   Long A, May S, Fung T. Specific directional exercises for patients with low back pain: a case series. *Physiother Can*. 2008;60:307–17.

McGill SM, Karpowicz A. Exercises for spine stabilization: motion/motor patters, stability progressions, and clinical technique. *Arch Phys Med Rehabil.* 2009;90(1):118–26.

Nau E, Hanney WJ, Kolber MJ. Spinal conditioning for athletes with lumbar spondylolysis and spondylolisthesis. *Strength Cond J.* 2008;30:43–52.

Riebe D, senior editor. *ACSM's Guidelines for Exercise Testing and Prescription.* 10th ed. Philadelphia (PA): Wolters Kluwer; 2018.

Surkitt LD, Ford JJ, Hahne AJ, Pizzari T, McMeeken JM. Efficacy of directional preference management for low back pain: a systematic review. *Phys Ther.* 2012:92:652–65.

CASE STUDY CPT.III(1)

Multiple-Choice Answers for Case Study CPT.III(1)

1—C. Class II obesity

Resource: Riebe D, senior editor. *ACSM's Guidelines for Exercise Testing and Prescription.* 10th ed. Philadelphia (PA): Wolters Kluwer; 2018.

Barbara is classified as "Class II Obesity" (35.0–39.9). BMI is calculated by using the following formula: kg / (m^2). Barbara's BMI is 37.1 $kg \cdot m^{-2}$.

2—B. 68 lb

Resources: Battista R, senior editor. *ACSM's Resources for the Personal Trainer.* 5th ed. Philadelphia (PA): Wolters Kluwer; 2018.

Riebe D, senior editor. *ACSM's Guidelines for Exercise Testing and Prescription.* 10th ed. Philadelphia (PA): Wolters Kluwer; 2018.

"Normal weight" is categorized by a BMI of 18.5–24.9. Because Barbara wants to lose the minimal amount of weight, 24.9 will be her goal BMI.

- Use the formula for BMI with Barbara's goal BMI and her current height to find what her new weight will be.

$24.9 = kg / (1.57^2)$
kg = 61.2 or 134.6 lb

- Subtract her goal weight from her current weight

203 lb − 134.6 lb = 68.4 lb

3—A. 0.4 lb

Resource: Riebe D, senior editor. *ACSM's Guidelines for Exercise Testing and Prescription.* 10th ed. Philadelphia (PA): Wolters Kluwer; 2018.

Barbara is reducing 1400 $kcal \cdot wk^{-1}$ at this rate. There are 3,500 kcal in 1 lb. She will lose approximately 0.4 lb each week.

4—C. 500–1,000 kcal

Resource: Riebe D, senior editor. *ACSM's Guidelines for Exercise Testing and Prescription.* 10th ed. Philadelphia (PA): Wolters Kluwer; 2018.

ACSM recommends weight loss of 1–2 $lb \cdot wk^{-1}$. This would mean a caloric deficit of 3,500–7,000 kcal each week or 500–1,000 kcal each day.

5—A. Extrinsic rewards; intrinsic rewards

Resource: Battista R, senior editor. *ACSM's Resources for the Personal Trainer.* 5th ed. Philadelphia (PA): Wolters Kluwer; 2018.

Extrinsic motivation is a motivation that helps to achieve a certain goal or reward. Extrinsic rewards are positive benefits that are often received through other people. Intrinsic rewards are rewards that are considered personal benefits because the goal achievement left the person feeling satisfied. Barbara expressed several times that she feels motivated/encouraged when she sees results in her weight. This is an example of an extrinsic reward. Being able to keep up with her grandson would be an example of an intrinsic reward.

Discussion Question Answers for Case Study CPT.III(1)

1. Barbara is contemplating change but still lacks self-esteem. You can use every motivational tool in the book to help Barbara. It is important to use active listening with Barbara and to encourage her strengths. Reflect what she tells you, and express that your concerns are the same as hers and provide nonthreatening feedback. Be sure that all praise and encouragement are genuine.

   Although it is important to point out the long-term benefits of exercise, including the possible reduction in all of her risk factors, Barbara is motivated most when she sees change. It is ideal to work with her on strategic planning. Work together to find several short-term goals that will help to motivate her as she slowly progresses toward her long-term goals. Set goals that are specific, measurable, achievable, realistic, and time-constrained (SMART).

Use motivational interviewing skills. Approach her nutritional habits in a way that is nonconfrontational. Ask her if she is willing to discuss general nutrition information and appropriate portion control. Focus as much as possible on intrinsic motivators. If she is still unwilling to discuss nutritional habits, point out small achievements such as increases in time on a machine or overall increase in energy.

> **Resources**: Battista R, senior editor. *ACSM's Resources for the Personal Trainer.* 5th ed. Philadelphia (PA): Wolters Kluwer; 2018.
>
> Riebe D, senior editor. *ACSM's Guidelines for Exercise Testing and Prescription.* 10th ed. Philadelphia (PA): Wolters Kluwer; 2018.

2. Give Barbara specific and realistic guidelines. Explain that American Heart Association and ACSM have recommended that she engage in at least 150 min each week of moderate intensity exercise. She will improve her cardiovascular and respiratory function, reduce her coronary artery disease risk factors, decrease morbidity and risk of early mortality, and improve quality of life. When she appears to have improved confidence, encourage her to engage in any appropriate group fitness classes or neighborhood walking programs. Offer other ways that Barbara can increase her overall physical activity. Use examples such as parking farther away, taking stairs whenever possible, taking short walks during commercial breaks, etc. Until she becomes fit enough to tolerate 30 min of nonstop aerobic activity, encourage her to engage in 10-min bouts of exercise that reach a moderate level of intensity. Without an HR monitor, you can describe moderate intensity as a level that makes her feel slightly short of breath or makes talking difficult. Find out what types of activities appeal to Barbara and provide examples of how she can incorporate physical activity into her daily life.

> **Resources**: Battista R, senior editor. *ACSM's Resources for the Personal Trainer.* 5th ed. Philadelphia (PA): Wolters Kluwer; 2018.
>
> Riebe D, senior editor. *ACSM's Guidelines for Exercise Testing and Prescription.* 10th ed. Philadelphia (PA): Wolters Kluwer; 2018.

CASE STUDY CPT.III(2)

Multiple-Choice Answers for Case Study CPT.III(2)

1—C. $31.8\ kg \cdot m^{-2}$

> **Resource**: Battista R, senior editor. *ACSM's Resources for the Personal Trainer.* 5th ed. Philadelphia (PA): Wolters Kluwer; 2018.
>
> BMI = weight (kg) / height (m²).

2—D. Class I obesity

> **Resource**: Battista R, senior editor. *ACSM's Resources for the Personal Trainer.* 5th ed. Philadelphia (PA): Wolters Kluwer; 2018.
>
> A BMI between 30.0 and 34.9 is categorized as class I obesity.

3—B. Preparation

> **Resource**: Battista R, senior editor. *ACSM's Resources for the Personal Trainer.* 5th ed. Philadelphia (PA): Wolters Kluwer; 2018.
>
> Carl has decided to make the change to be more physically active. He is seeking help to formulate a plan.

4—C. Emphasize self-liberation by helping Carl make a firm commitment to a goal and a start date

> **Resource**: Battista R, senior editor. *ACSM's Resources for the Personal Trainer.* 5th ed. Philadelphia (PA): Wolters Kluwer; 2018.

Commitment usually occurs at the beginning of the action stage. If Carl can set a firm time and date and stick to it, he will begin the action phase of adding exercise back into his life.

5—A. 460 protein, 1,600 carbohydrate, 540 fat

> One gram of carbohydrate has approximately 4 cal, 1 g of fat has approximately 9 cal, and approximately 1 g of protein has approximately 4 cal.
>
> **Resource**: Swain D, senior editor. *ACSM'S Resource Manual for Guidelines for Exercise Testing and Prescription,* 7th ed. Philadelphia (PA): Wolters Kluwer; 2014.

6—B. Mesosystem

> The mesosystem in the socioeconomic model includes environment, health agencies, community, competing sedentary activities, technology, mass media, and access to information. The proximity of a park to Carl's home would be a factor at the mesosystem level.
>
> **Resource**: Swain D, senior editor. *ACSM'S Resource Manual for Guidelines for Exercise Testing and Prescription,* 7th ed. Philadelphia (PA): Wolters Kluwer; 2014.

7—A. 2,386 cal

> If Carl wants to lose 1 lb a week and he will burn 2,000 extra calories each week with exercise, he will

need to create an additional 1,500 kcal deficit with his diet per week. In order to do that, he needs to decrease his caloric intake by approximately 214 kcal per day; this would equal 2,386 kcal each day.

Resource: Riebe D, senior editor. *ACSM's Guidelines for Exercise Testing and Prescription*. 7th ed. Philadelphia (PA): Wolters Kluwer; 2018.

Discussion Question Answers for Case Study CPT.III(2)

1. Answers might include family obligations, fatigue from work, and time management. Refer to his exam results and educate him about his six risk factors for disease. Ask him about how his health will affect his family and if he has support from his family and friends. Have him list ways he can overcome barriers such as working late, the boys' sports, and other family commitments. Make suggestions if he cannot think of anything. For example, he can walk or run while his boys are at practice. He can add in a short walk at lunch if he will not have time later for a longer exercise session.

   Resource: Battista R, senior editor. *ACSM's Resources for the Personal Trainer*. 5th ed. Philadelphia (PA): Wolters Kluwer; 2018.

2. Answers may include motivational interviewing and client-centered approach to questioning to determine SMART goals that Carl is ready to commit to. Agreeing with the client and not countering resistance, giving examples of specific SMART goals, and asking questions directed at determining which specific goal is most important, confidence in accomplishing that goal on a scale of 1–10, etc. Be sure to clarify the scale of 1–10 and ask why they feel they are not a 1. If they are a 6 or less, the goal needs to be adjusted so they are closer to an 8.

   Resource: Swain D, senior editor. *ACSM'S Resource Manual for Guidelines for Exercise Testing and Prescription*, 7th ed. Philadelphia (PA): Wolters Kluwer; 2014.

CASE STUDY CPT.IV

Multiple-Choice Answers for Case Study CPT.IV

1—D. Have physician consent formed signed

   Resource: Battista R, senior editor. *ACSM's Resources for the Personal Trainer*. 5th ed. Philadelphia (PA): Wolters Kluwer; 2018.

   Mrs. Kelly has two risk factors: no known disease and is asymptomatic. She will be participating in moderate exercise. Therefore, a GXT with a physician present is not required. Getting medical clearance is necessary unless she answers "yes" to any question under "General Health Questions" section on the Physical Activity Readiness Questionnaire + (PAR-Q+).

2—B. Explain to him the risks do not outweigh the benefits and how he can get hurt from this exercise

   Resource: Battista R, senior editor. *ACSM's Resources for the Personal Trainer*. 5th ed. Philadelphia (PA): Wolters Kluwer; 2018.

   The risks of this exercise vastly outweigh any benefit. It is within the scope of practice for a personal trainer to correct bad or incorrect posture during exercise. It is also within the code of ethics to help prevent injury to participants.

3—D. Use direct mail and host a fitness activity in the neighborhood park

   Resource: Battista R, senior editor. *ACSM's Resources for the Personal Trainer*. 5th ed. Philadelphia (PA): Wolters Kluwer; 2018.

   Because the fitness facility is new in town, a direct mail to that specific neighborhood would be helpful. In combination with community involvement at the neighborhood park, the two approaches would target that specific market in multiple ways.

4—C. Refer him to his physician or physical therapist

   Resources: Battista R, senior editor. *ACSM's Resources for the Personal Trainer*. 5th ed. Philadelphia (PA): Wolters Kluwer; 2018.

   Pire N. *ACSM's Career and Business Guide for the Fitness Professional*. Philadelphia (PA): Wolters Kluwer; 2012.

   Attempting to treat an injury is beyond the scope of practice of a personal trainer, and the client should be referred to someone who is qualified to care for this injury.

5—B. Write an incident report describing what happened and have her sign it

   Resource: Battista R, senior editor. *ACSM's Resources for the Personal Trainer*. 5th ed. Philadelphia (PA): Wolters Kluwer; 2018.

   Even though the member does not appear to have any serious injury, the incident needs to be documented to protect the facility from further claims on the part of the member.

6—B. Provide information to the client regarding participation options and risks

> **Resource**: Battista R, senior editor. *ACSM's Resources for the Personal Trainer*. 5th ed. Philadelphia (PA): Wolters Kluwer; 2018.

> The purpose of the informed consent form is to ensure the client has full knowledge of tests to be performed, understands the relative risks, is informed of alternative procedures, is given the chance to ask questions, and gives consent voluntarily. The informed consent document does not protect the trainer from liability.

7—C. Painful active contraction with limited range of motion

> **Resources**: Battista R, senior editor. *ACSM's Resources for the Personal Trainer*. 5th ed. Philadelphia (PA): Wolters Kluwer; 2018.

> Prentice W. *Principles of Athletic Training: A Competency Approach*. 14th ed. New York (NY): McGraw-Hill; 2011.

> Typically, a hamstring strain is not associated with loss of sensation. Contraction is possible but will be painful with a second-degree sprain. After 3 wk, point tenderness should not be present.

Discussion Question Answers for Case Study CPT.IV

1. Answers should include an ankle sprain of any degree, an injury to the peroneal tendons, or a fracture. She should stop working out, ice her injury, and stabilize with an elastic wrap. An incident report should be completed, and she should sign it. She should not participate in weight-bearing activities and not return to training without medical clearance.

> **Resources**: Battista R, senior editor. *ACSM's Resources for the Personal Trainer*. 5th ed. Philadelphia (PA): Wolters Kluwer; 2018.

> Prentice W. *Principles of Athletic Training: A Competency Approach*. 14th ed. New York (NY): McGraw-Hill; 2011.

2. Answers may include re-racking weights; checking bands for breaks; keeping the floor clear of debris and liquids; and checking stability balls, mats, and medicine balls for cleanliness and proper inflation. Machines should be in proper working order with no broken cables. Cardio equipment should be in proper working order with no broken pieces. Locker room floor should be dry and clear of clutter, and benches should be checked for stability. Locker rooms should be checked for members in distress. The group fitness floor should be dry, and equipment should be put away with the door locked so no one can enter without permission.

> **Resource**: Battista R, senior editor. *ACSM's Resources for the Personal Trainer*. 5th ed. Philadelphia (PA): Wolters Kluwer; 2018.

CPT Job Task Analysis

DOMAIN I: INITIAL CLIENT CONSULTATION AND ASSESSMENT

A. Provide instructions and initial documents to the client in order to proceed to the interview.		
Knowledge or Skill Statement	**Explanation/Examples**	**Resources**
Knowledge of components and preparation for the initial client consultation	• Use new Client Intake form to qualify client. • Assess compatibility, goals, scope, style, and schedule. • Exchange contact information (including emergency contact) and identify schedule preferences. • Discuss medical considerations and limitations; assess risk and need for medical doctor (MD) release form. • Schedule initial client consultation. • Provide service intro package.	*ACSM's Resources for the Personal Trainer*, 5th edition (9) • Chapter 10
Knowledge of the necessary paperwork to be completed by client prior to initial client interview	• American College of Sports and Medicine Exercise Pre-participation Health Screening Questionnaire for Exercise Professionals, Physical Activity Readiness Questionnaire + (PAR-Q+), informed consent, waiver • Medical clearance form (be sure to include Health Insurance Portability and Accountability Act [HIPAA] Release of Information Authorization Form) • Trainer–client contract • Organizational policies and procedures	*ACSM's Resources for the Personal Trainer*, 5th edition (9) • Chapters 10 and 11 • Figures 10.4, 11.1, and 11.2 *ACSM's Guidelines for Exercise Testing and Prescription* (GETP), 10th edition (14) • Chapter 2 U.S. Department of Health and Human Services, Health Insurance Portability and Accountability Act (41,42)
Skill in effective communication and in using multimedia resources (*i.e.*, e-mail, phone, text messaging) and/or in-person resources	• Provide information on the club's Web site dedicated to service introduction. • Verbal and nonverbal communication skills • Trainer contact information • Verbally explain process and preparation to client, such as attire, equipment, hydration, etc. • Remind client of day and time of next meeting and length of appointment. • Remind client to complete and return forms. • Give the opportunity to ask questions and/or to contact if concerns arise.	*ACSM's Resources for the Personal Trainer*, 5th edition (9) • Chapter 10

CPT

B. Interview client in order to gather and provide pertinent information to proceed to the fitness testing and program design.

Knowledge or Skill Statement	Explanation/Examples	Resources
Knowledge of the components and limitations of a health/medical history, preparticipation screening tools, informed consent, trainer–client contract, and organizational policies and procedures **Knowledge** of the use of medical clearance for exercise testing and program participation **Knowledge** of health behavior modification theories and strategies in order to determine client goals and expectations **Knowledge** of orientation procedures, including equipment use and facility layout **Skill** in obtaining a health/medical history, medical clearance, and informed consent	• Purpose, current health status, legal concerns, consent, administration, client commitment • Operational information concerning billing, cancellation, hours of operation, all policies and procedures • Review medical history form; stratify and establish trust and confidentiality; ask questions to clarify; document responses in a clear and concise manner. • Refer client to physician if warranted. • Review health/medical history for known disease, signs/symptoms, American College of Sports Medicine (ACSM) Preparticipation Screening Algorithm • Identify stage of change; use motivational interviewing; connect goal to core values plan for lapses in behavior, track changes, and progress. • Group or personal orientation session, which provides general guidelines on physical activity; personalized exercise regime; proper setup, usage, and safety of equipment; hands-on walk through of facility; identification of emergency exits and *phones with emergency numbers on them*, location of "public access" automated external defibrillator (AED) (in the cases of unstaffed facilities), or literature or Web site with available resources and services	*ACSM's Resources for the Personal Trainer*, 5th edition (9) • Chapters 7, 10, and 11 *ACSM's Health/Fitness Facility Standards and Guidelines*, 3rd edition (17) • Chapter 3

C. Review and analyze client data to assess risk, formulate a plan of action, and conduct physical assessments.

Knowledge or Skill Statement	Explanation/Examples	Resources
Knowledge of the risk factors for cardiovascular disease **Knowledge** of signs and symptoms suggestive of chronic cardiovascular, metabolic, and/or pulmonary disease **Knowledge** of the ACSM's model for determining the need for medical clearance prior to participation in fitness testing and exercise programs **Knowledge** of relative and absolute contraindications to exercise testing	• Utilize the algorithm in Chapter 2 of *ACSM's Guidelines for Exercise Testing and Prescription* (GETP), 10th edition, to determine if medical clearance is needed.	*ACSM's Resources for the Personal Trainer*, 5th edition (9) • Chapter 11 *ACSM's Guidelines for Exercise Testing and Prescription* (GETP), 10th edition (14) • Chapters 2 and 3

C. Review and analyze client data (*i.e.*, classify risk) to formulate a plan of action and/or conduct physical assessments. (cont.)

Knowledge or Skill Statement	Explanation/Examples	Resources
Skill in identifying modifiable major risk factors for cardiovascular disease and teaching clients about risk reduction **Skill** in determining fitness assessments based on the initial client consultation **Skill** in following protocols during fitness assessment administration	• Classify risk based on health/medical history for known disease, signs/symptoms, or coronary artery disease (CAD) risk factors; physician referral. • Choice of assessments based on risk, limiting orthopedic or metabolic conditions, goals, equipment availability, and physician recommendations. • Methods or procedures used for exercise clearance are left to the discretion of the medical provider.	*ACSM's Guidelines for Exercise Testing and Prescription* (GETP), 10th edition (14) • Chapter 3 • Table 3.1 and Box 3.1 *ACSM's Resources for the Personal Trainer*, 5th edition (9) • Chapter 12

D. Evaluate behavioral readiness to optimize exercise adherence.

Knowledge or Skill Statement	Explanation/Examples	Resources
Knowledge of behavioral strategies to enhance exercise and health behavior change (*e.g.*, reinforcement; specific, measurable, attainable, realistic and relevant, and time-bound [SMART] goal setting, social support)	• Help client create specific SMART goals. • Connect goals to deep motivation. • Determine between client-centered and behavior-oriented goals. • Create weekly manageable goals schedule. • Concentrate on what client is willing and able to do and works for them.	*ACSM's Resources for the Personal Trainer*, 5th edition (9) • Chapters 8 and 9 *ACSM's Guidelines for Exercise Testing and Prescription* (GETP), 10th edition (14) • Chapter 12
Knowledge of applications of health behavior change models (socioecologic model, readiness to change model, social cognitive theory, and theory of planned behavior, etc.) and effective strategies that support and facilitate behavioral change	• Raise consciousness through education. • Establish positive self-image. • Make formal commitment. • Create a structure of accountability. • Identify and eliminate cause of problem behavior from environment. • Substitute healthy behaviors for unhealthy ones. • Establish support and reinforcement. • Provide feedback.	*ACSM's Resources for the Personal Trainer*, 5th edition (9) • Chapters 7 and 8 *ACSM's Guidelines for Exercise Testing and Prescription* (GETP), 10th edition (14) • Chapter 12
Skill in setting effective client-oriented SMART behavioral goals **Skill** in choosing and applying health behavior modification strategies based on the client's skills, knowledge, and level of motivation	• Coach clients to set achievable goals and overcome potential obstacles.	*ACSM's Resources for the Personal Trainer*, 5th edition (9) *ACSM's Guidelines for Exercise Testing and Prescription* (GETP), 10th edition (14) • Chapter 12

CPT

| E. | Assess the components of health-related physical fitness (cardiorespiratory fitness, muscular strength, muscular endurance, flexibility, body composition) and the components of skill-related fitness (agility, balance, coordination, power, speed, reaction time) to establish baseline values, set goals, and develop individualized programs. |

Knowledge or Skill Statement	Explanation/Examples	Resources
Knowledge of the basic structures of bone, skeletal muscle, and connective tissue	• Identify types and classification of bone; structure and function; components of skeletal system; axial and appendicular skeletons, origins, and insertions of muscles.	*ACSM's Resources for the Personal Trainer*, 5th edition (9) • Chapter 3 • Figures 3.5 and 3.6
Knowledge of the basic anatomy of the cardiovascular (CV) and respiratory systems	• Location of and relationship between heart and lungs • Identify the structures of the heart. • Identify the structures of the upper and lower respiratory tract.	*ACSM's Resources for the Personal Trainer*, 5th edition (9) • Chapter 5
Knowledge of the terms describing human movement, planes of movement, spinal curvature, spinal curvature, and muscle function	• Anatomical locations and positions contained within Table 3.1 • Joint movements and lever systems	*ACSM's Resources for the Personal Trainer*, 5th edition (9) • Chapter 3 • Table 3.1
Knowledge of the interrelationships among center of gravity, base of support, balance, stability, and proper spinal alignment	• Line of gravity: defines proper body alignment and posture • Center of gravity: location of a theoretical point that can be used to represent the total weight of an object • Base of support: the area of the supporting surface of an object such as the feet standing • Balance: ability to maintain a position for a given period of time without moving — control center of mass with respect to base of support • Stability: ability to lean without changing the base of support • Spinal alignment and movements	*ACSM's Resources for the Personal Trainer*, 5th edition (9) • Chapter 3 • Figure 3.4
Knowledge of differences between aerobic and anaerobic energy systems and the effects of acute and chronic exercise on each	• Energy production with and without oxygen • Adaptations to exercise capacity and physiological systems	*ACSM's Resources for the Personal Trainer*, 5th edition (9) • Chapter 5 • Tables 5.1 and 5.2 • Figure 5.4
Knowledge of the differences between the aerobic and anaerobic energy systems and the effects of acute and chronic exercise on each	• Supply oxygenated blood to active tissues: effects on heart rate (HR), stroke volume (SV), cardiac output ($\dot{Q}$), blood flow and pressure, arteriovenous oxygen (a-v O_2) difference • Static and dynamic resistance training effects on muscle fibers and physiological systems	*ACSM's Resources for the Personal Trainer*, 5th edition (9) • Chapter 5 • Figure 5.3
Knowledge of the normal chronic physiologic adaptations associated with cardiovascular exercise and resistance training	• Benefits of CV training • Benefits of resistance training • Muscular hypertrophy, adaptations to muscle fibers, aerobic enzyme systems, nervous system	*ACSM's Resources for the Personal Trainer*, 5th edition (9) • Chapter 5 • Table 5.2

E. Assess the components of health-related physical fitness (cardiorespiratory fitness, muscular strength, muscular endurance, flexibility, body composition) and the components of skill-related fitness (agility, balance, coordination, power, speed, reaction time) to establish baseline values, set goals, and develop individualized programs. (cont.)		
Knowledge or Skill Statement	**Explanation/Examples**	**Resources**
Knowledge of the physiologic responses related to warm-up and cool-down	• Periods of metabolic and CV adjustments from rest to exercise and exercise to rest, respectively	*ACSM's Resources for the Personal Trainer*, 5th edition (9) • Chapters 15 and 18
Knowledge of the physiological basis of acute muscle fatigue and delayed onset muscle soreness (DOMS) vs. musculoskeletal injury or overtraining	• Use of Likert-type chart to determine appropriate muscle soreness ranges • Signs of muscle damage: swelling, pain, soreness, discoloration	*ACSM's Resources for the Personal Trainer*, 5th edition (9) • Chapter 14 • Box 14.1
Knowledge of the physiological adaptations that occur at rest and during submaximal and maximal exercise following chronic aerobic and anaerobic exercise training	• CV benefits of exercise: improvement in CV and respiratory function, decreased risk from premature death, reduction in death, increased health benefits	*ACSM's Resources for the Personal Trainer*, 5th edition (9) • Chapter 15 • Box 15.1 *ACSM's Guidelines for Exercise Testing and Prescription* (GETP), 10th edition (14) • Chapter 1 • Box 1.2
Knowledge of the physiological basis for improvements in muscular strength and endurance	• Adaptations to muscle fibers and contractile proteins, aerobic enzyme systems, capillary supply, and nervous system	*ACSM's Resources for the Personal Trainer*, 5th edition (9) • Chapter 5
Knowledge of expected blood pressure responses associated with postural changes, acute physical exercise, and adaptations resulting from long-term exercise training	• Acute: linear increase in systolic BP (SBP) with increased levels of exercise; diastolic BP (DBP) may decrease slightly or remain unchanged. • Chronic: resting SBP and DBP may decrease; lower BP at fixed submaximal work rate • Postural changes can produce hypotensive response.	*ACSM's Resources for the Personal Trainer*, 5th edition (9) • Chapters 5 and 12
Knowledge of the major bones and muscle groups of the human body, types of muscle contraction, joint classifications, the primary action, and joint range of motion specific to each major muscle group	• Isotonic: muscle contraction, which exerts a constant tension • Isometric (static): no change in muscle length • Isokinetic: muscle resistance throughout the range of motion (ROM) by controlling speed of movement • Concentric: muscle shortening (contraction) • Eccentric: muscle lengthening • Describe characteristics that comprise different types of joints.	*ACSM's Resources for the Personal Trainer*, 5th edition (9) • Chapter 14
Knowledge of the terms describing muscle growth or the lack thereof	• Hypertrophy: increase in muscular size • Atrophy: wasting away or loss of a part — usually muscle • Hyperplasia: increased cell production in a normal tissue	*ACSM's Resources for the Personal Trainer*, 5th edition (9) • Chapter 3

E.	Assess the components of health-related physical fitness (cardiorespiratory fitness, muscular strength, muscular endurance, flexibility, body composition) and the components of skill-related fitness (agility, balance, coordination, power, speed, reaction time) to establish baseline values, set goals, and develop individualized programs. (cont.)	
Knowledge or Skill Statement	**Explanation/Examples**	**Resources**
Knowledge of the physiologic basis of the components of health-related physical fitness: cardiovascular fitness, muscular strength, muscular endurance, flexibility, and body composition	• CV fitness: the ability of the circulatory and respiratory systems to supply oxygen during sustained physical activity • Muscular strength: the ability of muscle to exert force • Muscular endurance: the ability of muscle to continue to perform without fatigue • Body composition: the relative amounts of muscle, fat, bone, and other vital parts of the body • Flexibility: the ROM around a joint	*ACSM's Resources for the Personal Trainer*, 5th edition (9) • Chapters 5 and 15 • Box 15.1 • Table 5.2 *ACSM's Guidelines for Exercise Testing and Prescription* (GETP), 10th edition (14) • Chapter 1 • Box 1.1
Knowledge of the normal chronic physiologic adaptations associated with CV, resistance, and flexibility training	• Benefits of CV training • Muscular hypertrophy, adaptations to muscle fibers, aerobic enzyme systems, nervous system • Flex: improve ROM and joint mobility	*ACSM's Resources for the Personal Trainer*, 5th edition (9) • Chapter 5 • Table 5.2
Knowledge of test termination criteria and best practice procedures to be followed after cessation of an exercise test	• Relative contraindications — Box 5.2 may be tested only after careful evaluation of the risk/benefit ratio. • Absolute contraindications — Box 5.2 should not perform exercise tests until conditions are stabilized or adequately treated. • Test termination criteria — Box 4.4; volitional fatigue, predetermined endpoint, or general indications • Postexercise procedures includes passive cool-down, physiological observations continued for at least 5 min or longer of recovery, low-level exercise until HR and BP stabilize.	*ACSM's Guidelines for Exercise Testing and Prescription* (GETP), 10th edition (14) • Chapters 4 and 5 • Boxes 4.4 and 5.2
Knowledge of the advantages, disadvantages, and limitations of the various body measurements and body composition techniques	• Discuss basis of technique; reliability; sources of error; ease in administering, measuring, and calculating; pretest preparation; and client comfort.	*ACSM's Resources for the Personal Trainer*, 5th edition (9) • Chapter 12 • Box 12.2
Knowledge of fitness testing protocols, including pretest preparation and assessments of flexibility, cardiovascular fitness, muscular strength, muscular endurance, and body composition	• Selection of test dependent on population, mass testing vs. individual testing, ease and reliability in administering, orthopedic or metabolic restrictions, equipment availability	*ACSM's Resources for the Personal Trainer*, 5th edition (9) • Chapter 12
Knowledge of interpretation of fitness test results	• Use norm charts to classify results, application of knowledge of acute responses to exercise.	*ACSM's Resources for the Personal Trainer*, 5th edition (9) • Chapters 5 and 12

E.	Assess the components of health-related physical fitness (cardiorespiratory fitness, muscular strength, muscular endurance, flexibility, body composition) and the components of skill-related fitness (agility, balance, coordination, power, speed, reaction time) to establish baseline values, set goals, and develop individualized programs. (cont.)

Knowledge or Skill Statement	Explanation/Examples	Resources
Knowledge of the recommended order of fitness assessments (*e.g.*, CV test prior to strength assessment)	• HR • BP • Body composition • CV assessment • Muscular fitness • Flexibility	*ACSM's Resources for the Personal Trainer*, 5th edition (9) • Chapter 12
Knowledge of the documentation of unexpected signs or symptoms during an exercise session and when to refer to a physician	• Formal and informal means of evaluating health status • Recognizing situations, signs, symptoms, and injuries (shortness of breath, abnormal response to increase in intensity, etc.) • Stop training session and refer to physician.	*ACSM's Resources for the Personal Trainer*, 5th edition (9) • Chapter 11
Knowledge of various mechanisms for referral to a physician	• Significant change in frequency, intensity, or nature of existing signs and symptoms • Onset of new signs and symptoms associated with CV or metabolic disease (Table 11.2) • Serious joint injuries that do not resolve quickly; clients reporting muscular or joint problems, dizziness or nausea	*ACSM's Resources for the Personal Trainer*, 5th edition (9) • Chapter 11 • Table 11.2
Skill in locating/palpating pulse landmarks, accurately measuring HR, and obtaining rating of perceived exertion (RPE)	• Three common sites are radial, brachial, and carotid. • Start counting exercise HR with zero as reference. • Measure for 30 s and multiply by 2 to convert to minute value. • RPE: two scales used as a subjective measure to rate overall feelings of exertion instead of specific areas. Obtain rating during steady state.	*ACSM's Resources for the Personal Trainer*, 5th edition (9) • Chapters 12 and 15 • Figure 12.1 • Table 15.10
Skill in selecting and following best practice protocols while administering fitness assessments	• Selection of test dependent on population, mass testing vs. individual testing, ease and reliability in administering, orthopedic or metabolic restrictions, equipment availability • Ability to recognize signs of poor circulation and perfusion, failure for HR and SBP to increase with workload	*ACSM's Resources for the Personal Trainer*, 5th edition (9) • Chapters 12 and 15 *ACSM's Guidelines for Exercise Testing and Prescription* (GETP), 10th edition (14) • Chapter 4 • Box 4.4
Skill in locating anatomical sites for circumference and skinfold measurements	• Anatomical sites are located within the description of each site. • Waist-to-hip ratio identifies fat distribution; higher amount of abdominal fat associated with increased risk for CAD	*ACSM's Guidelines for Exercise Testing and Prescription* (GETP), 10th edition (14) • Chapter 4 • Tables 4.1 and 4.2

CPT

E. Assess the components of health-related physical fitness (cardiorespiratory fitness, muscular strength, muscular endurance, flexibility, body composition) and the components of skill-related fitness (agility, balance, coordination, power, speed, reaction time) to establish baseline values, set goals, and develop individualized programs. (cont.)		
Knowledge or Skill Statement	**Explanation/Examples**	**Resources**
Skill in selecting and administering cardiorespiratory fitness, muscular strength, and muscular endurance assessments and recognizing normal and abnormal responses during testing	• Selection of test dependent on population, mass testing vs. individual testing, ease and reliability in administering, orthopedic or metabolic restrictions, equipment availability, participant's skill level/limitations. • Ability to recognize volitional fatigue, poor form, muscle compensation, poor alignment, incomplete ROM	*ACSM's Resources for the Personal Trainer*, 5th edition (9) • Chapters 12 and 14
Skill in selecting and administering flexibility assessments for various muscle groups	• Selection of test dependent on population, mass testing vs. individual testing, ease and reliability in administering, orthopedic or metabolic restrictions, equipment availability • Knowledge of normal joint ROM • Ability to detect muscle tightness, breath and holding patterns	*ACSM's Resources for the Personal Trainer*, 5th edition (9) • Chapters 12 and 16
Skill in recognizing postural abnormalities that may affect exercise performance and body alignment	• Knowledge of deviations from normal spinal curvatures	*ACSM's Resources for the Personal Trainer*, 5th edition (9) • Chapter 3 • Figures 3.48 and 3.49
Skill in delivering test and assessment results in a positive manner in an effort to avoid negatively impacting client self-esteem	• Make client feel comfortable; be respectful; demonstrate professionalism, trust, and competence; maintain confidentiality, use as a baseline; accept client where they are; develop a plan for improvement; be empathetic, and nonjudgmental	*ACSM's Resources for the Personal Trainer*, 5th edition (9) • Chapters 9 and 12

F. Develop a comprehensive (*i.e.*, physical fitness, goals, behavior) reassessment plan/timeline.		
Knowledge or Skill Statement	**Explanation/Examples**	**Resources**
Knowledge of the development of fitness plans based on the information obtained in the client interview and the results of the physical fitness assessments	• Use frequency, intensity, time, type, volume, and progress (FITT-VP) framework for each component based on risk stratification, test results, goals, client availability, and commitment level.	*ACSM's Resources for the Personal Trainer*, 5th edition (9) • Chapter 13 • Box 13.1
Knowledge of effective and applicable health behavior modification strategies to meet client goals	• Use short-term goals based on specific, measurable, attainable, realistic and relevant, and time-bound (SMART) goals. • Behavior change pyramid	*ACSM's Resources for the Personal Trainer*, 5th edition (9) • Chapters 7–9
Knowledge of the purpose and timeline for reassessing each component of physical fitness included in the client's training plan	• Fitness changes dependent on time, frequency and intensity of training efforts, behavioral change status, physiological changes being measured • Standard follow-up 4 wk to 3 mo	*ACSM's Resources for the Personal Trainer*, 5th edition (9) • Chapters 5 and 12

DOMAIN II: EXERCISE PROGRAMMING AND IMPLEMENTATION

A. Review client goals, medical history, and assessment results to determine appropriate training program.		
Knowledge or Skill Statement	**Explanation/Examples**	**Resources**
Knowledge of the risks and benefits associated with guidelines for exercise training and programming for healthy adults, seniors, children and adolescents, and pregnant women	• Understanding of physiological changes of aging and growth • Effects of chronic exercise on physiological systems	*ACSM's Resources for the Personal Trainer*, 5th edition (9) • Chapter 20 *ACSM's Guidelines for Exercise Testing and Prescription* (GETP), 10th edition (14) • Chapters 6
Knowledge of the benefits and risks associated with exercise training and guidelines for exercise programming for individuals medically cleared to exercise with chronic disease	• American Heart Association (AHA) risk classification for exercise training (Class B) • Recognize abnormal responses to exercise and medication effects on exercise capacity. • Dose-response relationship between exercise and health outcomes • Activity needs to be individualized, with exercise prescription provided by qualified individuals and approved by primary health care provider. • Program modifications based on condition • Exercise capacity <6 metabolic equivalents (METs) • Target energy expenditure of 150–400 kcal · d^{-1}	*ACSM's Resources for the Personal Trainer*, 5th edition (9) • Chapter 20 *ACSM's Guidelines for Exercise Testing and Prescription* (GETP), 10th edition (14) • Chapters 9–11
Knowledge of health-related conditions that may require consultations with medical personnel prior to initiating physical activity	• Risks of exercise testing that outweigh the benefits need to be evaluated by a physician. • Review of preexercise test evaluation and careful review of medical history helps to identify potential contraindications and safety of testing and participation. • Absolute and relative contraindications of exercise	*ACSM's Guidelines for Exercise Testing and Prescription* (GETP), 10th edition (14) • Chapters 3 and 4
Knowledge of components of health-related physical fitness: cardiovascular fitness, muscular strength, muscular endurance, flexibility, and body composition	• Physical fitness components defined as a set of attributes or characteristics that people have or achieve that relates to the ability to perform physical activity. • Health-related and/or skill-related components	*ACSM's Guidelines for Exercise Testing and Prescription* (GETP), 10th edition (14) • Chapter 1 • Box 1.1

A. Review client goals, medical history, and assessment results to determine appropriate training program. (cont.)

Knowledge or Skill Statement	Explanation/Examples	Resources

Knowledge of program development for specific client needs (*i.e.*, specific sports, performance, lifestyle, functional, balance, agility, aerobic, and anaerobic)	• Program development based on the following:
	  • Needs assessment — screening and risk stratification
	  • Review of goals, motivation, and level of commitment
	  • Assessment results
	  • Client interview
		ACSM's Resources for the Personal Trainer, 5th edition (9)
		• Chapters 10–13
		"American College of Sports Medicine Position Stand. Quantity and Quality of Exercise for Developing and Maintaining Cardiorespiratory, Musculoskeletal, and Neuromotor Fitness in Apparently Healthy Adults: Guidance for Prescribing Exercise" (11)

Knowledge of special precautions and modifications of exercise programming for participation in various environmental conditions (altitude, different ambient temperatures, humidity, and environmental pollution)	• Basic understanding of how environmental conditions affect physiological systems during exercise • Tools used to evaluate environmental conditions • May need to adjust length of time exposed to the environment, decrease intensity, proper hydration, proper clothing, and adjust rest periods	*ACSM's Guidelines for Exercise Testing and Prescription* (GETP), 10th edition (14) • Chapter 8 • Tables 8.1 and 8.2 • Boxes 8.1 and 8.2 • Figure 8.1 *American Red Cross First Aid/CPR/ AED Participant Manual* (19) • Chapter 6
Knowledge of the importance and ability to record exercise sessions and perform periodic reevaluations to assess changes in fitness status	• Accurately track workouts and training sessions. Include observations (*i.e.*, holding breath, form deviations, reported pain) and performance parameters (*i.e.*, load, repetitions [reps]) • Accurately chart effects of exercise. • Reassessments 4 wk to 3 mo • Compare to baseline.	*ACSM's Resources for the Personal Trainer*, 5th edition (9) • Chapters 13 and 18

B. Select exercise modalities to achieve desired adaptations based on goals, medical history, and assessment results.

Knowledge or Skill Statement	Explanation/Examples	Resources
Knowledge of selecting appropriate exercises and training modalities based on age, functional capacity, and exercise test results	• Selection of modalities dependent on availability, client ability to perform specific exercise, client preference, client goal, medical and physical limitations, skill and fitness levels, and client commitment level	*ACSM's Resources for the Personal Trainer*, 5th edition (9) • Chapters 13–16
Knowledge of the principles of specificity and program progression	• Specificity: Only muscles that are trained will adapt and change in response to resistance or stimulus. • Progressive overload: As a body adapts to a given stimulus, an increase in stimulus is required for further adaptations or improvements. • Specific Adaptations to Imposed Demands (SAID), variation, and periodization	*ACSM's Resources for the Personal Trainer*, 5th edition (9) • Chapters 13 and 14

B. Select exercise modalities to achieve desired adaptations based on goals, medical history, and assessment results. (cont.)

Knowledge or Skill Statement	Explanation/Examples	Resources
Knowledge of the advantages, disadvantages, and applications of interval, continuous, and circuit training programs for cardiovascular fitness improvements	• Cardiovascular modes of training — selection of modalities dependent on availability, client ability to perform specific exercise, client preference, client goal, medical and physical limitations, skill and fitness levels, and client commitment level	*ACSM's Resources for the Personal Trainer*, 5th edition (9) • Chapter 15
Knowledge of activities of daily living (ADL) and their role in the overall health and fitness of the individual	• Ability to perform daily task such as self-care and essential household chores or essential work-related physical tasks • Exercise and activities that improve a person's overall physical functionality can enhance the ability to live independently.	*ACSM's Resources for the Personal Trainer*, 5th edition (9) • Chapters 13 and 18
Knowledge of differences between physical activity recommendations and training principles for general health benefits, weight management, fitness improvements, and athletic performance enhancement	• Adjustments in frequency, intensity, time, type, volume, and progress (FITT-VP) for different goals with greatest variation in intensity, time, and total number of kilocalorie per week; as goal along continuum increases, so does intensity. • Mode of training and variety are important factors.	*ACSM's Resources for the Personal Trainer*, 5th edition (9) • Chapters 13 and 18 • Table 13.5 *ACSM's Guidelines for Exercise Testing and Prescription* (GETP), 10th edition (14) • Chapter 6 • Tables 6.4–6.8
Knowledge of advanced resistance training exercises (*e.g.*, super setting, Olympic lifting, plyometric exercises, pyramid training) and when such techniques are contraindicated	• Advanced exercises are highly technical and intensive. • Exercises must not be completed with client if there are any preexisting conditions that may require medical clearance. • Client must be evaluated on form, technique, kinesthetic awareness, body alignment, skill, and experience.	*ACSM's Resources for the Personal Trainer*, 5th edition (9) • Chapters 14 and 19
Knowledge of the six motor skill–related physical fitness components and agility, balance, coordination, reaction time, speed and power	• Performance training based on core strength, conditioning level, functional training, and sport specifics • Use of plyometric exercises for upper and lower body to enhance ability to generate force	*ACSM's Resources for the Personal Trainer*, 5th edition (9) • Chapters 13 and 19

Knowledge of the benefits, risks, and contraindications for a wide variety of resistance training exercises specific to individual muscle groups (*e.g.*, for rectus abdominis performing crunches, supine leg raises, and plank exercises)	• Evaluate exercise based on the following:
	  • Biomechanical characteristics of the movement
	  • Exercise is designed to be primary or assistive.
	  • Single-joint vs. multijoint exercises
	  • Bilateral vs. unilateral
	  • Client's goal, fitness and skill level, and experience
		ACSM's Resources for the Personal Trainer, 5th edition (9)
		• Chapters 3, 4, and 14

B. Select exercise modalities to achieve desired adaptations based on goals, medical history, and assessment results. (cont.)

Knowledge or Skill Statement	Explanation/Examples	Resources

Knowledge of the benefits, risks, and contraindications for a wide variety of range of motion (ROM) exercises (*e.g.*, dynamic and passive stretching, tai chi, Pilates, yoga, proprioceptive neuromuscular facilitation, partner stretching)	• Benefits: improved ROM and improved performance of ADL
	• Risks: joint hypermobility, decreased strength, ineffectiveness
	• Evaluate based on the following:
	  • Anatomy and physical limitations
	  • Biomechanical characteristics
	  • Physical and psychological qualities of the client
	  • Client's goal, fitness and skill level, and experience
		ACSM's Resources for the Personal Trainer, 5th edition (9)
		• Chapter 16

Knowledge of the benefits, risks, and contraindications for a wide variety of cardiovascular training exercises and applications based on client experience, skill level, current fitness level, and goals (*e.g.*, progression example: walking, jogging, cross-country skiing, and racquet sports)	• Benefits: decreased risk from premature death, reduction in death, increased health benefits
	• Evaluate based on the following:
	  • Anatomy and physical limitations
	  • Biomechanical characteristics
	  • Physical and psychological qualities of the client
	  • Client's goal, fitness and skill level, and experience
		ACSM's Resources for the Personal Trainer, 5th edition (9)
		• Chapter 15
		• Box 15.1

C. Determine initial frequency, intensity, time (duration), and type (*i.e.*, the FITT principle of exercise prescription) of exercise based on goals, medical history, and assessment results.

Knowledge or Skill Statement	Explanation/Examples	Resources
Knowledge of the recommended frequency (F), intensity (I), and duration (T) of physical activity necessary for development of cardiovascular (CV) and musculoskeletal fitness in healthy adults, seniors, children/adolescents, and pregnant women	• Recommendations for healthy adults: Tables 6.5 and 6.6 • Seniors CV: F = minimum (min) five times a week moderate (mod), three times a week vigorous (vig), or combo; I = five to six times a week mod; seven to eight times a week vig (1–10 scale); T = 30–60 min mod, 20–30 min vig; T = any that does not impose excessive orthopedic stress • Senior resistance: F = two times a week min; I = mod to vig; T = progressive weight-training or weight-bearing calisthenics + balance • Children/adolescents: F = at least three to four times a week preferably all; I = mod to vig; T = 30 mod + 30 vig; T = variety • Pregnancy: adjust for symptoms, discomforts, and abilities; contraindications and considerations • F = at least three times a week, preferably four times; I = mod, RPE 12–14; T = 15–30 min (150 total per week); T = dynamic, rhythmic that use large muscle groups	*ACSM's Guidelines for Exercise Testing and Prescription* (GETP), 10th edition (14) • Chapters 6 and 7 • Tables 6.5 and 6.6 *ACSM's Resources for the Personal Trainer*, 5th edition (9) • Chapters 13 and 20

| | | |

C. Determine initial frequency, intensity, time (duration), and type (*i.e.*, the FITT principle of exercise prescription) of exercise based on goals, medical history, and assessment results. (cont.)

Knowledge or Skill Statement	Explanation/Examples	Resources
Knowledge of the recommended frequency, intensity, and duration of physical activity necessary for development of CV and musculo-skeletal fitness in clients with stable chronic diseases who are medically cleared for exercise, including stable coronary artery disease, other CV diseases, diabetes mellitus (DM), obesity, metabolic syndrome, hypertension (HTN), arthritis, chronic back pain, osteoporosis, chronic obstructive pulmonary disease (COPD), and chronic pain	• CV disease: Chapter 9, *ACSM's GETP* • Arthritis: Chapter 10, *ACSM's GETP* • DM: Chapter 10, *ACSM's GETP*; use Table 10.1 diagnostic criteria and special considerations • HTN: Chapter 10, *ACSM's GETP*; use exercise prescription (Ex R$_x$) + special considerations • Metabolic syndrome: Chapter 10, *ACSM's GETP*; use Table 10.2 clinical criteria and special considerations • Obesity: Chapter 10, *ACSM's GETP*; use Ex R$_x$, special considerations, and behavioral programs • Osteoporosis: Chapter 11, *ACSM's GETP*; use Ex R$_x$ + special considerations • COPD: Chapter 9, *ACSM's GETP*; use Table 9.3 for classification, Ex R$_x$ + special considerations	*ACSM's Guidelines for Exercise Testing and Prescription* (GETP), 10th edition (14) • Chapters 9–11 *ACSM's Resources for the Personal Trainer*, 5th edition (9) • Chapter 20
Knowledge of appropriate exercise modifications based on individual abilities, physical limitations, and other special considerations (*e.g.*, injury rehabilitation, neuromuscular and postural limitations, and scoliosis)	• Research condition through physical therapy and medical networks; use reputable sources for information. • Proper alignment and posture • Do not aggravate condition; avoid exercises that are contraindicated. • Train surrounding musculature to enhance strength and function of joint. • Injury rehabilitation: Determine primary site of injury and prior injury profile.	*ACSM's Resources for the Personal Trainer*, 5th edition (9) • Chapters 3 and 13
Knowledge of implementation of the components of an exercise program including warm-up, training stimulus, cool-down, and stretching	• Warm-up: 5–10 min of low- to moderate-intensity CV exercise and muscular endurance exercises • Training stimulus: 20–60 min of aerobic, resistance, neuromuscular, and/or sport activities • Cool-down: 5–10 min of low- to moderate-intensity CV and ms endurance exercises • Stretching: at least 10 min after warm-up and cool-down	*ACSM's Guidelines for Exercise Testing and Prescription* (GETP), 10th edition (14) • Chapter 6 • Box 6.1 *ACSM's Resources for the Personal Trainer*, 5th edition (9) • Chapters 13 and 18

CPT

C. Determine initial frequency, intensity, time (duration), and type (*i.e.*, the FITT principle of exercise prescription) of exercise based on goals, medical history, and assessment results. (cont.)		
Knowledge or Skill Statement	**Explanation/Examples**	**Resources**
Knowledge of applied biomechanics and exercises associated with movements of the major muscle groups (*e.g.*, seated knee extension — quadriceps)	• Evaluate muscle length, movement arm and resistance arm distances, exercise type, movement direction, and speed of movement for specific joint associated with exercise.	*ACSM's Resources for the Personal Trainer*, 5th edition (9) • Chapters 4 and 14
Knowledge of the application of various methods for establishing and monitoring levels of exercise intensity, including heart rate, rating of perceived exertion (RPE), pace, oxygen consumption and/or metabolic equivalents (METs)	• Determine appropriate method based on conditioning level, medications, information available (maximal volume of oxygen per unit of time [$\dot{V}O_{2max}$], etc.), and shortcomings of each method. • Use metabolic equations (*ACSM's GETP*) to estimate work rate for various modes of training.	*ACSM's Resources for the Personal Trainer*, 5th edition (9) • Chapter 15 • Table 15.2 *ACSM's Guidelines for Exercise Testing and Prescription* (GETP), 10th edition (14) • Chapter 6 • Table 6.3 • Boxes 6.2 and 6.3
Knowledge of the determination of target/training heart rates using predicted maximum heart rate and the heart rate reserve method (Karvonen formula) with recommended intensity percentages based on client fitness level, medical considerations, and goals	• HR_{max}: $220 -$ age • THR $= 220 -$ age $\times 0.64$ (low) • THR $= 220 -$ age $\times 0.94$ (high) • Intensity: 64/70% $-$ 94% • HRR: $HR_{max} -$ resting HR (HR_{rest}) • THR $= [(0.4) \times HRR] + HR_{rest}$ • THR $= [(0.85) \times HRR] + HR_{rest}$ • Intensity: 40%/50% $-$ 85%	*ACSM's Resources for the Personal Trainer*, 5th edition (9) • Chapter 15 *ACSM's Guidelines for Exercise Testing and Prescription* (GETP), 10th edition (14) • Chapter 6
Knowledge of periodization for CV, resistance training, and conditioning program design and progression of exercises when necessary to avoid training plateaus or injury	• Systematic variations in the prescribed volume and intensity during different phases of training program • Recognize signs of overtraining. • Make appropriate modifications for injuries and plateaus.	*ACSM's Resources for the Personal Trainer*, 5th edition (9) • Chapters 13–15 • Tables 13.5 and 16.1–16.3
Knowledge of repetitions (reps) sets, load, and rest periods necessary for desired outcome goals	• Intensity and reps are inversely related. • Reps and rest time are inversely related. • Muscle strength = 8–12 reps (60%–80% one repetition maximum [1-RM]) • Muscle endurance = 15–25 reps (no more than 50% of 1-RM)	*ACSM's Resources for the Personal Trainer*, 5th edition (9) • Chapter 14 *ACSM's Guidelines for Exercise Testing and Prescription* (GETP), 10th edition (14) • Chapter 6
Knowledge of using rep maximum test results procedure to determine resistance training loads	• Use a percentage of 1-RM (70%–85%). • RM: maximum load that can be lifted for a specific number of reps • Absolute resistance: only a specific number of reps	*ACSM's Resources for the Personal Trainer*, 5th edition (9) • Chapter 14

D. Review proposed program with client; demonstrate and instruct the client to perform exercises safely and effectively.

Knowledge or Skill Statement	Explanation/Examples	Resources
Knowledge of and ability to describe the unique adaptations to exercise training regarding strength, functional capacity (FC), and motor skills	• FC relates to physiological adaptations to aerobic exercise. • Strength adaptations related to physiological adaptations of resistance training • Motor skills adaptations occur through cardiovascular (CV) training (intervals); resistance and plyometric training; and flexibility, balance, and agility training.	*ACSM's Resources for the Personal Trainer*, 5th edition (9) • Chapters 13–16 "American College of Sports Medicine Position Stand: Progressive Models in Resistance Training" (15)
Knowledge of and the ability to safely demonstrate exercises designed to enhance CV endurance, muscular strength and endurance, balance, and range of motion	• Each exercise requires understanding of joint range of motion and surrounding muscle anatomy: different modes and techniques, biomechanics, precautions for individuals with health concerns, specifics concerning the movement, key points, details, and safety considerations. • Demonstration involves modeling the exercise accurately, precisely, and correctly — at normal speed and at slower speed/in phases.	*ACSM's Resources for the Personal Trainer*, 5th edition (9) • Chapters 3, 5, and 13–16
Knowledge of appropriate teaching techniques and the ability to demonstrate exercises for improving range of motion of all major joints	• Understanding of joint range of motion and surrounding muscle origins and insertions • Communicate clearly and accurately the guidelines or how to perform and check for understanding. • Model proper technique including alignment, position, breathing, and specifics concerning the technique used. • Engage client in exercise — practice. • Evaluate client performance. • Provide feedback to client. • Have client perform exercise again while cuing for corrections.	*ACSM's Resources for the Personal Trainer*, 5th edition (9) • Chapter 16 • Table 16.1 • Figure 16.2; all figures in chapter are useful *ACSM's Guidelines for Exercise Testing and Prescription* (GETP), 10th edition (14) • Chapter 6

CPT

D.	**Review proposed program with client; demonstrate and instruct the client to perform exercises safely and effectively. (cont.)**	
Knowledge or Skill Statement	**Explanation/Examples**	**Resources**
Knowledge of and the ability to safely demonstrate a wide range of resistance training modalities and activities including variable resistance devices, dynamic constant external resistance devices, kettlebells, static resistance devices, and other resistance devices	• Each exercise requires understanding of joint range of motion and surrounding muscle anatomy: different modes and techniques, biomechanics, precautions for individuals with health concerns, specifics concerning the movement, key points, details, and safety considerations. • Demonstration involves modeling the exercise accurately, precisely, and correctly — at normal speed and at slower speed/in phases. • Communicate clearly and accurately how to perform and check for understanding. • Model proper technique including alignment, position, breathing, and specifics concerning the technique used. • Choice of modality based on availability, needs, goals, experience, and limitations of the client	*ACSM's Resources for the Personal Trainer*, 5th edition (9) • Chapters 13, 14, and 19 • KettleBell Concepts (24)
Knowledge of and ability to safely demonstrate a wide variety of functional training exercises involving nontraditional equipment such as stability balls, balance boards, resistance bands, medicine balls, and foam rollers	• Each exercise requires understanding of joint range of motion and surrounding muscle anatomy: different modes and techniques, biomechanics, precautions for individuals with health concerns, specifics concerning the movement, key points, details, and safety considerations. • Demonstration involves modeling the exercise accurately, precisely, and correctly — at normal speed and at slower speed/in phases. • Communicate clearly and accurately how to perform and check for understanding. • Model proper technique including alignment, position, breathing, and specifics concerning the technique used. • Choice of modality based on availability, needs, goals, experience, and limitations of the client	*ACSM's Resources for the Personal Trainer*, 5th edition (9) • Chapters 13 and 19 ACSM Brochures (1) Perform Better (31) Thera-Band Academy (36)
Knowledge of the physiological effects of the Valsalva maneuver and the associated risks	• Forced exhalation against a closed glottis that results in increases in intrathoracic pressure • Increased blood pressure (BP) response; changes in cardiac physiology	

D. Review proposed program with client; demonstrate and instruct the client to perform exercises safely and effectively. (cont.)

Knowledge or Skill Statement	Explanation/Examples	Resources
Knowledge of the biomechanical principles for the performance of common physical activities (*e.g.*, walking, running, swimming, cycling, resistance training, yoga, Pilates, functional training)	• Understanding biomechanical laws and principles as it influences gait, ground force reaction, inertia, joint angles, body position, lifting and carrying, and external resistive forces (*e.g.*, water, wind)	*ACSM's Resources for the Personal Trainer*, 5th edition (9) • Chapter 4
Knowledge of the concept of detraining or reversibility of conditioning and effects on fitness and functional performance	• When physical training is stopped or reduced, systems readjust in accordance with diminished physiologic stimuli and adaptations to exercise are gradually reduced or lost.	
Knowledge of signs and symptoms of overreaching/overtraining and recommendations to prevent and/or reverse the detrimental effects	• Signs and symptoms — physical, metabolic, and physiological indicators • Proper program design, periodization (planned volume and variation of work), nutrition, and sufficient recovery time • Rest and/or decrease in volume can reverse effects.	
Knowledge of improper exercise form and/or techniques to modify/prevent musculoskeletal injury	• Intrinsic and extrinsic risk factors • Improper biomechanics, improper training techniques, excessive training, misuse of weight-training equipment, fatigue, high intensity, speed of movement, common lifting and movement errors • Teach proper alignment or technique and monitor rehearsal of movements.	
Knowledge of appropriate exercise attire (*e.g.*, footwear, layering for cold, light colored in heat) for specific activities, environments, and conditions	• Clothing should be comfortable, breathable, and allow movement. Footwear should fit properly, not show excessive wear, and be suitable for particular exercise and surfaces. • Clothing can restrict the maximum rate of evaporative cooling in the heat. Covered area, fabric weave, weight, color, air spaces, and *proper fit* are important. • Proper clothing is a primary mechanism for achieving thermal balance during *heat* and cold stress. Adequate layers of insulation, wind protection, and area covered are important.	

CPT

D. Review proposed program with client; demonstrate and instruct the client to perform exercises safely and effectively. (cont.)

Knowledge or Skill Statement	Explanation/Examples	Resources
Knowledge of communication techniques for effective teaching and client retention with awareness of visual, auditory, and kinesthetic learning styles	• Visual: learn through seeing; demonstration; images and diagrams, watching a video, use of imagery, visual cues for proper body alignment, use mirrors for feedback • Auditory: learn through hearing; verbal instruction and cuing, clear verbal presentation • Kinesthetic: learn by direct involvement after short and concise explanation; palpate muscle used, guide clients physically through movement, practice without resistance to review movement pattern	*ACSM's Resources for the Personal Trainer*, 5th edition (9) • Chapter 9
Knowledge of proper spotting positions and techniques for injury prevention and exercise assistance	• Goal of spotting is to prevent injury. • Be in a position to assist client with lift if unable to perform correctly, break form, or possible loss of balance. • Good communication • Know proper hand grip positions. • Know proper exercise technique. • Know number of reps lifter intends to do. • Know plan of action if serious injury occurs.	*ACSM's Resources for the Personal Trainer*, 5th edition (9) • Chapters 14 and 18

E. Monitor client technique and response to exercise modifying as necessary.

Knowledge or Skill Statement	Explanation/Examples	Resources
Knowledge of normal and abnormal responses to exercise and criteria for termination of exercise (*e.g.*, shortness of breath [SOB], unusual joint pain, dizziness, abnormal heart rate [HR] response)	• Normal response — HR, systolic blood pressure (SBP), and respiratory rate increase as work increases. • Termination: abnormal response in HR, blood pressure (BP), chest pain, or change in heart rhythm; poor perfusion; physical or verbal manifestations of severe fatigue, SOB, wheezing, leg cramps, etc.	*ACSM's Resources for the Personal Trainer*, 5th edition (9) • Chapters 5 and 15 *ACSM's Guidelines for Exercise Testing and Prescription* (GETP), 10th edition (14) • Chapter 4 • Box 4.4
Knowledge of proper and improper form and technique while using cardiovascular conditioning equipment (*e.g.*, stair-climbers, stationary cycles, treadmills, and elliptical trainers)	• Provide cues for proper alignment and posture based on biomechanics. • Review manufacturer's instructions and warranty information. • Provide safety instructions for mounting and dismounting equipment.	*ACSM's Resources for the Personal Trainer*, 5th edition (9) • Chapter 15

E. Monitor client technique and response to exercise modifying as necessary. (cont.)

Knowledge or Skill Statement	Explanation/Examples	Resources
Knowledge of proper and improper form and technique while performing resistance exercises (*e.g.*, resistance machines, stability balls, free weights, resistance bands, calisthenics/body weight)	• Proper posture, body alignment, and breathing • Line up joint with axis of rotation. • Exercises use full range of motion conducted in a deliberate, controlled manner and involve concentric and eccentric muscle actions. • Provide safety instructions. • Instruct, demonstrate, and provide feedback.	*ACSM's Resources for the Personal Trainer*, 5th edition (9) • Chapter 14 *ACSM's Guidelines for Exercise Testing and Prescription* (GETP), 10th edition (14) • Chapter 6
Knowledge of proper and improper form and technique for flexibility exercises (*e.g.*, static stretching, dynamic, partner stretching)	• Proper posture and alignment • Emphasize proper breathing. • Hold endpoints. • Exhale when you feel the muscle being stretched, relaxed, and softened. • Slowly reposition and allow muscle to recover. • Do not bounce or force a stretch while holding breath. • Do not stretch beyond limits.	*ACSM's Resources for the Personal Trainer*, 5th edition (9) • Chapters 13 and 16
Skill in interpreting client understanding/comprehension and body language during exercise	• Use established rapport. • Knowledge of common body language cues • Observe; confirm observations verbally with client.	*ACSM's Resources for the Personal Trainer*, 5th edition (9) • Chapters 9, 10, and 18
Skill in effective communication, including active listening, cuing, and providing constructive feedback during and after exercise	• Customer service skills on body language, communication, greeting • Feedback should be immediate, specific, and based on performance standards. It should also be objective, nonthreatening, clarifying, and supportive. • Cues can be verbal, visual, and/or physical.	*ACSM's Resources for the Personal Trainer*, 5th edition (9) • Chapters 9 and 18

F. Recommend appropriate exercise progressions to improve or maintain the client's fitness level.		
Knowledge or Skill Statement	**Explanation/Examples**	**Resources**
Knowledge of specific exercises and program modifications for healthy adults, seniors, children and adolescents, and pregnant women	• Once competency of basic exercises is established, add advanced exercises and progress by increasing intensity or duration. • Modifications for specific population based on structural, physiological effects of maturation and/or condition	*ACSM's Resources for the Personal Trainer*, 5th edition (9) • Chapters 12, 13, and 20 *ACSM's Guidelines for Exercise Testing and Prescription* (GETP), 10th edition (14) • Chapter 7
Knowledge of specific exercises and program modifications for individuals with chronic disease who are medically cleared to exercise — stable coronary artery disease, other cardiovascular (CV) diseases, diabetes mellitus, obesity, metabolic syndrome, hypertension, arthritis, chronic back pain, osteoporosis, chronic pulmonary disease, and chronic pain	• Once competency of basic exercises is established, add advanced exercises and progress by increase intensity or duration. • Modifications for specific population based on structural, physiological effects of maturation and/or condition	*ACSM's Resources for the Personal Trainer*, 5th edition (9) • Chapters 12, 13, and 20 *ACSM's Guidelines for Exercise Testing and Prescription* (GETP), 10th edition (14) • Chapters 9–11
Knowledge of principles of progressive overload, specificity, and program progression to avoid training plateaus and promote continued improvement and goal achievement	• Progressive overload: As the body adapts to a given stimulus, an increase in stimulus is required for further adaptation and improvement (increase load or volume). • Specificity: Only muscles that are trained will adapt and change (training two to three times per week for each body part). • Progression: Modify volume and add advanced exercises once competency is achieved. • Be wary of signs and symptoms of overtraining.	*ACSM's Resources for the Personal Trainer*, 5th edition (9) • Chapters 13 and 14
Knowledge of appropriate methods to teach progression of exercises for all major muscle groups (*e.g.*, progression of standing lunge to walking lunge to walking lunge with resistance)	• Progressions: Move from wide to smaller base of support, supported to unsupported movement, bilateral to unilateral, short to long lever, simple to complex, single joint to compound exercises.	*ACSM's Resources for the Personal Trainer*, 5th edition (9) • Chapters 13 and 14
Knowledge of modifications to periodized conditioning programs to increase or maintain muscular strength and/or endurance, hypertrophy, power, CV endurance, balance, and range of motion/flexibility	• Hypertrophy: high volume — short rest periods • Strength/power: reduced volume, increased load and rest periods • CV endurance: once frequency and baseline conditioning is established, increase intensity and vary modes (interval training). • Balance: vary base of support, use unstable surfaces, change perturbations • Flexibility: Use different modes and techniques; increase frequency.	*ACSM's Resources for the Personal Trainer*, 5th edition (9) • Chapters 14–16

G. Seek client feedback to ensure satisfaction and enjoyment of the program.		
Knowledge or Skill Statement	**Explanation/Examples**	**Resources**
Knowledge of effective techniques for program evaluation and client satisfaction (*e.g.*, survey, written follow-up, verbal feedback)	• Use of assessments • Feedback vehicles both written and verbal • Track response rate. • Establish best practices. • Track programs year over year (client database). • Timely follow-up and feedback • Positive reinforcement	*ACSM's Resources for the Personal Trainer*, 5th edition (9) • Chapters 8 and 13
Knowledge of client goals and appropriate review and modification	• Use of assessments on a periodic basis (4 wk to 3 mo) as a measure of success for achieving goals and motivation • Consistency of workouts; check motivation levels, self-efficacy	*ACSM's Resources for the Personal Trainer*, 5th edition (9) • Chapters 12, 13, and 18

DOMAIN III: EXERCISE LEADERSHIP AND CLIENT EDUCATION

A. Create a positive exercise experience in order to optimize participant adherence by applying effective communication techniques, motivation techniques, and behavioral strategies.		
Knowledge or Skill Statement	**Explanation/Examples**	**Resources**
Knowledge of effective and timely uses of a wide variety of communication modes (*i.e.*, e-mail, telephone, Web site, newsletters)	• Analyze effectiveness, timeliness, cost, return on investment, number of people reached, audience, and number of responses. • Monitor consistency, reliability, and credibility of message delivery.	
Knowledge of verbal and nonverbal behaviors that communicate positive reinforcement and encouragement (*i.e.*, eye contact, targeted praise, empathy)	• Positive body language, facial expressions, head movements, positive client-centered approach, eye contact • Accept clients.	*ACSM's Resources for the Personal Trainer*, 5th edition (9) • Chapters 9 and 10
Knowledge of and skill in enhancing client engagement utilizing active listening techniques	• Use of reflective statements to clarify and summarize client issues • Nonjudgmental • Undivided attention • Eye contact • Empathy	*ACSM's Resources for the Personal Trainer*, 5th edition (9) • Chapters 9 and 10
Knowledge of different types of learners (auditory, visual, kinesthetic) and how to apply teaching and training techniques to optimize a client's training session	• Visual: learn through seeing; demonstration; alignment cuing • Auditory: learn through hearing; verbal instruction • Kinesthetic: learn by direct involvement; moving, experiencing	*ACSM's Resources for the Personal Trainer*, 5th edition (9) • Chapters 7–9 and 18

CPT

A. Create a positive exercise experience in order to optimize participant adherence by applying effective communication techniques, motivation techniques, and behavioral strategies. (cont.)

Knowledge or Skill Statement	Explanation/Examples	Resources
Knowledge of different types of feedback (*i.e.*, evaluative, supportive, descriptive) and the ability to use feedback to optimize a client's training session	• Corrective feedback should be immediate • All feedback should be nonthreatening, objective, clarifying, reflective, and supportive.	*ACSM's Resources for the Personal Trainer*, 5th edition (9) • Chapter 9
Knowledge of and the application of health behavior change models (socioecological model, readiness to change model, social cognitive theory, and theory of planned behavior, etc.) and effective strategies that support and facilitate exercise adherence	• Behavior change pyramid moves clients through stages to their goal. • Action-oriented process of making a commitment, identifying and eliminating cues that produce problem behavior; provide healthy substitutions; elicit social support and provide reinforcement	*ACSM's Resources for the Personal Trainer*, 5th edition (9) • Chapters 7 and 8 *ACSM's Guidelines for Exercise Testing and Prescription* (GETP), 10th edition (14) • Chapter 12
Knowledge of barriers to exercise adherence and compliance (*e.g.*, time management, injury, fear, lack of knowledge, weather)	• Identify solutions to common barriers: personal, behavioral, environmental, social, and programmatic. • Discuss and brainstorm solutions such as scheduling workouts, alternative training environments, progressive plans, educating clients, home exercise recommendations, and incentives.	*ACSM's Resources for the Personal Trainer*, 5th edition (9) • Chapter 8 *ACSM's Guidelines for Exercise Testing and Prescription* (GETP), 10th edition (14) • Chapter 12 • Table 12.3
Knowledge of triggers to relapse and prevention strategies	• Plan for common lapses in healthy behavior such as work pressures, travel, and boredom. • Prevention strategies: stress management skills, goal setting, variety of activities, places to exercise, and competitive events	*ACSM's Resources for the Personal Trainer*, 5th edition (9) • Chapters 8 and 9
Knowledge of specific techniques to facilitate motivation (*e.g.*, goal setting, incentive programs, achievement recognition, social support)	• Use goal setting to establish level of concern. • Pleasant training environment • Tracking progress and knowledge of results to establish success; rewarding achievement	*ACSM's Resources for the Personal Trainer*, 5th edition (9) • Chapters 8 and 9
Knowledge of extrinsic and intrinsic reinforcement strategies (*e.g.*, T-shirt, improved self-esteem)	• Extrinsic: Identify outside factors that support a desire to attain a goal. • Intrinsic: Remain important long after goal is achieved. • Strategies: motivational interviewing, disadvantages of current behavior, and advantage to change	*ACSM's Resources for the Personal Trainer*, 5th edition (9) • Chapters 8 and 9

A. Create a positive exercise experience in order to optimize participant adherence by applying effective communication techniques, motivation techniques, and behavioral strategies. (cont.)		
Knowledge or Skill Statement	**Explanation/Examples**	**Resources**
Knowledge of strategies to increase nonstructured physical activity levels (*e.g.*, stair walking, parking farther away, bike to work)	• Walking or biking short distances when one would normally drive a car • Take the stairs instead of elevator or escalator. • Park at far end of parking lot when shopping. • Take a walk for half of your lunch hour. • Get off one stop before destination and walk the rest of the way. • Pace while talking on the phone. • Walk to the next office instead of sending an e-mail or phoning. • Get up and walk around for 10 min out of every hour while at work. • Use a pedometer to track the number of steps taken per day. • Physical activity can be part of the routine activities of day-to-day living, such as farming, gardening, walking or cycling to work, walking to catch a bus, house cleaning, or doing household chores.	"Physical Activity and Public Health: Updated Recommendation for Adults from the American College of Sports Medicine and the American Heart Association" (12)
Knowledge of health coaching principles and lifestyle management techniques related to behavior change	• Goal setting; connecting goals to deeper motivation; adopt a being curious attitude; ask clients what they are willing to do; create manageable weekly goals between sessions; focus on what's working.	*ACSM's Resources for the Personal Trainer*, 5th edition (9) • Chapters 7 and 8
Knowledge of specific, age-appropriate leadership techniques, and educational methods to increase client engagement	• Social support and participation of similar niches • Community-based programs • Appropriate music and intensity level • Fun	

B. Educate clients using scientifically sound resources to enhance knowledge, enjoyment, and adherence.		
Knowledge or Skill Statement	**Explanation/Examples**	**Resources**
Knowledge of the influence of lifestyle factors, including nutrition and physical activity habits, on lipid and lipoprotein profiles	• Chronic adaptations to cardiovascular exercise • Fundamentals of nutrition and fat metabolism • Good sources of fats	*ACSM's Resources for the Personal Trainer*, 5th edition (9) • Chapters 5 and 6 • Table 5.2

B. Educate clients using scientifically sound resources to enhance knowledge, enjoyment, and adherence. (cont.)		
Knowledge or Skill Statement	**Explanation/Examples**	**Resources**
Knowledge of the value of carbohydrates, fats, and proteins as fuels for exercise and physical activity	• Explain the functions of carbohydrates as preferred fuel, quick energy source, protein sparing, oxidation of fat, and storage forms. • Explain the functions of fats as an insulation from extreme temperatures, cushion for concussion forces, satiety, and carrier of essential nutrients. • Explain the functions of protein in hormone production, acid–base balance, growth and tissue maintenance, transport of nutrients, and fluid balance enzyme synthesis.	*ACSM's Resources for the Personal Trainer*, 5th edition (9) • Chapter 6
Knowledge of the following terms: body composition, body mass index (BMI), lean body mass, anorexia nervosa, bulimia nervosa, and body fat distribution	• Body composition: Explain the relative proportion of fat and fat-free mass. • BMI: technique of using weight relative to height • Lean body mass: term used to describe a collection of tissues (muscle, bone, etc.) other than fat, which make up total body weight • Anorexia nervosa: eating disorder characterized by restrictive eating due to being afraid of gaining weight, even though at least 15% below expected weight for age and height • Bulimia nervosa: eating disorder of usually normal weight individuals characterized by cycles of overeating and purging or other compensatory behaviors	*ACSM's Resources for the Personal Trainer*, 5th edition (9) • Chapter 12 "American College of Sports Medicine Position Stand. The Female Athlete Triad" (13)
Knowledge of the relationship between body composition and health	• Explanation of the strong correlation between obesity and the increased risk of chronic diseases	*ACSM's Resources for the Personal Trainer*, 5th edition (9) • Chapter 12
Knowledge of the effectiveness of diet, exercise, and behavior modification as a method for modifying body composition	• Explain the effectiveness a healthy and balanced diet, consisting of portion control, healthy food choices and food preparation, caloric intake on weight, and body composition. • Explain the relationship between type, intensity, frequency, and duration of exercise and caloric expenditure. • Explain the common behavioral strategies such as nonsupervised and supervised exercise and occupational and leisure time activities as mean to increase physical activity.	"American College of Sports Medicine Position Stand. Appropriate Physical Activity Intervention Strategies for Weight Loss and Prevention of Weight Regain for Adults" (10)

B. Educate clients using scientifically sound resources to enhance knowledge, enjoyment, and adherence. (cont.)

Knowledge or Skill Statement	Explanation/Examples	Resources
Knowledge of the importance of maintaining hydration before, during, and after exercise	• Explain the goal of prehydration is to start activity hydrated and with normal plasma electrolyte levels. • Explain the goal of drinking during physical activity is to prevent dehydration. • Explain the goal of hydration after exercise is to replace any electrolyte fluid deficit. • Explain individual fluid replacement rate is based on individual sweat rates, choice of beverages, length and intensity of activity, and environmental conditions.	"American College of Sports Medicine Position Stand. Exercise and Fluid Replacement" (16) *ACSM's Resources for the Personal Trainer*, 5th edition (9) • Chapter 6
Knowledge of the USDA 2015-2020 Edition of the Dietary Guidelines for Americans	• Guidelines explaining the different food groups, sources, and portions of a balanced and healthy eating plan • USDA Dietary Guidelines 2010 is the federal government's evidence-based nutritional guidance to promote health, reduce the risk of chronic diseases, and reduce the prevalence of overweight and obesity through improved nutrition and physical activity. • American Dietetic Association is the world's largest organization of food and nutrition professionals.	ChooseMyPlate, formerly known as USDA Food Guide Pyramid (38) "USDA Dietary Guidelines for Americans" (39) Academy of Nutrition and Dietetics, formerly known as American Dietetic Association (18)
Knowledge of the Female Athlete Triad	• Explain the interrelationships between energy availability, menstrual cycle, and bone mineral density of women and girls who participate in athletics on the clinical manifestations of eating disorders, amenorrhea, and osteoporosis and possible interventions and/or educational measures used to prevent or mitigate the effects.	"American College of Sports Medicine Position Stand. The Female Athlete Triad" (13)
Knowledge of the myths and consequences associated with inappropriate weight loss methods (*e.g.*, fad diets, dietary supplements, overexercising, starvation diets)	• Explain scientifically based safe methods of weight loss using the proper eating habits and appropriate physical activity guidelines and issues associated with diets based on extreme or exclusive principles.	*ACSM's Resources for the Personal Trainer*, 5th edition (9) • Chapter 6
Knowledge of the number of kilocalories in 1 g of carbohydrate, fat, protein, and alcohol	• Carbohydrate = $4 \text{ kcal} \cdot \text{g}^{-1}$ • Fat = $9 \text{ kcal} \cdot \text{g}^{-1}$ • Protein = $4 \text{ kcal} \cdot \text{g}^{-1}$ • Alcohol = $7 \text{ kcal} \cdot \text{g}^{-1}$	*ACSM's Resources for the Personal Trainer*, 5th edition (9) • Chapter 6

CPT

B. Educate clients using scientifically sound resources to enhance knowledge, enjoyment, and adherence. (cont.)

Knowledge or Skill Statement	Explanation/Examples	Resources
Knowledge of the ACSM's guidelines for caloric intake for individuals desiring to lose or gain weight	• Weight loss = calories out > calories in • Weight gain = calories in > calories out • Explain the physical activity expenditure recommendations for weight loss and weight maintenance in minutes and the associated caloric equivalent.	"American College of Sports Medicine Position Stand. Appropriate Physical Activity Intervention Strategies for Weight Loss and Prevention of Weight Regain for Adults" (10) *ACSM's Resources for the Personal Trainer*, 5th edition (9) • Chapter 6
Knowledge of accessing and dissemination of scientifically based, relevant health, exercise, and wellness-related resources and information	• Identify competent and reputable sources of current information such as ACSM Web site, National Institutes of Health (NIH) Web site, peer-reviewed journals, and others.	ACSM's Web site and resources (1–3) National Institutes of Health (28,29) WebMD Healthy Living (43) Mayo Clinic Health Information (25)
Knowledge of community-based exercise programs that provide social support and structured activities (*e.g.*, walking clubs, intramural sports, golf leagues, cycling clubs)	• Identify national and local programs targeted toward specific conditions, age, sponsoring organizations, sport categories, and level of fitness. • Contact chamber of commerce, rotary club, or civic organizations.	"National Blueprint: Increasing Physical Activity among Adults Aged 50 and Older" (27) President's Council on Fitness, Sports & Nutrition (32) Exercise is Medicine (22) National Physical Activity Plan (30) The Community Guide to Promoting Physical Activity (23)
Knowledge of stress management and relaxation techniques (*e.g.*, progressive relaxation, guided imagery, massage therapy)	• Explain the differences between common relaxation and stress management techniques. • Knowledge of proper breathing techniques	WebMD Stress Management Health Center (44) "Stress Management Techniques" (35) "Relaxation Technique for Stress Relief" (34)

DOMAIN IV: LEGAL, PROFESSIONAL, BUSINESS, AND MARKETING

A. Perform a pre-exercise readiness assessment as delineated in the current edition of ACSM's Guidelines for Exercise Testing and Prescription.

Knowledge or Skill Statement	Explanation/Examples	Resources
Knowledge of pre-exercise readiness assessment as delineated in the current edition of ACSM's Guidelines for Exercise Testing and Prescription in order to minimize client injury and/or medical complications.	• Properly identify those who pose an increased risk of experiencing exercise-related cardiovascular incident.	*ACSM's Resources for the Personal Trainer*, 5th edition (9) • Chapters 11, 20, and 22 *ACSM's Health/Fitness Facility Standards and Guidelines*, 3rd edition (17) • Chapter 2 • Table 2.1

A. Perform a pre-exercise readiness assessment as delineated in the current edition of ACSM's Guidelines for Exercise Testing and Prescription. (cont.)

Knowledge or Skill Statement	Explanation/Examples	Resources
Knowledge of the appropriate level of supervision and monitoring recommended for individuals with known disease based on disease-specific risk stratification guidelines and current health status	• High-risk clients: recommended medical exam and graded exercise test (GXT) prior to exercise program for moderate and vigorous exercise; medical doctor (MD) supervision of exercise test recommended • Moderate-risk clients: recommended medical exam and GXT with medical supervision prior to exercise program for vigorous exercise. • Medical examination and GXT not necessary for moderate exercise for moderate-risk clients	*ACSM's Resources for the Personal Trainer*, 5th edition (9) • Chapter 11 • Figures 11.5 and 11.6 • Tables 11.1 and 11.2
Skill in the application of the ACSM pre-exercise readiness assessment and associated medical clearance guidelines prior to exercise testing and program participation.	• May need to use a facility with medically qualified staff	*ACSM's Resources for the Personal Trainer*, 5th edition (9) • Chapter 11 • Figure 11.2

B. Collaborate with healthcare professionals and organizations in order to create a network of providers that can assist in maximizing program effectiveness, minimizing risk of liability, and provide services outside the scope of practice of the ACSM Certified Personal Trainer.

Knowledge or Skill Statement	Explanation/Examples	Resources
Knowledge of reputable professional resources and referral sources to ensure client safety and program effectiveness	• Establish a local network of health care professionals. • Establish policies, procedures, and forms for matching clients with appropriate professionals, services, appraisals, programs, and referrals.	*ACSM's Resources for the Personal Trainer*, 5th edition (9) • Chapter 11
Knowledge of the scope of practice for the Certified Personal Trainer and the need to practice within this scope	• Scope: fitness professional who develops and implements safe and sound programs through an individualized approach to exercise leadership in healthy populations and/or those individuals with medical clearance to exercise • Minimize risk of exposure to liability.	ACSM Web site (7) *ACSM's Resources for the Personal Trainer*, 5th edition (9) • Chapters 1 and 21
Knowledge of effective and professional communication with allied health and fitness professionals	• Proper spelling and grammar used • Confidential cover sheet • Contact prior to sending fax. • Secure network if using e-mail. • Up-to-date self-credentials and contact information	*ACSM's Resources for the Personal Trainer*, 5th edition (9) • Chapter 9 U.S. Department of Health and Human Services, Health Insurance Portability and Accountability Act (41,42)

CPT

B. Collaborate with healthcare professionals and organizations in order to create a network of providers that can assist in maximizing program effectiveness, minimizing risk of liability, and provide services outside the scope of practice of the ACSM Certified Personal Trainer. (cont.)

Knowledge or Skill Statement	Explanation/Examples	Resources
Knowledge of identifying individuals requiring referral to a physician or allied health services such as physical therapy, dietary counseling, stress management, weight management, and psychological and social services	• Knowledge of conditions, signs, or indicators that fall outside of scope of practice • Establish local network of health care professionals. • Establish policies, procedures, and forms for matching clients with appropriate services, appraisals, programs, and referrals.	*ACSM's Resources for the Personal Trainer*, 5th edition (9) • Chapter 11

C. Develop a comprehensive risk management program (including emergency action plan and injury prevention program) to enhance the standard of care and reflect a client-focused mission.

Knowledge or Skill Statement	Explanation/Examples	Resources
Knowledge of local resources available to obtain basic life support, automated external defibrillator (AED), and cardiopulmonary resuscitation (CPR) certification	• Current certification that includes demonstration of practical skills	*American Red Cross First Aid/CPR/AED Participant Manual* (19) American Heart Association Basic Life Support (BLS) or Lifesaver Certification (20)
Knowledge of appropriate emergency procedures (*i.e.*, telephone procedures, written emergency procedures, personnel responsibilities) in a health and fitness setting	• Written plan that addresses major emergency situations • Explicit steps and instructions on how each emergency situation is handled and the roles of responders • Emergency medical services (EMS) contact information, emergency equipment location • Rehearsal of plan four times a year • Proper follow-up and documentation	*ACSM's Resources for the Personal Trainer*, 5th edition (9) • Chapter 22 *ACSM's Health/Fitness Facility Standards and Guidelines*, 3rd edition (17) • Chapter 4 • Appendix D and Form 26
Knowledge of basic first aid procedures for exercise-related injuries, such as bleeding, strains/sprains, fractures, and exercise intolerance (dizziness, syncope, heat injury)	• Rest, ice, compression, and elevation (RICE) for strains/sprains • Direct pressure for bleeding • Let professionals treat fractures and serious injuries out of scope of training. • Supine with legs elevated for fainting	*American Red Cross First Aid/CPR/AED Participant Manual* (19)
Knowledge of precautions taken in an exercise setting to ensure participant safety (*e.g.*, equipment placement, facility cleanliness, floor surface)	• Signage for potential risk; conform to relevant laws, regulations, and published standards • Americans with Disabilities Act requirements for passageway width, signage, and clear floor space • Circulation areas adjacent to physical activity areas • Proper signage on any equipment or areas of facility that are out of order or unusable	*ACSM's Resources for the Personal Trainer*, 5th edition (9) • Chapter 22 *ACSM's Health/Fitness Facility Standards and Guidelines*, 3rd edition (17) • Chapters 6 and 7 *Risk Management for Health/Fitness Professionals* (21) • Chapter 10

C. Develop a comprehensive risk management program (including emergency action plan and injury prevention program) to enhance the standard of care and reflect a client-focused mission. (cont.)		
Knowledge or Skill Statement	**Explanation/Examples**	**Resources**
Knowledge of the following terms related to musculoskeletal injuries (*e.g.*, shin splints, sprain, strain, bursitis, fractures, tendonitis, patellofemoral pain syndrome, low back pain, plantar fasciitis)	• Sprain: injury to a ligament • Strain: injury to a muscle • Bursitis: inflammation of bursa • Tendonitis: inflammation of tendon • Fracture: broken bone • Plantar fasciitis: chronic inflammatory condition that results in pain at the calcaneal insertion • Patellofemoral pain syndrome: common disorder in young athletes that produces anterior knee pain	*ACSM's Resources for the Personal Trainer*, 5th edition (9) • Chapter 3
Knowledge of contraindicated exercises/postures and potential risks associated with certain exercises (*e.g.*, straight-leg sit-ups, double-leg raises, full squats, hurdler's stretch, cervical and lumbar hyperextension, and standing bent-over-toe touch)	• Potential risks: Correct body alignment and joint position are critical for maximum results and minimal risk of injury. • Potentially harmful postures/exercises should be modified to safer joint positions. • Any exercises which are contraindicated by physician should be avoided.	*ACSM's Resources for the Personal Trainer*, 5th edition (9) • Chapter 16
Knowledge of the responsibilities, limitations, and the legal implications for the Certified Personal Trainer of carrying out emergency procedures	• Duty of care • Current certifications, including CPR/AED; familiarity of facility emergency plan; documentation of incident; professional liability insurance	*ACSM's Resources for the Personal Trainer*, 5th edition (9) • Chapter 22 *Risk Management for Health/Fitness Professionals* (21) • Chapter 11
Knowledge of potential musculoskeletal injuries (*e.g.*, knowledge of contusions, sprains, strains, fractures), cardiovascular/pulmonary complications (*e.g.*, chest pain, palpitations/arrhythmias, tachycardia, bradycardia, hypotension/hypertension, hyperventilation), and metabolic abnormalities (*e.g.*, fainting/syncope, hypoglycemia/hyperglycemia, hypothermia/hyperthermia)	• Cardiovascular/pulmonary complications: identification —Table 37.5; basic first aid guidelines —Table 37.6 • Potential musculoskeletal injuries —Table 37.2 • Metabolic abnormalities: basic first aid guidelines —Table 37.6 • Environmental conditions: basic first aid —Table 37.8; Box 37.11	*ACSM's Resources for the Personal Trainer*, 5th edition (9) • Chapter 3 *American Red Cross First Aid/CPR/AED Participant Manual* (19)
Knowledge of the initial management and first aid techniques associated with open wounds, musculoskeletal injuries, cardiovascular/pulmonary complications, and metabolic disorders	• Open wounds — Chapter 7 • Musculoskeletal injuries — Chapter 8 • Breathing and cardiac emergencies — Chapters 2–4 • Sudden illness — Chapter 5	*American Red Cross First Aid/CPR/AED Participant Manual* (19) • Chapter 2–5, 7, and 8 *ACSM's Guidelines for Exercise Testing and Prescription* (GETP), 10th edition (14) • Appendix B
Knowledge of the need for and components of an equipment service plan/agreement and how it may be used to evaluate the condition of exercise equipment to reduce the potential risk of injury	• Daily, weekly, and monthly care for all equipment • Regular inspection and preventative maintenance of equipment and documentation of inspection and repairs • Knowledge of equipment warranty and repair information • Follow manufacturer's recommendations.	*ACSM's Health/Fitness Facility Standards and Guidelines*, 3rd edition (17) • Chapter 7 • Tables 7.3 and 7.4 • Appendix A • Supplements 3 and 4 *Risk Management for Health/Fitness Professionals* (21) • Chapter 9

C. Develop a comprehensive risk management program (including emergency action plan and injury prevention program) to enhance the standard of care and reflect a client-focused mission. (cont.)

Knowledge or Skill Statement	Explanation/Examples	Resources
Knowledge of the need for and use of safety policies and procedures (*e.g.,* incident/accident reports, emergency procedure training) and legal necessity thereof	• Duty to public to provide safe facility and programs • Emergency response system critical to providing safe environment • Address major emergency situation. • Elicit instructions and roles of how to respond. • Document system (training, instructions) • Rehearsal four times a year • Available first aid and emergency equipment • Coordination with local EMS	*ACSM's Resources for the Personal Trainer*, 5th edition (9) • Chapter 22 *ACSM's Health/Fitness Facility Standards and Guidelines*, 3rd edition (17) • Chapter 4 *Risk Management for Health/Fitness Professionals* (21) • Chapter 11
Knowledge of the need for and components of an emergency action plan.	• Written emergency action plan with explicit steps and instructions on how each emergency situation is handled and the roles of responders • EMS contact information, emergency equipment location • Rehearsal • Knowledge of fire safety and facility evacuation procedures • Proper follow-up and documentation	*ACSM's Resources for the Personal Trainer*, 5th edition (9) • Chapter 22 *ACSM's Health/Fitness Facility Standards and Guidelines*, 3rd edition (17) • Chapter 4 *ACSM's Guidelines for Exercise Testing and Prescription* (GETP), 10th edition (14) • Appendix B *Risk Management for Health/Fitness Professionals* (21) • Chapter 11
Knowledge of effective communication skills and the ability to inform staff and clients of emergency policies and procedures for the facility or program	• Establish who is responsible for communication to EMS and within facility as part of the emergency action plan. • Telephone number for emergency assistance should be clearly posted near all phones. Emergency communication devices must be readily available and working properly. • Plans should include medical, fire, evacuations, and other emergencies. • Rehearse plan, including communication portion every 3 mo. • Unsupervised facility: signage of what steps members should take in the event of a witnessed emergency situation.	*Risk Management for Health/Fitness Professionals* (21) • Chapter 11 *ACSM's Health/Fitness Facility Standards and Guidelines*, 3rd edition (17) • Chapter 8 *ACSM's Guidelines for Exercise Testing and Prescription* (GETP), 10th edition (14) • Appendix B
Skill in demonstrating and carrying out emergency procedures during exercise testing and/or training	• Emergency drills convened four times a year • Follow-up evaluation of personnel and response and documentation of drills	*ACSM's Health/Fitness Facility Standards and Guidelines*, 3rd edition (17) • Chapter 4 *ACSM's Guidelines for Exercise Testing and Prescription* (GETP), 10th edition (14) • Appendix B

C. Develop a comprehensive risk management program (including emergency action plan and injury prevention program) to enhance the standard of care and reflect a client-focused mission. (cont.)

Knowledge or Skill Statement	Explanation/Examples	Resources
Skill in assisting, spotting, and monitoring a client safely and effectively during exercise testing and/or training	• Knowledge of exercise being performed, possible adverse effects, common errors in performing, proper positioning to assist lift, being alert, good communication	*ACSM's Resources for the Personal Trainer*, 5th edition (9) • Chapters 14 and 18

D. Participate in approved continuing education programs on a regular basis to maximize effectiveness, increase professionalism, and enhance knowledge and skills in the field of health and fitness.

Knowledge or Skill Statement	Explanation/Examples	Resources
Knowledge of the role of continuing education, professional resources, and requirements for certification and recertification	• Obligation to public and clients to keep current with science and practice-related research • Certification requirements: 18 yr old; high school diploma (general education developmental [GED]); adult cardiopulmonary resuscitation (CPR) certification • American College of Sports Medicine (ACSM) Certification is valid for 3 yr. • Recertification: 45 credits	ACSM Web site (5,6) *ACSM's Resources for the Personal Trainer*, 5th edition (9) • Chapters 1 and 2
Knowledge of the requirements for obtaining and maintaining continuing education credits (CEC) and where one can obtain ACSM-approved CEC **Knowledge** of the continually evolving field of health and fitness and the need for Certified Personal Trainers to keep abreast of new research and applications in the field of exercise science	• Identify ACSM-approved providers for CEC. • Identify credible health/fitness resources to obtain CEC in person (workshops) and via Internet.	ACSM Web site (5,6) *ACSM's Resources for the Personal Trainer*, 5th edition (9) • Chapters 1 and 2 ACSM Journals (4)

E. Adhere to ACSM Certification's Code of Ethics by practicing in a professional manner within the scope of practice of an ACSM Certified Personal Trainer.

Knowledge or Skill Statement	Explanation/Examples	Resources
Knowledge of the components of both the ACSM's Code of Ethics as well as the ACSM Certified Personal Trainer scope of practice	• Code of Ethics: Improve knowledge and skill, maintain high professional and scientific standards, safeguard the public, and improve both the health and well-being of the individual and the community. • Scope: fitness professional who develops and implements an individualized approach to exercise leadership in healthy populations and/or those individuals with medical clearance to exercise	ACSM Web site (8) *ACSM's Resources for the Personal Trainer*, 5th edition (9) • Chapters 1 and 2

CPT

E. Adhere to ACSM Certification's Code of Ethics by practicing in a professional manner within the scope of practice of an ACSM Certified Personal Trainer. (cont.)

Knowledge or Skill Statement	Explanation/Examples	Resources
Knowledge of appropriate work attire and professional behavior	• Work attire may be dictated by professional work environments. • Professional behavior established via code of ethics and scope of practice; good communication skills, ability to build relationships	*ACSM's Resources for the Personal Trainer*, 5th edition (9) • Chapters 1 and 2
Skill in conducting all professional activities within the scope of practice of the ACSM Certified Personal Trainer	• Leading and demonstrating safe and effective methods of exercise by applying the fundamental principles of exercise science • Writing appropriate exercise recommendations • Motivating individuals to begin and to continue with their healthy behaviors	ACSM Web site (1,4) *ACSM's Resources for the Personal Trainer*, 5th edition (9) • Chapters 1 and 2

F. Develop a business plan to establish mission, business, budgetary, and sales objectives.

Knowledge or Skill Statement	Explanation/Examples	Resources
Knowledge of implementation methods for effective, ethical, and professional business practices	• Create vision, mission statement, core business values, services, and operational policies. • Collect and review the most recent publications of standards and guidelines by national organizations.	*ACSM's Resources for the Personal Trainer*, 5th edition (9) • Chapter 21
Knowledge of various business structures (*e.g.*, sole proprietorship, independent contractor, partnership, various corporation types)	• Sole: one person owned business • Individual contractor: provides services for an individual or business • Partner: two or more people with a contract filed with local or state government • Corporation: formal business entity subject to laws, regulations, and demands of stockholders • Limited liability corporation (LLC): similar to a corporation, owners have limited personal liability for the debts and actions of the LLC. Other features of LLCs are more like a partnership, providing management flexibility, and the benefit of pass-through taxation. (from Internal Revenue Service [IRS] Web site: http://www.irs.gov/businesses /small/article/0,,id=98277,00.html) • S corporation: alternative for small business that combines advantages of the other business models.	*ACSM's Resources for the Personal Trainer*, 5th edition (9) • Chapter 21

F. Develop a business plan to establish mission, business, budgetary, and sales objectives. (cont.)

Knowledge or Skill Statement	Explanation/Examples	Resources
Skill in the development of a basic business plan, which includes establishing a budget (*i.e.*, billing, cancellation policy, late arrival policy, payment methods/plans)	• Demographic and competitive analysis • Establish a budget. • Revenue and expense management • Develop management policies, marketing, sales, and pricing.	*ACSM's Resources for the Personal Trainer*, 5th edition (9) • Chapter 21
Skill in the development of business objectives (*i.e.*, clearly define business mission statement, business, goals, benchmarks, membership/ financial goals, program evaluation)	• Define philosophy and purpose of program or center. • Use mock business plans as a template. • Knowledge of industry standards for goals and benchmarks • Results outcomes expected/ projected for all categories • Measure key performance indicators.	*ACSM's Resources for the Personal Trainer*, 5th edition (9) • Chapter 21
Skill in market niches and the components of a mission statement (*i.e.*, vision, values, service description)	• Using demographics to identify niches based on client type, training needs, or location	*ACSM's Resources for the Personal Trainer*, 5th edition (9) • Chapter 21
Skill in using spreadsheet software to develop and manage budget	• Use QuickBooks or Mind Your Own Business (MYOB) software programs.	Microsoft Excel (26)
Skill in career development practices (*i.e.*, hiring, setting training standards)	• Steps to hiring personal trainers • Establish training standards. • Train and empower staff. • Manage staff and business. • Provide education to staff.	*ACSM's Resources for the Personal Trainer*, 5th edition (9) • Chapters 2 and 21

G. Develop marketing materials and engage in networking/business exchanges to build client base, promote services, and increase resources.

Knowledge or Skill Statement	Explanation/Examples	Resources
Knowledge of management policies, marketing, sales, and pricing	• Operational policies such as billing, cancellation, payment methods • Marketing: lead boxes, referrals, advertising, direct mail, and multimedia • Sales: eight-step sales generation process and sales checklist • Pricing based on education, experience, environment/location, and expenses	*ACSM's Resources for the Personal Trainer*, 5th edition (9) • Chapter 21
Knowledge of marketing materials to promote the business (*i.e.*, brochures, business cards, web pages, blogs, video clips, e-marketing)	• Converts leads to prospects and prospects to members. • Create positive image. • Web sites, print/video brochures	*ACSM's Resources for the Personal Trainer*, 5th edition (9) • Chapter 21

G. Develop marketing materials and engage in networking/business exchanges to build client base, promote services, and increase resources. (cont.)

Knowledge or Skill Statement	Explanation/Examples	Resources
Knowledge of various methods for distribution and promotion of the personal training business (*i.e.*, social networking, press releases, feature newspaper articles)	• External signage, Web sites, radio, TV, billboards, community involvement • Create a positive image and educate consumers.	*ACSM's Resources for the Personal Trainer*, 5th edition (9) • Chapter 21
Skill in the development of various marketing materials via computer applications (*i.e.*, Microsoft Word, Microsoft Power Point, PDF, Publisher)	• Use online assistance for each application. • Marketing should not be too busy, eye-catching, colorful, and targeted.	*ACSM's Resources for the Personal Trainer*, 5th edition (9) • Chapter 21

H. Obtain personal training and liability insurance and follow industry-accepted professional, ethical, and business standards to optimize safety and reduce liability risk.

Knowledge or Skill Statement	Explanation/Examples	Resources
Knowledge of professional liability and common types of negligence seen in training environments	• Negligence is failing to do something that a reasonable, prudent person would have done under same or similar circumstances or doing something that a reasonable, prudent person would not have done. • Types: gross, contributory, comparative, omission • Duty of care, breach of duty, causation, damages • Level of responsibility to protect from harm • Safe premises, equipment usage, scope of practice, qualifications, emergency preparedness	*ACSM's Resources for the Personal Trainer*, 5th edition (9) • Chapter 22 *Risk Management for Health/Fitness Professionals* (21) • Chapter 2
Knowledge of legal issues pertinent to health care delivery by licensed and nonlicensed health care professionals providing rehabilitative services and exercise testing and legal risk management techniques	• Higher standard level of care expected at medical facilities • Refer to appropriate health care professional if not within scope of practice. • Establish strategic alliances.	*ACSM's Resources for the Personal Trainer*, 5th edition (9) • Chapter 22
Knowledge of equipment maintenance such to decrease risk of injury and liability (*i.e.*, maintenance plan, service schedule, safety considerations for each piece)	• Follow manufacturer's recommendations. • Regular inspection and preventative cleaning and maintenance • Documentation of maintenance for each piece of equipment • Out of order sign if not in proper working condition • Signage for proper usage of equipment with varying degrees (danger, warning, caution)	*ACSM's Resources for the Personal Trainer*, 5th edition (9) • Chapter 22 *ACSM's Health/Fitness Facility Standards and Guidelines*, 3rd edition (17) • Chapter 7 • Tables 7.3 and 7.4 *Risk Management for Health/Fitness Professionals* (21) • Chapter 9

I. Engage in healthy lifestyle practices in order to be a positive role model for all clients.

Knowledge or Skill Statement	Explanation/Examples	Resources
Knowledge of appropriate professional behavior (*i.e.*, not smoking, substance-free, nonoffensive dress, courtesy, politeness, active listening skills)	• Model healthy lifestyle. • Be prompt and prepared. • Customer service skills • Educated • Current certifications	*ACSM's Resources for the Personal Trainer*, 5th edition (9) • Chapters 1, 2, and 9
Knowledge of environmental influences that may negatively impact client satisfaction/compliance (*i.e.*, music choice/volume level, personal hygiene, scent sensitivity)	• Use facility standards and guidelines to ensure proper range of environmental factors. • Ask for feedback through surveys, comment cards, feedback books, etc. • Create facility policies to ensure comfortable, safe atmosphere for all.	*ACSM's Resources for the Personal Trainer*, 5th edition (9) • Chapters 8 and 18 *ACSM's Health/Fitness Facility Standards and Guidelines*, 3rd edition (17)
Knowledge of the need to avoid distractions during a training session (*i.e.*, texting, cell phone calls, in-person conversation with others)	• Client deserves and pays for your full attention. • Manage your energy level through proper sleep, eating well, regular exercise, and good self-care. • Administrative time used for correspondence • If unavoidable, temporarily excuse yourself, keep it brief, and refer to other floor staff.	*ACSM's Resources for the Personal Trainer*, 5th edition (9) • Chapters 1, 9, and 18

J. Respect copyright laws by obtaining permission before using protected materials and other covered intellectual property.

Knowledge or Skill Statement	Explanation/Examples	Resources
Knowledge of and application of national and international copyright laws	• Copyright, a form of intellectual property law, protects original works of authorship including literary, dramatic, musical, and artistic works, such as poetry, novels, movies, songs, computer software, and architecture. Copyright does not protect facts, ideas, systems, or methods of operation, although it may protect the way these things are expressed.	*ACSM's Resources for the Personal Trainer*, 5th edition (9) • Chapter 1 United States Copyright Office (37)
Knowledge of the referencing of non-original work	• Part of code of ethics: Credentialed professionals take credit, including authorship, only for work they have actually performed and give credit to the contributions of others if warranted. • All nonoriginal ideas must be cited. Parenthetically, most common: authors last name and year of publication. On the reference page, list all authors for works with three, four, or five authors.	*ACSM's Resources for the Personal Trainer*, 5th edition (9) • Chapter 1 Purdue Online Writing Lab: MLA In-Text Citations (33)

CPT

J. Respect copyright laws by obtaining permission before using protected materials and other covered intellectual property. (cont.)		
Knowledge or Skill Statement	**Explanation/Examples**	**Resources**
Skill in developing original educational material	• Research a variety of sources. • Discuss in laymen's terms. • Highlight important points. • Length of material will vary based on space and audience. • Create an eye-appealing format and a catchy title. • Use templates as a starting point.	ACSM Web site (1–3)

K. Safeguard client confidentiality and privacy rights unless formally waived or in emergency situations.		
Knowledge or Skill Statement	**Explanation/Examples**	**Resources**
Knowledge of practices/systems for maintaining client confidentiality with electronic and hard copy files	• American College of Sports Medicine (ACSM) guideline: A facility should ensure that fitness testing, health promotion, and wellness have a system that provides for and protects the complete confidentiality of all user records and meetings. • Permitting only certain authorized individuals access to information, with the understanding that they will disclose it only to authorized individuals • User records should only be released with an individual's signed authorization.	*ACSM's Resources for the Personal Trainer*, 5th edition (9) • Chapters 10 and 22 *Risk Management for Health/Fitness Professionals* (21) • Chapter 6
Knowledge of the importance of client privacy (*i.e.*, client personal safety, legal liability, client credit protection, client medical disclosure)	• Protection against theft or injury, prevention of potential harm to a client's reputation, maintain trust and provide a safe environment, prevent litigation	*ACSM's Resources for the Personal Trainer*, 5th edition (9) • Chapters 10 and 22
Knowledge of the Family Educational Rights and Privacy Act (FERPA) and Health Insurance Portability and Accountability Act (HIPAA) laws depending on setting and state that the personal training business resides in	• HIPAA: strict policies regarding safety and security of private records • FERPA: policy for the stewards of education data to ensure students' personal information is properly safeguarded and is used only for legitimate purposes and only when absolutely necessary	*ACSM's Resources for the Personal Trainer*, 5th edition (9) • Chapter 22 U.S. Department of Health and Human Services, Health Insurance Portability and Accountability Act (41,42) U.S. Department of Education: Family Educational Rights and Privacy Act (40) *Risk Management for Health/Fitness Professionals* (21) • Chapter 6
Skill in obtaining and maintaining rapid access to client health history and emergency contact information	• Create a secure, accurate, current, and alphabetized filing system for active client files.	*ACSM's Resources for the Personal Trainer*, 5th edition (9) • Chapter 22

REFERENCES

ACSM REFERENCES:

1. American College of Sports Medicine. ACSM brochures. American College of Sports Medicine [Internet]. [cited December 2016]. Available from: http://www.acsm.org/access-public-information/brochures-fact-sheets/brochures

2. American College of Sports Medicine. ACSM current comment fact sheet. American College of Sports Medicine [Internet]. [cited 2011 Sep 22]. Available from: http://www.acsm.org/access-public-information/brochures-fact-sheets/fact-sheets

3. American College of Sports Medicine. ACSM fit society page. American College of Sports Medicine [Internet]. [cited 2011 Sep 22]. Available from: http://www.acsm.org/access-public-information/newsletters/fit-society-page

4. American College of Sports Medicine. ACSM journals. American College of Sports Medicine [Internet]. [cited 2012 Mar 4]. Available from http://www.acsm.org/access-public-information/acsm-journals

5. American College of Sports Medicine. Certified personal trainer ACSM certification/renewal form. American College of Sports Medicine [Internet]. [cited 2011 Sep 22]. Available from: http://forms.acsm.org/_frm/crt/New/certification_renewal_form.asp

6. American College of Sports Medicine. Certified personal trainer renewing your ACSM certification. American College of Sports Medicine [Internet]. [cited 2011 Sep 22]. Available from: http://certification.acsm.org/renew-your-certification

7. American College of Sports Medicine. Certified personal trainer scope of practice. American College of Sports Medicine [Internet]. [cited 2011 Sep 22]. Available from: http://certification.acsm.org/acsm-certified-personal-trainer

8. American College of Sports Medicine. Code of ethics of American College of Sports Medicine. American College of Sports Medicine [Internet]. [cited 2011 Sep 22]. Available from: http://www.acsm.org/Content/NavigationMenu/MemberServices/MemberResources/CodeofEthics/Code_of_Ethics.htm

9. Battista R, senior editor. *ACSM's Resources for the Personal Trainer*. 5th ed. Philadelphia (PA): Wolters Kluwer; 2018. p.

10. Donnelly JE, Blair SN, Jakicic JM, et al. American College of Sports Medicine position stand. Appropriate physical activity intervention strategies for weight loss and prevention of weight regain for adults. *Med Sci in Sports Exerc*. 2009;41(2):459–71.

11. Garber CE, Blissmer B, Deschenes MR, et al. American College of Sports Medicine position stand. Quantity and quality of exercise for developing and maintaining cardiorespiratory, musculoskeletal, and neuromotor fitness in apparently healthy adults: guidance for prescribing exercise. *Med Sci Sports Exerc*. 2011;43(7):1334–59.

12. Haskell WL, Lee IM, Pate RR, et al. Physical activity and public health: updated recommendation for adults from the American College of Sports Medicine and the American Heart Association. *Med Sci Sports Exerc*. 2007;39(8):1423–34.

13. Nattiv A, Loucks AB, Manore MM, et al. American College of Sports Medicine position stand. The female athlete triad. *Med Sci Sports Exerc*. 2007;39(10):1867–82.

14. Riebe D, editor. *ACSM's Guidelines for Exercise Testing and Prescription*. 10th ed. Philadelphia (PA): Wolters Kluwer; 2018. p.

15. Ratamess NA, Alvar BA, Evetock TK, et al. American College of Sports Medicine position stand. Progressive models in resistance training. *Med Sci Sports Exercise*. 2009;41(3):687–708.

16. Sawka MN, Burke LM, Eichner ER, et al. American College of Sports Medicine position stand. Exercise and fluid replacement. *Med Sci Sports Exerc*. 2007;39(2):377–90.

17. Tharrett SJ, McInnis KJ, Peterson JA. *ACSM's Health/Fitness Facility Standards and Guidelines*. 3rd ed. Champaign (IL): Human Kinetics; 2007. 203 p.

NON-ACSM REFERENCES:

18. Academy of Nutrition and Dietetics Web site [Internet]. Chicago (IL): Academy of Nutrition and Dietetics. [cited 2012 Mar 4]. Available from: http://www.eatright.org

19. American Red Cross. *American Red Cross First Aid/CPR/AED Participant Manual*. Yardley (PA): Staywell; 2011. 181 p.

20. Bureau of Labor Statistics. Occupational outlook handbook, 2010–2011 edition, fitness workers. Bureau of Labor Statistics [Internet]. [cited 2011 Sep 22]. Available from: http://www.bls.gov/oco/ocos296.htm

21. Eickhoff-Schemek J, Herbert DL, Connaughton DP. *Risk Management for Health/Fitness Professionals: Legal Issues and Strategies*. Philadelphia (PA): Lippincott Williams & Wilkins; 2009. 407 p.

22. Exercise is Medicine. Additional resources. Exercise is Medicine [Internet]. [cited 2011 Sep 22]. Available from: http://exerciseismedicine.org/resources.htm

23. The Guide to Community Preventive Services. Community guide topics. Promoting physical activity. The Guide to Community Preventive Services [Internet]. [cited 2012 Mar 4]. Available from: http://www.thecommunityguide.org/pa/index.html

24. KettleBell Concepts Web site [Internet]. New York (NY): KettleBell Concepts; [cited 2012 Mar 4]. Available from: http://www.kettlebellconcepts.com/index.php

25. Mayo Clinic. Health information. Diseases and conditions. Mayo Clinic [Internet]. [cited 2012 Mar 4]. Available from: http://www.mayoclinic.com/health-information/

26. Microsoft Excel. Manage your personal budget with Excel. Microsoft Office [Internet]. [cited 2012 Mar 4]. Available from: http://office.microsoft.com/en-us/excel-help/manage-your-personal-budget-with-excel-HA001045087.aspx

27. National blueprint: increasing physical activity among adults aged 50 and older. Active aging partnerships. Blueprint Partners [Internet]. [cited 2012 Mar 4]. Available from: http://www.agingblueprint.org/partnership.cfm

28. National Institute of Health. Health information, health topics. National Institute of Health [Internet]. [cited 2012 Mar 4]. Available from: http://health.nih.gov/see_all_topics.aspx

29. National Institute of Health. Research and training. Science education. National Institute of Health [Internet]. [cited 2012 Mar 4]. Available from: http://www.nih.gov/science/education.htm

30. National Physical Activity Plan Web site [Internet]. Columbia (SC): National Physical Activity Plan [cited 2012 Mar 4]. Available from: http://www.physicalactivityplan.org

31. Perform Better. Balance and stabilization training exercises. Perform Better [Internet]. [cited 2012 Mar 4]. Available from: http://www.performbetter.com

32. President's Council on Fitness, Sports & Nutrition. Resources. President's Council on Fitness, Sports & Nutrition [Internet]. [cited 2012 Mar 4]. Available from: http://www.fitness.gov/resources-and-grants/resources/

33. Purdue Online Writing Lab. MLA In-Text Citations: the basics. Purdue University [Internet]. [cited 2012 Sep 8]. Available from: http://owl.english.purdue.edu/owl/resource/747/02/

34. Robinson L, Segal R, Segal J, et al. Relaxation technique for stress relief. Helpguide [Internet]. [cited 2012 Mar 4]. Available from: http://helpguide.org/mental/stress_relief_meditation_yoga_relaxation.htm

35. Stoppler MC, Sheil WC, editor. Stress management techniques. MedicineNet [Internet]. [cited 2012 Mar 4]. Available from: http://www.medicinenet.com/stress_management_techniques/page3.htm

36. Thera-Band Academy. Theraband exercises. Thera-Band Academy [Internet]. [cited 2012 Mar 4]. Available from: http://www.thera-bandacademy.com/

37. U.S. Copyright Office Web site [Internet]. Washington (DC): U.S. Copyright Office; [cited 2012 Mar 4]. Available from: http://www .copyright.gov/

38. U.S. Department of Agriculture. USDA center for nutrition policy and promotion. United States Department of Agriculture [Internet]. [cited 2011 Sep 26]. Available from: http://www.choosemyplate.gov/index.html

39. U.S. Department of Agriculture. USDA dietary guidelines for Americans. United States Department of Agriculture [Internet]. [cited 2011 Sep 26]. Available from: http://www.cnpp.usda.gov /DietaryGuidelines.htm

40. U.S. Department of Education. Family educational rights and privacy act. U.S. Department of Education [Internet]. [cited 2012 Mar 4]. Available from: www2.ed.gov/offices/OM/fpco/ferpa/index.html

41. U.S. Department of Health and Human Services. Health information privacy. U.S. Department of Health & Human Services [Internet]. [cited 2012 Mar 4]. Available from: http://www.hhs.gov/ocr/privacy/

42. U.S. Department of Health and Human Services. Summary of the HIPPA privacy rule. U.S. Department of Health & Human Services [Internet]. [cited 2011 Sep 22]. Available from: http://www.hhs.gov /ocr/privacy/hipaa/understanding/summary/privacysummary.pdf

43. WebMD. Healthy living A–Z. WebMD [Internet]. [cited 2012 Mar 4]. Available from: http://www.webmd.com/a-to-z-guides/healthy -living/default.htm

44. WebMD. Stress management health center. WebMD [Internet]. [cited 2012 Mar 4]. Available from: http://www.webmd.com/balance/stress -management/stress-management-relieving-stress

DIRECTIONS: Each of the numbered items or incomplete statements in this section is followed by answers or by completions of the statement. Select the ONE lettered answer or completion that is BEST in each case.

1. Which of the following exercise modes allows buoyancy to reduce the potential for musculoskeletal injury?
   A) Cycling
   B) Walking
   C) Skiing
   D) Water exercise

2. In which stage of motivational readiness is a person who is an irregular exerciser?
   A) Precontemplation
   B) Contemplation
   C) Preparation
   D) Action

3. Which of the following medications is designed to modify blood cholesterol levels?
   A) Nitrates
   B) β-Blockers
   C) Antihyperlipidemics
   D) Aspirin

4. Which of the following represents more than 90% of the fat stored in the body and is composed of a glycerol molecule connected to three fatty acids?
   A) Phospholipids
   B) Cholesterol
   C) Triglycerides (TG)
   D) Free fatty acids

5. Limited flexibility of which of the following muscle groups increases the risk of low back pain?
   A) Quadriceps
   B) Hamstrings
   C) Hip flexors
   D) Gluteus maximus

6. Calcium, phosphorus, magnesium, potassium, sulfur, sodium, and chloride are examples of _____.
   A) Macrominerals
   B) Microminerals
   C) Proteins
   D) Vitamins

7. Which of the following terms represents an imaginary horizontal plane passing through the midsection of the body and dividing it into upper and lower portions?
   A) Sagittal
   B) Frontal
   C) Transverse
   D) Superior

8. A personal trainer fails to spot a client performing heavy incline dumbbell presses, and the client injures himself when the dumbbell is dropped on his face. Which of the following identifies the appropriate type of negligence displayed in this scenario?
   A) Admission
   B) Commission
   C) Omission
   D) Legal

9. The preparticipation health screening process is based upon _____.
   A) How long the client has been physically active; presence of signs or symptoms and/or known metabolic, renal, or cardiovascular disease; and exercise intensity at which individual desires to exercise
   B) Individual's current physical activity level; presence of signs or symptoms and/or known metabolic, renal, or cardiovascular disease; and exercise intensity at which individual desires to exercise
   C) How long the client has been exercising, number of cardiovascular disease risk factors, and how long the individual has been physically active
   D) The current level of physical activity the individual is engaging in; how long client has been physically active; and presence of signs or symptoms and/or known metabolic, renal, or cardiovascular disease

10. Which of the following stages defines people having the greatest risk of relapse?
    A) Precontemplation
    B) Contemplation
    C) Preparation
    D) Action

CPT

11. Uncoordinated gait, headache, dizziness, vomiting, and elevated body temperature are signs and symptoms of _____.
    A) Acute exposure to the cold
    B) Hypothermia
    C) Heat exhaustion and heat stroke
    D) Acute altitude sickness

12. The informed consent document provides all of the following *except* _____.
    A) The opportunity to choose to withdraw involvement at any point
    B) Protection of personal trainer against lawsuits of negligence
    C) Information regarding risks and benefits of participation
    D) The opportunity for potential client to ask questions

13. Which of the following are part of the initial client consultation?
    A) Discussion of current health status and health history and/or Physical Activity Readiness Questionnaire + (PAR-Q+)
    B) Health and fitness assessments
    C) Informed consent document
    D) All of the above

14. You are conducting an initial client consultation. Your potential client has walked for $1 \text{ h} \cdot \text{d}^{-1}$, $6 \text{ d} \cdot \text{wk}^{-1}$ for the previous 10 yr. She informs you that three times over the previous 6 mo she has been becoming dizzy during her walks and had one episode of syncope during a walk. She has not spoken with her physician about these episodes and attributes them to her not having eaten enough prior to her exercise bout. As her personal trainer, what would be the most prudent course of action?
    A) Explain the potential causes of dizziness before, during, and after exercise and continue with the consultation.
    B) Tell her it is nothing to be worried about but to mention it to her physician at her next appointment.
    C) Tell her to discontinue all exercise and make an appointment with her physician for medical clearance.
    D) Tell her to slow her walking pace and be sure to drink enough fluids.

15. How many calories are contained in a food bar that contains 5 g of fat, 30 g of carbohydrates including 4 g of fiber, and 3 g of protein?
    A) 161 kcal
    B) 168 kcal
    C) 177 kcal
    D) 193 kcal

16. Verbal encouragement, material incentives, self-praise, and use of specific contingency contracts are examples of _____.
    A) Shaping
    B) Reinforcement
    C) Antecedent control
    D) Setting goals

17. Which physiologic response(s) would be expected to occur under conditions of high ambient temperature?
    A) Decreased maximal oxygen uptake
    B) Decreased heart rate (HR) at rest
    C) Increased HR at submaximal workload
    D) Decreased maximal HR

18. Regular exercise will result in what chronic adaptation in cardiac output (CO) during exercise at the same workload?
    A) Increase
    B) Decrease
    C) No change
    D) Increase during dynamic exercise only

19. Which of the following conditions is characterized by a decrease in bone mass and density, producing bone porosity and fragility?
    A) Osteoarthritis
    B) Osteomyelitis
    C) Epiphyseal osteomyelitis
    D) Osteoporosis

20. Studies designed to measure the success of a program based on some quantifiable data that can be analyzed examine _____.
    A) Incomes
    B) Outcomes
    C) Client progress notes
    D) Attendance records

21. When using the original Borg scale (6–20) for the general public, exercise intensity should be maintained between _____.
    A) 7 and 10
    B) 12 and 16
    C) 17 and 18
    D) 19 and 20

22. Rotation of the anterior surface of a bone toward the midline of the body is called _____.
    A) Medial rotation
    B) Lateral rotation
    C) Supination
    D) Pronation

23. Your new client is 6 ft tall and weighs 275 lb. What is his body mass index (BMI) classification?
    A) $37.3 \text{ kg} \cdot \text{m}^{-2}$; class I obesity
    B) $40.0 \text{ kg} \cdot \text{m}^{-2}$; class III obesity
    C) $40.0 \text{ kg} \cdot \text{m}^{-2}$; class II obesity
    D) $37.3 \text{ kg} \cdot \text{m}^{-2}$; class II obesity

24. During the preparticipation screening process, you learn that your new client has previously had a stent and also has diabetes. You also learn that he has been regularly physically active for the previous 2 yr, are asymptomatic, and compliant with medication use as prescribed by his physician. Your client would like to engage in vigorous-intensity exercise. How do you advise your new client?
    A) Advise the new client to halt all exercise and seek medical clearance before resuming activity
    B) Advise the new client to begin vigorous-intensity exercise (*i.e.*, rating of perceived exertion [RPE] ≥14 or ≥60% heart rate reserve [HRR]) without medical clearance
    C) Advise the new client to pursue medical clearance, and once obtained, your client may then begin adding in bouts of vigorous-intensity exercise
    D) Advise the new client not to engage in vigorous-intensity exercise for safety

25. A new client is sedentary, has no known disease, but does possess signs and symptoms that suggest presence of cardiovascular, metabolic, or renal disease. Is medical clearance recommended prior to beginning any intensity (*i.e.*, light, moderate, or vigorous) of exercise?
    A) Medical clearance is recommended for moderate to vigorous but not light-intensity exercise.
    B) Medical clearance is recommended prior to beginning any intensity exercise.
    C) Medical clearance is recommended for vigorous-intensity exercise only.
    D) Medical clearance is not necessary.

26. Which of the following water-soluble vitamins must be consumed on a daily basis?
    A) Vitamins A and C
    B) Vitamins A, D, E, and K
    C) Vitamins B complex and C
    D) Vitamins A, B complex, D, and K

27. You have a new client, a 47-yr-old male who is a current smoker. He would like to quit smoking and adopt a more active lifestyle. He is currently not regularly exercising, has a blood pressure (BP) of 136/88 mm Hg, total cholesterol of 182 mg · dL^{-1}, waist circumference of 38 in, fasting plasma glucose of 92 mg · dL^{-1}, and no known family history of cardiovascular disease (CVD). How many positive risk factors for CVD does he have?
    A) Two
    B) Three
    C) Four
    D) Five

28. What is angina pectoris?
    A) Discomfort associated with myocardial ischemia
    B) Discomfort associated with hypertension
    C) Discomfort associated with heartburn
    D) Discomfort associated with papillary necrosis

29. Which of the following BP readings would be considered prehypertensive for an adult?
    A) 126/80 mm Hg
    B) 118/78 mm Hg
    C) 144/94 mm Hg
    D) 156/92 mm Hg

30. According to the Adult Treatment Panel III (ATP III), which of the following would be considered an *optimal* level of low-density lipoprotein cholesterol (LDL-C)?
    A) 130 mg · dL^{-1}
    B) 105 mg · dL^{-1}
    C) 95 mg · dL^{-1}
    D) 120 mg · dL^{-1}

31. Which of the following is an appropriate method of monitoring exercise intensity for a pregnant client?
    A) RPE
    B) Target $\dot{V}O_{2max}$
    C) Percentage of maximal heart rate (%HR$_{max}$)
    D) Percentage of HRR

32. Which of the following is a warning sign to terminate exercise during pregnancy?
    A) Increased fetal movement
    B) Dyspnea prior to exertion
    C) Dizziness
    D) Both B and C

33. When exercise training children, _____.
    A) Exercise programs should increase physical fitness in the short term and strength and power in the long term.
    B) Strength training should be avoided for safety reasons.
    C) Increasing the rate of training intensity more than approximately 10% per week increases the likelihood of overuse injuries of bone.
    D) Children with exercise-induced asthma are often unable to lead active lives.

34. Which of the following appropriately defines SMART goals?
    A) Specialized, meticulous, accurate, reasonable, time-oriented
    B) Specific, measurable, achievable, realistic, time-oriented
    C) Specialized, meticulous, achievable, realistic, time-oriented
    D) Specific, measurable, assessable, reasonable, time-oriented

35. A client is using a pedometer to measure the amount of steps taken each day and then writes it in a daily journal. This would be an example of _____.
    A) Goal setting
    B) Self-monitoring
    C) Problem solving
    D) Goal measuring

36. Which of the following components of the exercise prescription (Ex R$_x$) work inversely with each other?
    A) Intensity and duration
    B) Mode and intensity
    C) Mode and duration
    D) Mode and frequency

37. Which of the following types of muscle stretching can cause residual muscle soreness, is time-consuming, and typically requires a partner?
    A) Static
    B) Ballistic
    C) Proprioceptive neuromuscular facilitation (PNF)
    D) All of the above

38. Failure of a Certified Personal Trainer (CPT) to perform in a generally acceptable standard is called _____.
    A) Malpractice
    B) Malfeasance
    C) Negligence
    D) None of the above

39. Which of the following statements is *not* true about synovial joints?
    A) The joint cavity is enclosed by the joint capsule.
    B) They are the most common type of joint found in the human body.
    C) A synovial membrane lines the joint cavity.
    D) They are the least common type of joint found in the human body.

40. Which of the following is an example of a social barrier?
    A) A single parent with no child care
    B) A friend encouraging you to skip your afternoon walk and have dinner with them instead
    C) Family members discouraging you to join a gym
    D) All of the above

41. Feeling good about being able to perform an activity or skill, such as finally being able to run a mile or to increase the speed of walking a mile, is an example of an _____.
    A) Extrinsic reward
    B) Intrinsic reward
    C) External stimulus
    D) Internal stimulus

42. An important safety consideration for exercise equipment in a fitness center includes _____.
    A) Flexibility of equipment to allow for different body sizes
    B) Ability of equipment to restrict range of motion (ROM)
    C) Affordability of equipment to allow for changing out equipment periodically
    D) Mobility of equipment to allow for easy rearrangement

43. The social cognitive theory (SCT) posits which of the following as the most important factor relating to behavior change?
    A) Perception of risk of untoward health outcomes
    B) Self-efficacy and expectation of outcome related to behavior changes
    C) Belief that behavior change is worth the improvement in health
    D) None of the above

44. A method of strength and power training that involves an eccentric loading of muscles and tendons followed immediately by an explosive concentric contraction is called _____.
    A) Plyometrics
    B) Periodization
    C) Supersets
    D) Isotonic reversals

45. Which of the following personnel is responsible for program design as well as implementation of that program?
    A) Administrative assistant
    B) Personal trainer
    C) Manager or director
    D) Health fitness specialist

46. What is the purpose of agreements, releases, and consent forms?
    A) To inform the client of participation risks as well as the rights of the client and the facility
    B) To inform the client what he or she can and cannot do in the facility
    C) To define the relationship between the facility operator and the personal trainer
    D) Body composition, flexibility, cardiorespiratory fitness, and muscular fitness

47. After 30 yr of age, skeletal muscle strength begins to decline primarily because of which of the following?
    A) A gain in fat tissue
    B) A gain in lean tissue
    C) A loss of muscle mass caused by a loss of muscle fibers
    D) Myogenic precursor cell inhibition

48. The health belief model assumes that people will engage in a behavior, such as exercise, when _____.
    A) There is a perceived threat of disease.
    B) External motivation is provided.
    C) Optimal environmental conditions are met.
    D) Internal motivation outweighs external circumstances.

49. The informed consent document _____.
    A) Is a legal document
    B) Provides immunity from prosecution
    C) Provides an explanation of the test to the client
    D) Legally protects the rights of the client

50. A measure of muscular endurance is _____.
    A) One repetition maximum
    B) Three repetition maximum
    C) Number of curl-ups in 1 min
    D) Number of curl-ups in 3 min

51. If a client exercises too much without rest days or develops a minor injury and does not allow time for the injury to heal, what can occur?
    A) An overuse injury
    B) Shin splints
    C) Sleep deprivation
    D) Decreased physical conditioning

52. Which of the following is *not* a sign of exertional heat stroke?
    A) Hypoventilation
    B) Hyperventilation
    C) Disorientation
    D) Vomiting

53. Which of the following is an absolute aerobic exercise contraindication during pregnancy?
    A) Preeclampsia
    B) Restrictive lung disease
    C) Persistent third trimester bleeding
    D) All of the above

54. Which of the following is a change seen as a result of regular chronic exercise?
    A) Decreased HR at rest
    B) Increased stroke volume at rest
    C) No change in CO at rest
    D) All of the above

55. A client has expressed to you that she has set a goal of wearing a particular dress size in time for the wedding of her son. This is an example of _____.
    A) Intrinsic motivation
    B) Self-efficacy
    C) Extrinsic motivation
    D) Self-worth

56. Which of the following is an example of a biological barrier to exercise?
    A) Obesity
    B) Pregnancy
    C) Disease
    D) Injury

57. Print brochures, video brochures, and Web sites are all examples of _____.
    A) Strategic alliances
    B) Reputation management
    C) Promotional materials
    D) Community involvement

58. Which of the following is the first step in constructing a business plan?
    A) Determine sales goals
    B) Conduct a comprehensive demographic analysis
    C) Establish a budget
    D) Evaluate the competition

59. You are a personal trainer providing your services to various health clubs in your region. Although you set your own fees, the percentage of those fees you receive is determined by the health clubs with which you work. What type of business model does this represent?
    A) Sole proprietorship
    B) S corporation
    C) Partnership
    D) Independent contractor

60. All of the following are major agonist muscles involved in knee flexion *except* _____.
    A) Gracilis
    B) Gastrocnemius
    C) Soleus
    D) Popliteus

61. Nodding your head, clarifying what your client has told you, and making eye contact are all examples of _____.
    A) Rapport development
    B) Active listening
    C) Appreciative inquiry
    D) Motivational interviewing

62. Which of the following is *not* an example of social support?
    A) Encouragement from a friend to join their walking group
    B) A family member requesting to join you on your daily walks
    C) Spouses synchronizing schedules so they can attend the same group fitness classes
    D) A friend inquiring why you have not been in exercise class lately

63. In commercial settings, clients should be more extensively screened for potential health risks. The information solicited should include which of the following?
    A) Personal medical history
    B) Present medical status
    C) Medication
    D) All of the above

64. Which of the following is an appropriate measure to take in an effort to counteract dehydration?
    A) Drink excessive amounts of water prior to exercise, even if euhydrated
    B) Consume a low-sodium meal prior to and postexercise bout
    C) Take snack breaks during longer training sessions
    D) Consume a high-protein meal prior to exercise bout

65. What is the planning tool that addresses the organization's short- and long-term goals; identifies the steps needed to achieve the goals; and gives the time line, priority, and allocation of resources to each goal?
    A) Financial plan
    B) Strategic plan
    C) Risk management plan
    D) Marketing plan

66. After 6 mo of personal training and coaching sessions, your client expresses to you that she believes she can now implement what you have taught her and exercise on her own. This is an example of enhanced _____.
    A) Self-worth
    B) Self-esteem
    C) Self-regulation
    D) Self-efficacy

67. Which of the following marketing strategies is the most costly and generates the lowest return on investment?
    A) Lead boxes
    B) Direct mail
    C) Reputation management
    D) Television advertising

68. Which of the following is considered an abnormal curve of the spine with lateral deviation of the vertebral column in the frontal plane?
    A) Lordosis
    B) Scoliosis
    C) Kyphosis
    D) Primary curve

69. Which of the following is not true regarding the Health Insurance Portability and Accountability Act (HIPAA)?
    A) The patient must provide written authorization prior to disclosure or use of information by a third party.
    B) It assures the individual will have access to his or her own personal health information.
    C) Copies of the HIPAA privacy rule do not need to be provided to the individual.
    D) It provides protection of privacy of one's personal health care information.

70. Which of the following BMI values would classify an individual as class I obesity?
    A) $29.9 \text{ kg} \cdot \text{m}^{-2}$
    B) $35.0 \text{ kg} \cdot \text{m}^{-2}$
    C) $32.5 \text{ kg} \cdot \text{m}^{-2}$
    D) $36.0 \text{ kg} \cdot \text{m}^{-2}$

71. Which of the following is an adaptation to resistance training?
    A) Increased capillary density
    B) Decreased aerobic enzyme activity
    C) Increased lactate removal
    D) Both A and C

72. Specifically, muscle shortening under a load is a type of muscle action referred to as _____.
    A) Concentric action
    B) Isometric action
    C) Eccentric action
    D) Dynamic action

73. Why is it important for an individual to perform a cool-down following an exercise bout?
    A) In order to avoid postexercise hypotension and dizziness
    B) In order to avoid postexercise hypertension and dizziness
    C) In order to decrease HR and metabolic end products
    D) Both A and C

74. Which of the following conditions refers to the loss of skeletal muscle mass typically observed with aging?
    A) Osteopenia
    B) Osteoporosis
    C) Sarcopenia
    D) Rheumatoid arthritis

75. Adults age physiologically at individual rates. Therefore, adults of any specified age will vary widely in their physiologic responses to exercise testing. Special considerations should be given to the older adult when giving a fitness test because _____.
    A) Age may be accompanied by deconditioning and disease.
    B) Age automatically predisposes the older adult to clinical depression and neurologic diseases.
    C) The older adult cannot be physically stressed beyond 75% of age-adjusted maximum HR.
    D) The older adult is not as motivated to exercise as a younger person.

76. All of the following are rotator cuff muscles except _____.
    A) Infraspinatus
    B) Teres minor
    C) Subscapularis
    D) Trapezius

77. Compared with running, swimming will result in _____ even if exercise intensity is the same.
    A) A higher HR
    B) A lower HR
    C) A lower CO
    D) A higher CO

78. Attempting to decrease sweating via clothing insulation adjustments and use of clothing vents are recommended during exercise in what type of environment?
    A) High-altitude environment
    B) Cold weather environment
    C) Dry-heat environment
    D) Wet environment

79. Which condition is commonly associated with a progressive decline in bone mineral density (BMD) and calcium content in postmenopausal women?
    A) Osteoarthritis
    B) Osteoporosis
    C) Arthritis
    D) Epiphysitis

80. Which of the following is a result of an older person participating in an exercise program?
    A) Overall improvement in the quality of life and increased independence
    B) No changes in the quality of life but an increase in longevity
    C) Increased longevity but a loss of bone mass
    D) Loss of bone mass with a concomitant increase in bone density

81. In response to regular resistance training, _____.
    A) Older men and women demonstrate similar or even greater strength gains when compared with younger individuals.
    B) Younger men have greater gains in strength than older men.
    C) Younger women have greater gains in strength than older women.
    D) Younger men and women demonstrate similar or greater strength gains compared with older persons.

82. Which of the following statements about confidentiality is *not* correct?
    A) All records must be kept by the program director/manager under lock and key.
    B) Data must be available to all individuals who need to see it.
    C) Data should be kept on file for at least 1 yr before being discarded.
    D) Sensitive information (*e.g.*, participant's name) needs to be protected.

83. Which of the following statements best describes capital budgets?
    A) Include the costs of equipment and building or facility expense
    B) Include the costs to operate a program
    C) Are not necessary with fitness programs
    D) Are included as part of the balance sheet in financial reports

84. Emergency procedures and safety planning should address which of the following?
    A) Injury prevention
    B) Basic principles for exercise training
    C) Metabolic calculations
    D) Common exercise scenarios

85. Which of the following examples is correct regarding appropriate sequencing of resistance exercises?
    A) Perform exercises for strong areas before those for weak areas
    B) Perform least intense exercises prior to most intense exercises
    C) Perform small muscle group exercises prior to large group exercises
    D) Perform multijoint exercises prior to single-joint exercises

86. Within a skeletal muscle fiber, large amounts of calcium are stored in the _____.
    A) Nuclei
    B) Mitochondria
    C) Myosin
    D) Sarcoplasmic reticulum

87. Which of the following is not within the scope of practice of an American College of Sports Medicine (ACSM) CPT?
    A) Determination of current level of client fitness through fitness assessment and testing
    B) Development of client Ex R_x
    C) Aiding clients in setting realistic goals
    D) Providing the client a written detailed dietary plan in conjunction with the Ex R_x

88. All of the following are isotonic resistance exercises *except* _____.
    A) Dumbbell biceps curls
    B) Pull-ups
    C) Box squat jumps
    D) The half-squat wall-sit

89. Which of the following is an adaptation to aerobic conditioning?
    A) Maximal HR will decrease at maximal effort exercise.
    B) CO will increase during submaximal effort exercise.
    C) Lactic acid production will decrease during submaximal effort exercise.
    D) All of the above

90. Which of the following types of stretching involves both contraction and relaxation of a muscle group?
    A) Dynamic stretching
    B) PNF
    C) Ballistic stretching
    D) Static stretching

91. A transient deficiency of blood flow to the myocardium resulting from an imbalance between oxygen demand and oxygen supply is known as _____.
    A) Infarction
    B) Angina
    C) Ischemia
    D) Thrombosis

92. Special precautions for patients with hypertension include all of the following *except* _____.
    A) Avoiding muscle-strengthening exercises that involve low resistance
    B) Avoiding activities that involve the Valsalva maneuver
    C) Monitoring for arrhythmias in a person taking diuretics
    D) Avoiding exercise if resting systolic blood pressure (SBP) is >200 mm Hg or diastolic blood pressure (DBP) is >115 mm Hg

93. A 62-yr-old, obese factory worker complains of pain in his right shoulder on arm abduction; on evaluation, decreased ROM and strength are noted. You also notice that he is beginning to use accessory muscles to substitute movements and to compensate. These symptoms may indicate _____.
    A) A referred pain from a herniated lumbar disk
    B) Rotator cuff strain or impingement
    C) Angina
    D) Advanced stages of multiple sclerosis

94. Which of the following is an exercise program goal for an obese individual?
    A) Improve metabolic profile
    B) Decrease sedentary behavior
    C) Maximize caloric expenditure
    D) All of the above

95. Older adults who have a mobility disability or are at increased risk for falls should incorporate neuromuscular exercise *at least* _____.
    A) $5 \text{ d} \cdot \text{wk}^{-1}$
    B) $1–2 \text{ d} \cdot \text{wk}^{-1}$
    C) $2–3 \text{ d} \cdot \text{wk}^{-1}$
    D) $7 \text{ d} \cdot \text{wk}^{-1}$

96. Which of the following transtheoretical model (TTM) stages of change is correctly defined?
    A) Action: Individual has been regularly active for less than 6 mo.
    B) Preparation: Individual has been making behavior changes for less than 30 d.
    C) Action: Individual has been regularly active and making positive behavior changes for more than 6 mo.
    D) None of the above

97. Which of the following is false about goal setting?
    A) Goal setting can increase motivation and effort to maintain positive behavior changes.
    B) It is an important tool that can help the client adhere to and maintain newly adopted behavior change.
    C) Goal setting can help clients plan for potential barriers.
    D) Goals are most effective when the trainer selects them and the client agrees to them.

98. All of the following are major agonist muscles involved hip flexion *except* _____.
    A) Rectus femoris
    B) Sartorious
    C) Iliopsoas
    D) Quadratus lumborum

99. A type of negligence action that involves claims brought against a defined professional is referred to as _____.
    A) Risk management
    B) Liability
    C) Malpractice
    D) Assumption of risk

100. The acronym HIPAA stands for _____.
    A) Health Insurance Privacy and Accountability Association
    B) Health Insurance Portability and Accountability Act
    C) Health Insurance Privacy and Accountability Act
    D) Health Information Portability and Accountability Association

CPT EXAMINATION ANSWERS AND EXPLANATIONS

1—D. Water exercise

Water exercise has gained in popularity because the buoyancy properties of water help to reduce the potential for musculoskeletal injury and may even allow injured people an opportunity to exercise without further injury. Various activities may be offered in a water-exercise class. Walking, jogging, and dance activity all may be adapted for water. Water-exercise classes typically should combine the benefits of the buoyancy properties of water with the resistive properties of water. In this regard, both an aerobic stimulus as well as activity to enhance muscular strength and endurance may be provided.

2—C. Preparation

Preparation is an individual who is planning for or irregularly exercising, whereas the stage of action represents a person who is currently exercising.

3—C. Antihyperlipidemics

Nitrates and nitroglycerine are antianginals (used to reduce chest pain associated with angina pectoris). β-Blockers are antihypertensives (used to reduce BP by inhibiting the action of adrenergic neurotransmitters at the β-receptor, thereby promoting peripheral vasodilation). β-Blockers also are designed to reduce BP by inhibiting the action of adrenergic neurotransmitters at the β-receptors, thereby decreasing CO. Antihyperlipidemics control blood lipids, especially cholesterol and LDL. Aspirin helps lower blood platelet coagulation making the blood less "sticky."

4—C. Triglycerides (TG)

Dietary fats include TG, sterols (*e.g.*, cholesterol), and phospholipids. TG represent more than 90% of the fat stored in the body. A TG is a glycerol molecule connected to three fatty acid molecules. The fatty acids are identified by the amount of "saturation" or the number of single or double bonds that link the carbon atoms. Saturated fatty acids only have single bonds. Monounsaturated fatty acids have one double bond, and polyunsaturated fatty acids have two or more double bonds.

5—B. Hamstrings

An adequate ROM or joint mobility is requisite for optimal musculoskeletal health. Specifically, limited flexibility of the low back and hamstring regions may relate to an increased risk for development of chronic low back pain and disability. Activities that will enhance or maintain musculoskeletal flexibility should be included as a part of a comprehensive preventive or rehabilitative exercise program.

6—A. Macrominerals

Minerals are inorganic substances that perform various functions in the body. Many play an important role in assisting enzymes (or coenzymes) that are necessary for the proper functioning of body systems. They also are found in cell membranes, hormones, muscles, and connective tissues as well as electrolytes in body fluids. Minerals are considered to be either macrominerals (needed in relatively large doses), such as calcium, phosphorus, magnesium, potassium, sulfur, sodium, and chloride, or microminerals (needed in very small amounts), such as iron, zinc, selenium, manganese, molybdenum, iodine, copper, chromium, and fluoride.

7—C. Transverse

The body has three cardinal planes, and each individual plane is perpendicular to the other two. Movement occurs along these planes. The sagittal plane divides the body into right and left parts, and the midsagittal plane is represented by an imaginary vertical plane passing through the midline of the body, dividing it into right and left halves. The frontal plane is represented by an imaginary vertical plane passing through the body, dividing it into front and back halves. The transverse plane represents an imaginary horizontal plane passing through the midsection of the body and dividing it into upper and lower portions.

8—C. Omission

Negligence is a failure to conform one's conduct to a generally accepted standard or duty. *Gross negligence* (also referred to as reckless conduct or willful/wanton conduct) is a conscious, voluntary act (commission), or failure to act (omission), in reckless disregard of the legal duty and of the consequences to the plaintiff. In this situation, the trainer failed to spot (omission) the client, which resulted in injury.

9—B. Individual's current physical activity level; presence of signs or symptoms and/or known metabolic, renal, or cardiovascular disease; and exercise intensity at which individual desires to exercise. Please see *ACSM's Guidelines for Exercise Testing and Prescription*, 10th edition, Chapter 2 for details on the preparticipation health screen process.

10—D. Action

People in the action stage are at the greatest risk of relapse. Instruction about avoiding injury, exercise boredom, and burnout is important for those who have recently begun an exercise program. Providing social support and praise are the most important contributors to maintained activity. Planning for high-risk, relapse situations (*e.g.*, vacations, sickness, bad weather, increased demands on time) is also important. The exercise professional can emphasize that a short lapse in activity can be a learning opportunity and is not failure. Planning can help to develop coping strategies and to eliminate the "all-or-none" thinking sometimes typical of people who have missed several exercise sessions and think they need to give it up.

11—C. Heat exhaustion and heat stroke

Heat exhaustion and heat stroke are serious conditions that result from a combination of the metabolic heat generated from exercise accompanied by dehydration and electrolyte loss from sweating. Signs and symptoms include uncoordinated gait, headache, dizziness, vomiting, and elevated body temperature. If these conditions are present, exercise must be stopped. Attempts to rehydrate, perhaps intravenously, should be attempted, and the body must be cooled by any means possible. The person should be placed in the supine position with the feet elevated.

12—B. Protection of personal trainer against lawsuits of negligence

The informed consent document does not provide protection against negligence lawsuits. It provides the subject the opportunity to choose to withdraw involvement at any point, the information regarding the risks and benefits of participation, and the opportunity for the individual to ask questions. Greater detail on informed consent can be found in *ACSM's Resources for the Personal Trainer.*

13—D. All of the above

Discussion of current health status and health history, PAR-Q+, health and fitness assessments, and informed consent documentation are all part of the initial client consultation.

14—C. Tell her to discontinue all exercise and make an appointment with her physician for medical clearance.

Irrespective of other factors, the potential client is expressing having symptoms suggestive of metabolic, cardiovascular, or pulmonary disease, and medical clearance is needed prior to continuing with an exercise program prescription. Please refer to Chapter 2, Figure 2.2 in the 10th edition of *ACSM's Guidelines for Exercise Testing and Prescription.*

15—A. 161 kcal

There are 4 kcal $\cdot$ g^{-1} of carbohydrate and protein and 9 $\cdot$ kcal g^{-1} of fat.

5 g $\times$ 9 kcal = 45 kcal from fat

3 g $\times$ 4 kcal = 12 kcal from protein

26 g $\times$ 4 kcal = 104 kcal from carbohydrate

Total calories in the bar is 161 kcal.

Fiber is a carbohydrate but, because it is not absorbed, there are no absorbable carbohydrates, and it should not be used in determining calorie content of food.

16—B. Reinforcement

Reinforcement is the positive or negative consequence for performing or not performing a behavior. *Positive consequences* are rewards that motivate behavior. This can include both intrinsic and extrinsic rewards. *Intrinsic rewards* are the benefits gained because of the rewarding nature of the activity. *Extrinsic or external rewards* are the positive outcomes received from others, which may include encouragement and praise or material reinforcements such as T-shirts and money.

17—C. Increased HR at submaximal workload

Compared with a cool and dry environment, a higher metabolic cost exists at submaximal workloads when exercising in the heat and humidity. Thus, the exercise prescription should be altered by lowering the work intensity. Evaporation of sweat cools the skin; therefore, wiping away sweat would decrease evaporative cooling and heat loss. Heat loss by convection, such as that which occurs when a breeze is created by running, can be beneficial but not unless the workload of activity is reduced. It is necessary in the heat and humidity to become acclimated to the environment; it will not occur by being sedentary.

18—C. No change

CO does not change significantly primarily because the person is performing the same amount of work and, thus, responds with the same CO. It should be noted, however, that the same CO is now being generated with a lower HR and higher stroke volume compared with when the person was untrained.

19—D. Osteoporosis

Every population that has been studied exhibits a decline in bone mass with aging. Therefore, bone loss is considered by most clinicians to be an inevitable consequence of aging. *Osteoporosis* refers to a condition that is characterized by a decrease in bone mass and density, producing bone porosity and fragility, and it refers to the clinical condition of low bone mass and the accompanying increase in susceptibility to fracture from minor trauma. The age at which bone loss begins and the rate at which it occurs vary greatly between males and females. Risk factors for age-related bone loss and development of clinical osteoporosis include being a white or Asian female, being thin-boned or petite, having a low peak bone mass at maturity, having a family history of osteoporosis, premature or surgically induced menopause, alcohol abuse and/or cigarette smoking, sedentary lifestyle, and inadequate dietary calcium intake.

20—B. Outcomes

Outcomes are designed to measure the success of a program based on the outcome for a patient or client. Outcome studies require quantifiable data that can be analyzed — data that study the success of a program in terms of quantifiable measures (*e.g.*, change in body composition). Measuring client satisfaction, level of change, length of time for change to occur, or percentage of clients who reach their goals are other examples of outcomes. Outcomes can be very helpful in marketing programs as well as in comparing one facility with another.

21—B. 12 and 16

Although some learning is required on the part of the participant, the RPE should be considered an adjunct to HR measures. The RPE can be used as a reliable barometer of exercise intensity. The RPE is particularly useful when participants are incapable of monitoring their pulse accurately or when medications such as β-blockers alter the HR response to exercise. The ACSM recommends an exercise intensity that will elicit an RPE within a range of 12–16 on the original Borg scale of 6–20.

22—A. Medial rotation

Rotation is the turning of a bone around its own longitudinal axis or around another bone. Rotation of the anterior surface of the bone toward the midline of the body is *medial rotation*, whereas rotation of the same bone away from the midline is *lateral rotation*. *Supination* is a specialized rotation of the forearm that results in the palm of the hand being turned forward (anteriorly). *Pronation* (the opposite of supination) is the rotation of the forearm that results in the palm of the hand being directed backward (posteriorly).

23—D. $37.3 \text{ kg} \cdot \text{m}^{-2}$; class II obesity

$6 \text{ ft} = 72 \text{ in} = 182.88 \text{ cm} = 1.83 \text{ m}$

$275 \text{ lb} = 125 \text{ kg}$

$1.83^2 = 3.35$

$\text{BMI} = \text{weight (kg)} / \text{height (m}^2\text{)} = 125 / 3.35 = {\sim}37.3 \text{ kg} \cdot \text{m}^{-2}$

24—C. Advise the new client to pursue medical clearance, and once obtained, your client may then begin adding in bouts of vigorous-intensity exercise.

Please refer to the algorithm in Chapter 2, Figure 2.2 of *ACSM's Guidelines for Exercise Testing and Prescription*. This individual would be clear to exercise at light- and moderate-intensity activities; however, due to his history of stenting procedure and having diabetes, it is recommended that he pursues medical clearance prior to engaging in vigorous-intensity physical activity.

25—B. Medical clearance is recommended prior to beginning any intensity exercise.

Medical clearance is recommended for any sedentary individual with signs or symptoms suggestive of cardiovascular, metabolic, or renal disease irrespective of his or her disease status. Following medical clearance, this individual should begin an exercise program of light-to-moderate intensity exercise, progressing as tolerated following ACSM guidelines.

26—C. Vitamins B complex and C

Fat-soluble vitamins are composed of vitamins A, D, E, and K and are stored in body fat after consumption. Vitamins C and B complex are water-soluble vitamins, must be consumed on a regular basis, and excess amounts are excreted. Water-soluble vitamins are found in citrus fruits, broccoli, cauliflower, brussels sprouts, whole grain breads and cereals, and organ meats. They serve as antioxidants as well as coenzymes in carbohydrate metabolism, metabolic pathways, amino acid metabolism, and nucleic acid metabolism.

27—B. Three

Positive risk factors for this client include age (men ≥45 yr old), current smoker, and not currently regularly physically active. This client is also on borderline for hypertension and obesity. Table 3.1 in *ACSM's Guidelines for Exercise Testing and Prescription* lists each of the negative and positive risk factors for CVD.

28—A. Discomfort associated with myocardial ischemia

Angina pectoris is a heart-related chest pain caused by ischemia, which is insufficient blood flow that results from a temporary or permanent reduction of blood flow in one or more coronary arteries. Angina-like symptoms often are felt in the chest area, neck, shoulder, or arm.

29—A.   126/80 mm Hg

Prehypertension is considered an SBP of 120–139 mm Hg *or* DBP of 80–89 mm Hg.

30—C.   95 mg · dL^{-1}

An LDL-C level of <100 mg · dL^{-1} is considered *optimal*. An LDL-C level of ≥130 mg · dL^{-1} is considered high. Please see Table 3.3 in *ACSM's Guidelines for Exercise Testing and Prescription.*

31—A.   RPE

RPE and the talk test are both appropriate measures of exercise intensity for the pregnant individual. HR at rest and during maximal exertion can vary greatly over the course of a pregnancy and should not be used in as a method of monitoring exercise intensity.

32—D.   Both B and C

Exercise should be stopped immediately and medical counsel should be pursued if any of the following signs or symptoms are present: dyspnea prior to exertion, dizziness, vaginal bleeding, headache, muscle weakness, chest pain, preterm labor, calf pain or swelling, detection of decreased fetal movement, or amniotic fluid leakage (*ACSM's Resources for the Personal Trainer* and the American Congress of Obstetricians and Gynecologists, Committee Opinion).

Resource: ACOG Committee on Obstetric Practice. ACOG Committee Opinion No. 650: physical activity and exercise during pregnancy and the postpartum period. *Obstet Gynecol.* 2015;126:e135–e142.

33—C.   Increasing the rate of training intensity more than approximately 10% per week increases the likelihood of overuse injuries of bone.

Increasing the rate of progression of training more than approximately 10% per week is a risk factor for overuse injuries of bone. Exercise programs for children and adolescents should increase physical fitness in the short term and lead to adoption of a physically active lifestyle in the long term. Strength training in youth carries no greater risk of injury than comparable strength training programs in adults if proper instruction, exercise prescription, and supervision are provided. Children who have exercise-induced asthma often are physically unfit because of restriction of activity imposed by the child, parents, or physicians.

34—B.   Specific, measurable, achievable, realistic, time-oriented

Resource: Bovend'Eerdt TJH, Botell RE, Wade DT. Writing SMART rehabilitation goals and achieving goal attainment scaling: a practical guide. *Clin Rehabil.* 2009;23(4):352–61.

35—B.   Self-monitoring

The client is using the pedometer as a measurement device; he is self-monitoring his daily steps. Other examples of self-monitoring may include a daily food intake journal, accelerometer use, tracking workout days in a journal, etc.

36—A.   Intensity and duration

Intensity and duration of exercise must be considered together and are inversely related. Similar improvements in aerobic fitness may be realized if a person exercises at a low intensity for a longer duration or at a higher intensity for less time.

37—C.   Proprioceptive neuromuscular facilitation (PNF)

Three different stretching techniques typically are practiced and have associated risks and benefits. Static stretching is the most commonly recommended approach to stretching. It involves slowly stretching a muscle to the point of individual discomfort and holding that position for a period of 10–30 s. Minimal risk of injury exists, and it has been shown to be effective. Ballistic stretching uses repetitive bouncing-type movements to produce muscle stretch. These movements can produce residual muscle soreness or acute injury. PNF stretching alternates contraction and relaxation of both agonist and antagonist muscle groups. This technique is effective, but it can cause residual muscle soreness and is time-consuming. Additionally, a partner typically is required, and the potential for injury exists when the partner-assisted stretching is applied too vigorously.

38—C.   Negligence

Legal issues abound for fitness professionals involved in exercise testing, exercise prescription, and program administration. Legal concerns can develop with the instructor–client relationship, the exercises involved, the exercise setting, the purpose of the programs and exercises used, and the procedures used by the staff. A tort law is simply a type of civil wrong. *Negligence* is the failure to perform on the level of a generally accepted standard. Fitness professionals have certain documented and understood responsibilities to ensure the client's safety and to succeed in reaching predetermined goals. If these responsibilities are not followed, it is possible that a person could be considered negligent.

39—D. They are the least common type of joint found in the human body.

Synovial joints are the most common, not the least common, joints found in the human body. Please see *ACSM's Resources for the Personal Trainer* for greater detail on joint characteristics throughout the body.

40—D. All of the above

Social barriers relate to barriers that arise from one's social network of friends and family. Social barriers have the potential to significantly decrease one's adherence to an exercise program if ways to overcome such barriers are not discussed and implemented. It is important for the personal trainer to discuss any type of barrier a client may have in meeting his or her fitness goals.

41—B. Intrinsic reward

Reinforcement is the positive or negative consequence for performing or not performing a behavior. Positive consequences are rewards that motivate behavior. This can include both intrinsic and extrinsic rewards. Intrinsic rewards are the benefits gained because of the rewarding nature of the activity. Extrinsic or external rewards are the positive outcomes received from others, which may include encouragement and praise or material reinforcements such as T-shirts and money.

42—A. Flexibility of equipment to allow for different body sizes

Creating a safe environment in which to exercise is a primary responsibility for any fitness facility. In developing and operating facilities and equipment for use by exercisers, the managers and staff are obligated to meet a standard of care for exerciser safety. The equipment to be used includes not only testing, cardiovascular, strength, and flexibility pieces but also rehabilitation, pool, locker room, and emergency equipment. You must evaluate a number of criteria when selecting equipment. These criteria include correct anatomic positioning, ability to adjust to different body sizes, quality of design and materials, durability, repair records, and then price.

43—B. Self-efficacy and expectation of outcome related to behavior changes

Both A and C relate closer to the health belief model. Self-efficacy and expectation of outcome are those factors that are most important in behavior change according to the SCT.

44—A. Plyometrics

Plyometrics is a method of strength and power training that involves an eccentric loading of muscles and tendons followed immediately by an explosive concentric contraction. This stretch-shortening cycle may allow an enhanced generation of force during the concentric (shortening) phase. Most well-controlled studies have shown no significant difference in power improvement when comparing plyometrics with high-intensity strength training. The explosive nature of this type of activity may increase the risk for musculoskeletal injury. Plyometrics should not be considered a practical resistance exercise alternative for health/fitness applications but may be appropriate for select athletic or performance needs.

45—C. Manager or director

The characteristics of a good manager or director include designing programs and monitoring the implementation of programs. He or she also guides the staff or clients through the program. He or she is a good communicator who also purchases equipment and supplies. A good manager monitors the safety of the program or facility and surveys clients and staff to assess the success and value of the program.

46—A. To inform the client of participation risks as well as the rights of the client and the facility

Agreements, releases, and consents are documents that clearly describe what the client is participating in, the risks involved, and the rights of the client and the facility. If signed by the client, he or she is accepting some of the responsibility and risk by participating in this program. All fitness facilities are strongly encouraged to have program or service agreements and informed consents drafted by a lawyer for their protection.

47—C. A loss of muscle mass caused by a loss of muscle fibers

After 30 yr of age, skeletal muscle strength begins to decline. However, the loss of strength is not linear, with most of the decline occurring after 50 yr of age. By 80 yr of age, strength loss usually is in the range of 30%–40%. The loss of strength with aging results primarily from a loss of muscle mass, which, in turn, is caused by both the loss of muscle fibers and the atrophy of the remaining fibers.

48—A. There is a perceived threat of heart disease.

The health belief model assumes that people will engage in a behavior (*e.g.*, exercise) when there exist a perceived threat of disease and a belief of susceptibility to disease and the threat of disease is severe. This model also incorporates cues to action as critical to adopting and maintaining behavior. The concept of self-efficacy (confidence) is also added to this model. Motivation and environmental considerations are not a part of the health belief model.

49—C.   Provides an explanation of the test to the client

Informed consent is not a legal document. It does not provide legal immunity to a facility or individual in the event of injury to a client nor does it legally protect the rights of the client. It simply provides evidence that the client was made aware of the purposes, procedures, and risks associated with the test or exercise program. The consent form does not relieve the facility or individual of the responsibility to do everything possible to ensure the safety of the client. Negligence, improper test administration, inadequate personnel qualifications, and insufficient safety procedures all are items that are not expressly covered by informed consent. Because of the limitations associated with informed consent documents, legal counsel should be sought during the development of the document.

50—C.   Number of curl-ups in 1 min

Three common assessments for muscular endurance include the bench press, for upper body endurance (a weight is lifted in cadence with a metronome or other timing device; the total number of lifts performed correctly and in time with the cadence); the push-up, for upper body endurance (the client assumes a standardized beginning position with the body held rigid and supported by the hands and toes for men and the hands and knees for women; the body is lowered to the floor and then pushed back up to the starting position; the score is the total number of properly performed push-ups completed without a pause by the client, with no time limit); and the curl-up (crunch), for abdominal muscular endurance (the client begins in the bent-knee sit-up with knees at 90 degrees, the arms at the side, and palms facing down with middle fingers touching masking tape. A second piece of tape is placed 10-cm apart. OR set a metronome to 50 bpm and the client performs slow, controlled curl-ups to lift the shoulder blades off the mat with the trunk making a 30-degree angle, in time with the metronome at a rate of 25 per minute done for 1 min. OR the client performs as many curl-ups as possible in 1 min).

51—A.   An overuse injury

Overuse injuries become more common when people participate in greater amounts of exercise by increasing time, duration, or intensity too quickly. For example, a client exercises too much without allowing appropriate time for rest and recovery, or a client develops a minor injury and does not reduce or change that exercise allowing the injury to heal.

52—A.   Hypoventilation

Hypoventilation is an indication of heat syncope. Exertional heat stroke signs and symptoms include the following: disorientation, dizziness, irrational behavior, apathy, headache, nausea, vomiting, hyperventilation, and wet skin. Please see Table 8.2 in *ACSM's Guidelines for Exercise Testing and Prescription.*

53—D.   All of the above

There are relative and absolute contraindications to aerobic exercise during pregnancy. These can be found in *ACSM's Complete Guide to Fitness & Health.* Absolute contraindications include restrictive lung disease, hemodynamically significant heart disease, incompetent cervix, women with multiple gestation at risk for premature labor, persistent second or third trimester bleeding, placenta previa after 26 wk of gestation, premature labor during current pregnancy, ruptured membranes, and pregnancy-induced hypertension or preeclampsia. Relative contraindications include those with severe anemia, unelevated maternal cardiac arrhythmia, chronic bronchitis, poorly controlled Type 1 diabetes, extreme morbid obesity or extremely underweight (BMI $<12\ kg \cdot m^{-2}$), a history of sedentary lifestyle, intrauterine growth restriction in current pregnancy, poorly controlled hypertension, orthopedic limitations, poorly controlled seizure disorder, poorly controlled hyperthyroidism, or are a heavy smoker.

54—D.   All of the above

The effects of regular (chronic) exercise can be classified or grouped into those that occur at rest, during moderate (or submaximal) exercise, and during maximal effort work. For example, you can measure an untrained individual's resting heart rate (HR_{rest}), train the person for several weeks or months, and then measure HR_{rest} again to see what change has occurred. HR_{rest} declines with regular exercise, probably because of a combination of decreased sympathetic tone, increased parasympathetic tone, and decreased intrinsic firing rate of the sinoatrial node. Stroke volume increases at rest as a result of increased time for ventricular filling and an increased myocardial contractility. Little or no change occurs in CO at rest because the decline in HR is compensated for by the increase in stroke volume.

55—C.   Extrinsic motivation

Factors such as losing weight and desire to look a certain way externally are examples of extrinsic motivation; individuals are pursing activities in order to achieve an external result. Intrinsic motivation may include activities that an individual pursues because he or she enjoys the internal result of feeling as though he or she accomplished a goal or enjoyed participating in an activity. Self-efficacy refers to one's belief that he or she is capable and able to complete a given task or activity. Self-worth refers to how well an individual perceives he or she is accomplishing or performing what he or she has set out to do.

56—B. Pregnancy

Pregnancy is a biological barrier to exercise, whereas obesity, disease, and injury are all considered physical barriers to exercise.

57—C. Promotional materials

Print brochures, video brochures, and Web sites are all examples of promotional materials and are marketing strategies aimed at developing prospective clients. Strategic alliances comprise relationships built between organizations that are trying to reach the same audience of clientele and, through this relationship, increase prospective clients. Reputation management is a type of marketing strategy used to increase a business's reputation within its community via positive rapport building with local media outlets and providing information about the business via methods such as press kits. Community involvement is a marketing strategy that may be used by a personal trainer to make a name for oneself within the community he or she hopes to serve. Building individual relationships with their current clients and providing high-quality training so much so that their clients refer them to others, volunteering for speaking engagements in the community, and volunteering at other organizations within the community they serve are all examples of community involvement.

58—B. Conduct a comprehensive demographic analysis

The following are the steps that should be taken when an individual sets out to establish his or her personal training business: Perform a demographic and competitor analysis, develop and establish a budget, develop and establish management policies, and determine what type of marketing is most appropriate as well as sales goals and pricing of services. Please see *ACSM's Resources for the Personal Trainer* for a greater depth of discussion on each of the aforementioned factors.

59—D. Independent contractor

A sole proprietorship represents a business model where only one person owns the business. S corporations are businesses where there is no double taxation on salary and business income, each partner in the corporation has the autonomy to distribute dividends, and risk to personal assets

is significantly reduced. Business partnerships may be formed between two or more individuals and is beneficial in that all parties are able to combine resources together for the growth of the business.

60—C. Soleus

Hamstrings, gracilis, sartorius, popliteus, gastrocnemius are all major agonist muscles involved in knee flexion. Please see *ACSM's Resources for Personal Trainer* for more detailed information.

61—B. Active listening

Other examples of active listening include restating, repeating, and summarizing information your client has discussed with you.

62—D. A friend inquiring why you have not been in exercise class lately

If the friend were encouraging you to attend the exercise class, or offering to pick you up and carpool to the exercise class, etc., it would be an example of social support. Simply asking why you are not attending class would not be an example of social support.

63—D. All of the above

Different types of health screenings are used for various purposes. In commercial settings, clients should be screened more extensively for potential health risks. At minimum, a personal medical history should be taken. In addition, present medical status should be examined and questions asked regarding the use of medications (both prescription and over-the-counter).

64—C. Take snack breaks during longer training sessions

Drinking excessive amounts of water may lead to hyponatremia (a below-normal blood sodium level) which may affect cognitive function. Consuming a meal containing sodium will aid in thirst production, and consuming a high-protein meal prior to exercise may contribute to dehydration during activity.

65—B. Strategic plan

The strategic plan addresses strategic decisions of the organization in defining short- and long-term goals and serves as the overarching planning tool. Health and fitness programs, financial plans, risk management efforts, and marketing plans only address subsegments within the overall strategic plan.

66—D. Self-efficacy

What this client is expressing is that she now has a belief that she is able to competently implement the exercises you have taught her on her own; this is an example of self-efficacy. This client's improved self-efficacy will aid in improving her self-regulation of exercise. Self-worth would include how well she perceives herself carrying out the exercises you have taught her, and self-esteem simply refers to how one views himself or herself overall.

67—D. Television advertising

Lead boxes and direct mail both provide much lower rate of return compared to television advertising. Reputation management is costly in time (building relationships with local media outlets) and effort (maintaining contact and following up with local media outlets) and is typically used to enhance the reputation of the business in the community.

68—B. Scoliosis

The vertebral column serves as the main axial support for the body. The adult vertebral column exhibits four major curvatures when viewed from the sagittal plane. *Scoliosis* is an abnormal lateral deviation of the vertebral column. *Kyphosis* is an abnormal increased posterior curvature, especially in the thoracic region. *Lordosis* is an abnormal, exaggerated anterior curvature in the lumbar region. A primary curve refers to the thoracic and sacral curvatures of the vertebral column that remain in the original fetal positions.

69—C. Copies of HIPAA privacy rule do not need to be provided to the individual.

The patient must provide written authorization prior to disclosure or use of information by a third party, the individual is assured that he or she will have access to his or her own personal health information, and the individual is provided protection of his or her personal health care information.

70—C. 32.5 kg · m^{-2}

Underweight is a BMI less than 18.5 kg · m^{-2}, normal weight is a BMI between 18.5 and 24.9 kg · m^{-2}, overweight is a BMI between 25.0 and 29.9 kg · m^{-2}, class I is a BMI between 30.0 and 34.9 kg · m^{-2}, class II obesity is a BMI between 35.0 and 39.9, and class III obesity is a BMI greater than or equal to 40.0 kg · m^{-2}. Please see *ACSM's Guidelines for Exercise Testing and Prescription*, Chapter 4 and Table 4.1 for greater detail on body composition and BMI.

71—D. Both A and C

Aerobic enzyme activity is increased, not decreased, as a result of resistance training. Both capillary density and lactate removal are increased as an adaptation to resistance training.

72—A. Concentric action

Eccentric action is muscle lengthening under a load; isometric (static) action is when a muscle attempts to shorten under load but is unable to overcome the resistance placed on it; therefore, it does not shorten or lengthen but does generate force. Dynamic muscle action encompasses both concentric (muscle shortening under load) and eccentric (muscle lengthening under load) muscle actions.

73—D. Both A and C

The cool-down phase allows blood to return to the heart and brain instead of pooling in the lower extremities, potentially causing hypotension and dizziness.

74—C. Sarcopenia

Osteoporosis: BMD is severely reduced, significantly increasing risk of fracture. BMD >2.5 standard deviations < mean peak value for young normal adults.

Osteopenia: low bone mass; BMD between 1.0 and 2.5 standard deviations < mean peak value for young normal adults.

Sarcopenia: loss of skeletal muscle mass. This is commonly seen during the process of aging.

Rheumatoid arthritis: autoimmune disease; body attacks and eventually destroys the surface of the joint

For more in depth on each of the aforementioned, please see the source: *ACSM's Resources for the Personal Trainer*.

75—A. Age may be accompanied by deconditioning and disease.

Age is often accompanied by deconditioning and disease, and these factors must be taken into consideration when selecting appropriate fitness test protocols. In addition, adaptation to a specific workload is often prolonged in older adults (a prolonged warm-up, followed by small increments in workload are recommended). Test stages in graded exercise tests should be prolonged, lasting at least 3 min, to allow the participant to reach steady state. An appropriate test protocol should be selected to accommodate these special needs.

76—D. Trapezius

SITS = Subscapularis, infraspinatus, teres minor, and subscapularis encompass the rotator cuff muscles.

77—B. A lower HR

At any given intensity, HR will be lower during swimming than exercise performed in a standing position, such as running, because of postural differences. While swimming, the body is in a prone position so that the heart's pumping action does not have to overcome the full effects of gravity. Thus, even at rest, stroke volume is at its maximal value. Because of the higher stroke volume evident during submaximal swimming compared with running, the same CO can be achieved with a lower HR during swimming.

78—B. Cold weather environment

In an effort to better insulate against colder temperatures, multiple light layers should be worn instead of one heavy layer. Multiple layers allow body heat generated during activity to be trapped between the layers of insulation. Clothing vents allow the body to dissipate heat from sweating and not wet the clothing.

79—B. Osteoporosis

Advancing age brings a progressive decline in BMD and calcium content. This loss is accelerated in women immediately after menopause. As a result, older adults are more susceptible to osteoporosis and bone fractures.

80—A. Overall improvement in the quality of life and increased independence

Most older adults are not sufficiently active. This population can benefit greatly from regular participation in a well-designed exercise program. Benefits of such a program include increased fitness, improved health status (reduction in risk factors associated with various diseases), increased independence, and overall improvement in the quality of life.

81—A. Older men and women demonstrate similar or even greater strength gains when compared with younger individuals.

Muscle strength peaks in the mid-20s for both genders and remains fairly stable through the mid-40s. Muscle strength declines by approximately 15% per decade in the sixth and seventh decades and by approximately 30% per decade thereafter. However, older men and women demonstrate similar or even greater strength gains when compared with younger individuals in response to resistance training. These strength gains are related to improved neurologic function and, to a lesser extent, increased muscle mass.

82—C. Data should be kept on file for at least 1 yr before being discarded.

There is no accepted minimal or maximal amount of time that data should be stored. Clearly, however, data must be stored in a confidential (lock-and-key) manner, and discretion must be used when sharing data.

83—A. Include the costs of equipment and building or facility expense

Capital budgets refer to the budgeting of program implementation or facility. How much does it cost to start the program and to implement the first stage? Capital budgets usually include equipment, facility expense, staffing, initial marketing, and so on in the start-up. Operating a program is part of the operating budget, not the capital budget. Capital budgets are critical in determining whether to start a program. Capital budgets are not included in the balance sheet.

84—A. Injury prevention

Injury prevention often is overlooked, but it is an important part of a facility's emergency procedures and safety program. All exercise professionals should understand how to avoid emergencies. Basic principles for exercise training are important for general day-to-day operations but not for emergency procedures.

85—D. Perform multijoint exercises prior to single-joint exercises

Exercising large muscles and muscle groups and multijoint exercises prior to smaller muscles and muscle groups and single-joint exercises is recommended due to their requiring greater amounts of energy to perform. One is also able to use a greater amount of weight due to the assisting muscles of multijoint exercises not being as fatigued as they would be if they had been exercised early in the workout. Exercises for weak areas should be performed prior to those for strong areas, and intensity of exercises should begin with higher intensity working to lower intensity.

86—D. Sarcoplasmic reticulum

Within skeletal muscle fibers, the endoplasmic (sarcoplasmic) reticulum is particularly well developed so that it can store large amounts of calcium. When the motor neuron excites the membrane (sarcolemma) of the fiber, calcium is released from the sarcoplasmic reticulum, which triggers the fiber to twitch or contract.

87—D. Providing the client a written detailed dietary plan in conjunction with the Ex R$_x$

The ACSM CPT should understand the laws in their state regarding the practice of dietetics. Providing a detailed written dietary plan is within the scope of practice of a registered dietician and medical physician; however, this does not mean that the CPT cannot have conversations about healthy food options and encourage his or her clients to consume an overall healthy diet.

88—D. The half-squat wall-sit

The half-squat wall-sit exercise is an example of an isometric exercise; muscle is contracted and strengthened but only at the joint angle the exercise is performed in. Biceps curls, pull-ups, and box squat jumps are all isotonic (dynamic) exercises involving both concentric and eccentric muscle action.

89—C. Lactic acid production will decrease during submaximal effort exercise.

Maximal heart rate will stay the same at both submaximal and maximal exercise, and CO will decrease during submaximal exercise and increase during maximal exercise.

90—B. PNF

Static stretching involves performing a stretch until minor discomfort is reached and holding the stretch. Ballistic stretching involves a bouncing movement during the performance of a stretch and is typically not recommended due to the risk of possible tissue injury. Dynamic stretching involves performing a stretch throughout the entire ROM and gradually increasing the reach of the stretch through movement. Dynamic stretching is not a jerky movement like ballistic stretching but is a controlled movement that may gradually increase in speed.

91—C. Ischemia

Myocardial ischemia occurs when the oxygen supply does not meet oxygen demand resulting from decreased blood flow to the myocardium. This is usually owing to atherosclerotic lesions reducing blood flow or coronary artery spasm, both of which are the result of atherosclerosis. This process often leads to angina (symptoms) or myocardial infarction (MI) caused by a thrombosis.

92—A. Avoiding muscle-strengthening exercises that involve low resistance

Low-resistance muscle-strengthening exercises can be performed by those diagnosed with hypertension if they follow appropriate lifting techniques

and avoid the Valsalva maneuver. In addition, hemodynamic parameters (HR and BP) and medications should be controlled.

93—B. Rotator cuff strain or impingement

The subdeltoid bursa, supraspinatus muscle, and nerves become impinged between the coracoid and acromion process with shoulder abduction. The resulting pain leads to decreased ROM, disuse, and muscle atrophy. Such impingement of the rotator cuff is common in assembly line workers performing repetitive overhead tasks.

94—D. All of the above

In addition to improving metabolic profile, decreasing sedentary behavior, and maximizing caloric expenditure, maintaining and increasing lean body mass and resting metabolic rate, addressing behavior (*e.g.*, assessing dietary habits, environmental or social barriers to exercise adherence), lowering risk of mortality and associated comorbidities are all pertinent goals for exercise programming in those with obesity.

95—C. $2–3 \text{ d} \cdot \text{wk}^{-1}$

Individuals who are at increased risk for falls or have a mobility disability are encouraged to participate in at least $2–3 \text{ d} \cdot \text{wk}^{-1}$ of neuromuscular exercise.

96—A. Action: Individual has been regularly active for less than 6 mo.

The TTM stages are correctly defined as follows:

Precontemplation: Individual is neither intending on making behavior change nor considering the benefits the change may bring.

Contemplation: Individual is weighing the pros and cons of behavior change and is considering implementing changes in <6 mo.

Preparation: Individual has developed a behavior change plan and intends to implement it within the next month.

Action: Individual has been making positive activity and behavior changes for 6 mo or less.

Maintenance: Individual is maintaining positive behavior changes for ≥6 mo and is working on relapse prevention strategies.

97—D. Goals are most effective when the trainer selects them and the client agrees to them.

Goals are most effective and adhered to when the client is the one to identify and set his or her own goals. It is the responsibility of the personal trainer to provide the client with the education and tools for success in how to reach those goals and identify potential barriers.

98—D. Quadratus lumborum

The quadratus lumborum is a major agonist muscle involved in lateral flexion of the lumbar spine. The rectus femoris, sartorius, and iliopsoas are all major agonist muscles involved in hip flexion.

99—C. Malpractice

Negligence is defined as a failure to conform one's conduct to a generally accepted standard or duty.

Risk management is simply the identification of risks and the implementation of procedures to reduce those risks, and assumption of risk is a waiver or form an individual signs relinquishing his or her legal right to collect damages in the event of an injury.

100—B. Health Insurance Portability and Accountability Act

HIPAA stands for the Health Insurance Portability and Accountability Act.

CPT EXAMINATION QUESTIONS BY DOMAIN

Use the following table as a guide to assist you in your studying process. It is important to note that some questions can be classified as testing multiple domains by the knowledge and skills (KSs).

Domain Number	I	II	III	IV
Domain Name	Initial Client Consultation and Assessment	Exercise Programming and Implementation	Exercise Leadership and Client Education	Legal, Professional, Business, and Marketing
Percentage of Test Questions	21%	33%	25%	21%
Question Numbers	9, 12, 13, 14, 23, 24, 25, 26, 27, 28, 29, 30, 50, 60, 63, 72, 73, 76, 88, 89, 98	1, 3, 4, 5, 6, 7, 15, 17, 18, 19, 21, 31, 32, 36, 39, 47, 52, 53, 64, 70, 71, 74, 75, 77, 78, 85, 86, 90, 91, 92, 93, 94, 95	2, 10, 11, 16, 22, 33, 34, 35, 37, 40, 41, 43, 48, 54, 55, 56, 61, 62, 66, 68, 79, 80, 81, 96, 97	8, 20, 38, 42, 44, 45, 46, 49, 51, 57, 58, 59, 65, 67, 69, 82, 83, 84, 87, 99, 100

2

ACSM Certified Exercise Physiologist (EP-C)

ANDREW BOSAK, PhD, ACSM EP-C
Associate Editor

EP-C Case Studies

Note: EP-C certification candidates may also review the case studies found in Part 1, ACSM Certified Personal Trainer (CPT).

DOMAIN I: HEALTH AND FITNESS ASSESSMENT

CASE STUDY EP-C.I	Author: **Will Peveler, PhD**

You are working as a personal trainer at a university recreation facility. You have been assigned a new client, Mike. He has been relatively active but has never worked with a trainer or been on a structured program. He is a prior college football player but has been inactive since graduation (6 yr prior). He plays softball a couple times a week and walks two to three times a week. He is a software programmer and sits at a desk all day during his working hours. Although he feels fatigued, his overall goal is to become healthier and get in better shape.

Mike completes an informed consent and health status questionnaire. Mike is a 40-yr-old Caucasian, with a body mass of 95.24 kg and a height of 181 cm. His blood pressure (BP) is 112/78 mm Hg, total cholesterol is 221 mg $\cdot$ dL^{-1} (high-density lipoprotein [HDL] and low-density lipoprotein [LDL] are unknown), and fasting blood glucose is unknown. Both his father and his paternal grandfather have known cardiovascular disease. There are no known cardiovascular or metabolic diseases on his mother's side.

1. In addition to the given question's variables, if Mike mentioned to you that he was also recently diagnosed with a pulmonary disorder, such as chronic bronchitis, would you automatically refer him to a physician for medical clearance?
   A. Yes, he must be referred to a physician immediately due to the new recent diagnosis.
   B. No, he does not need to be automatically referred for medical clearance.

   Answer: A

2. Is a medical exam recommended prior to participation in moderate exercise?
   A. Yes
   B. No

   Answer: B

3. Is a medical exam recommended prior to participation in vigorous exercise?
   A. Yes
   B. No

   Answer: A

4. Is exercise testing recommended prior to exercise for participation in vigorous exercise?
   A. Yes
   B. No

   Answer: B

Once you have determined that Mike is clear to participate using the most recent ACSM guidelines, you then conduct a fitness assessment in order to establish baseline data.

1. Cardiovascular measures — Resting heart rate (HR_{rest}) was found to be 77 bpm and BP was found to be 118/78 mm Hg.
2. Body composition — After using skinfold calipers, a three-site formula was used to determine body composition: chest = 14 mm, abdomen = 28 mm, and thigh = 19 mm.
3. Cardiovascular endurance — The 1.5-mi walk/run test was chosen because it allows Mike to pace himself. He completed the distance in 14 min and 0 s.
4. Muscular endurance — The push-up and curl-up tests were conducted because they are the most common muscular endurance test used in the field. Both tests were conducted per ACSM guidelines. Mike successfully completed 30 push-ups and 40 curl-ups.
5. Muscular strength — Bench press one repetition maximum (1-RM) and leg press 1-RM were chosen to determine Mike's muscular strength, per ACSM guidelines. Mike was able to bench press 225 lb and leg press 455 lb.
6. Flexibility — Mike's trunk flexion was measured using a sit-and-reach box. He scored 18 cm.

MULTIPLE-CHOICE QUESTIONS FOR CASE STUDY EP-C.I

1. What is Mike's body mass index (BMI)?
   Note: BMI = weight (kg) divided by height (m)^2.
   A) $14.43 \text{ kg} \cdot \text{m}^{-2}$
   B) $39.71 \text{ kg} \cdot \text{m}^{-2}$
   C) $29.07 \text{ kg} \cdot \text{m}^{-2}$
   D) $52.62 \text{ kg} \cdot \text{m}^{-2}$

2. Using the correct answer from question 1, what is Mike's BMI classification?
   A) Underweight
   B) Normal
   C) Overweight
   D) Obese

3. Assuming Mike did complete the 1.5-mi walk/run test in 14 min, please calculate Mike's estimated maximal volume of oxygen consumed per unit time ($\dot{V}O_{2max}$) using the below equation:

   $\dot{V}O_{2max} (\text{mL} \cdot \text{kg}^{-1} \cdot \text{min}^{-1}) = 3.5 + 483/1.5\text{-mi}$ time (min)
   A) $34.5 \text{ mL} \cdot \text{kg}^{-1} \cdot \text{min}^{-1}$
   B) $52.8 \text{ mL} \cdot \text{kg}^{-1} \cdot \text{min}^{-1}$
   C) $29.5 \text{ mL} \cdot \text{kg}^{-1} \cdot \text{min}^{-1}$
   D) $38.0 \text{ mL} \cdot \text{kg}^{-1} \cdot \text{min}^{-1}$

4. Using the table ("Fitness Categories for Maximal Aerobic Power for Men and Women by Age") from the most recent edition of the guidelines, the 1.5-mi walk/run test would place Mike in which of the following categories?
   A) Superior
   B) Good
   C) Fair
   D) Poor

5. The push-up result for Mike would place him in which of the following fitness categories?
   A) Excellent
   B) Very good
   C) Good
   D) Fair

6. The curl-up result for Mike would place him in which of the following fitness categories?
   A) Above average
   B) Average
   C) Below average
   D) Well below average

7. The bench press 1-RM result for Mike would place him in which of the following fitness categories?
   A) Superior
   B) Excellent
   C) Fair
   D) Poor

8. The leg press 1-RM result for Mike would place him in which of the following fitness categories?
   A) Well above average
   B) Above average
   C) Average
   D) Below average

9. The trunk flexion result for Mike would place him in which of the following fitness categories?
   A) Excellent
   B) Very good
   C) Good
   D) Fair

EP-C

DISCUSSION QUESTIONS FOR CASE STUDY EP-C.I

1. Mike expressed a desire to have his muscular strength assessed on the bench press exercise and you determined that using the 1-RM test would be a good choice. Identify the necessary steps that are needed to successfully conduct this specific test on Mike.

2. You have decided to assess Mike's cardiorespiratory endurance and have selected the 1.5-mi run test. How would you conduct the 1.5-mi run test for Mike?

DOMAIN II: EXERCISE PRESCRIPTION, IMPLEMENTATION, AND ONGOING SUPPORT

CASE STUDY EP-C.II

Author: **Shawn Drake, PT, PhD**
Author's Certifications: **ACSM-RCEP, ACSM-PD, ACSM-CEP**

Mr. McCain is a 36-yr-old, African American male, who works as a construction worker. He is not participating in any exercise program because he is tired after working in the hot sun all day. At work, he is getting more than 30 min of physical activity 5 d · wk^{-1}. His father died of a heart attack at the age of 40 yr. Now that he is approaching the age of 40 yr, he wants to take steps to improve his health.

Mr. McCain is interested in a cross-fit program that he has heard about at work. He states that he would like to start that program but wants to make sure he is fit enough to begin the high-intensity program. Mr. McCain takes a β-blocker for hypertension. He is a nonsmoker and otherwise healthy.

On today's visit, his HR$_{rest}$ was 65 bpm and his resting BP was 140/84 mm Hg. Mr. McCain mentioned that he forgot to take his β-blocker today. He weighs 202 lb and is 72 in tall, and his body fat is 22%. His fasting blood lipid profile results were as follows: total cholesterol = 230 mg · dL^{-1}; HDL-cholesterol (HDL-C) = 46 mg · dL^{-1}; LDL = 140 mg · dL^{-1}; triglycerides = 220 mg · dL^{-1}. Fasting blood glucose results was 80 mg · dL^{-1}.

Mr. McCain completed a max Bruce treadmill exercise test in 11 min and 55 s (estimated $\dot{V}O_{2max}$ = 45.5 mL · kg^{-1} · min^{-1}). His maximal heart rate (HR$_{max}$) reached 185 bpm, and his BP was 186/98 mm Hg. Other health-related physical fitness parameters included sit and reach at 40 cm (the sit-and-reach box has a zero point at 23 cm), 50 curl-ups, and 21 push-ups.

MULTIPLE-CHOICE QUESTIONS FOR CASE STUDY EP-C.II

1. What is Mr. McCain's BP classification?
   A) Normal
   B) Prehypertension
   C) Stage I hypertension
   D) Stage II hypertension

2. Based on his $\dot{V}O_{2max}$, Mr. McCain would fall within which of the following fitness categories?
   A) Superior
   B) Excellent
   C) Good
   D) Fair

3. Based on the results of the trunk forward flexion (assume the sit-and-reach box has a zero point at 23 cm) test, Mr. McCain would fall in which of the following fitness categories?
   A) Excellent
   B) Very good
   C) Good
   D) Fair

4. What is Mr. McCain's target $\dot{V}O_2R$ if prescribing at 60% intensity level?
   A) 29.4 mL · kg^{-1} · min^{-1}
   B) 31.9 mL · kg^{-1} · min^{-1}
   C) 28.7 mL · kg^{-1} · min^{-1}
   D) 34.3 mL · kg^{-1} · min^{-1}

5. How many kilocalories would Mr. McCain burn if exercising at the 60% $\dot{V}O_2R$ for 30 min?
   A) 90 kcal
   B) 396 kcal
   C) 454 kcal
   D) 560 kcal

DISCUSSION QUESTIONS FOR CASE STUDY EP-C.II

1. Design an exercise program for Mr. McCain using the frequency, intensity, time, and type (FITT) framework based on his current health/fitness status.

2. Should Mr. McCain begin a high-intensity exercise program?

DOMAIN III: EXERCISE COUNSELING AND BEHAVIORAL STRATEGIES

CASE STUDY EP-C.III

Author: **Melissa Conway-Hartman MEd, LAT, ATC**
Author's Certifications: **ACSM EP-C**

Mrs. Kelly is a 55-yr-old female who has come to your fitness center looking for help with her workout. Her goals include becoming more active, losing a few pounds, and increasing strength and endurance for enhanced ability to carry out activities of daily living (ADL). She walks her dog around the block for approximately 15 min $\cdot$ d^{-1}. She has worked out in the past in a fitness center and is familiar with cardiovascular equipment and prefers the treadmill. She is not as familiar with resistance training but is comfortable if she has someone to instruct her. She does not like to work out with her husband because he intimidates her. She has also expressed her dislike of coming to the gym during busy hours because she feels as though people are watching her.

As you are interviewing her, she tells you she takes medication for high BP and her doctor wants her to work out to improve her cardiovascular health. She has problems periodically with her right knee. Her doctor diagnosed her with a tear in her medial meniscus. She is also in physical therapy for a sore left shoulder and has a history of adhesive capsulitis. She also reveals that she has struggled to keep her weight down over the last 5 yr; she currently weighs 210 lb and is 5 ft 6 in tall. Her results from her latest physical include the following:

Total cholesterol	202 mg $\cdot$ dL^{-1}
Triglycerides	155 mg $\cdot$ dL^{-1}
HDL-C	40 mg $\cdot$ dL^{-1}
LDL-cholesterol (LDL-C)	131 mg $\cdot$ dL^{-1}
Fasting glucose	105 mg $\cdot$ dL^{-1}
BP	122/78 mm Hg

Mrs. Kelly expresses to you that she knows she needs to make changes and feels ready to succeed this time but is still afraid to fail due to her intermittent success in the past. Fear of having severe cardiovascular issues is a big motivator for her this time around. She does not currently work outside of the home, spends much of her time caring for her sick nephew and mother, and frequently travels to visit family on the West coast.

Assume you have addressed her medical issues with proper medical clearance forms and assessments.

MULTIPLE-CHOICE QUESTIONS FOR CASE STUDY EP-C.III

1. According to the stages of change model or the transtheoretical model (TTM) of behavior change, which stage is Mrs. Kelly in?
   A) Precontemplation
   B) Action
   C) Maintenance
   D) Preparation

2. Given Mrs. Kelly's fear of developing severe cardiovascular issues, what behavior model would you use to help progress her behavior change?
   A) TTM
   B) Health belief model
   C) Social ecological model
   D) Self-efficacy model

3. Given that Mrs. Kelly has been unable to maintain her exercise plan, what strategy would you use to find out how you can best help her adhere to her program this time and facilitate behavior change?
   A) Goal setting
   B) Client-centered approach
   C) Decisional balance sheet
   D) Creating an exercise plan for her

4. You noticed that Mrs. Kelly has some self-efficacy issues due to her injuries. What is one way you can increase her self-efficacy so she will feel comfortable with her resistance training exercises?
   A) Include Mrs. Kelly in a small group resistance training session with women of similar age and interests
   B) Educate her on the benefits of resistance training
   C) Help her identify her barriers
   D) Ask what made her successful in the past

5. As Mrs. Kelly begins to have success in her program and enters the maintenance stage of the TTM, what strategies can you use to help her maintain her program?
   A) Enlist social support (e.g., working out with a friend)
   B) Inform her of the benefits of being active
   C) Help her replace her bad habits with good ones
   D) Help her see that the pros outweigh the cons

6. Based on the initial information given, which of the following would be an appropriate initial goal you would suggest for Mrs. Kelly?
   A) Decrease caloric intake
   B) Increase total volume of cardiovascular exercise as tolerated until she meets the ACSM recommended amount of a minimum of 150 min of moderate-to-vigorous intensity activity each week
   C) Incorporate abdominal exercises into her program
   D) Because she does not like to work out with her husband, suggest she get a friend to work out with

7. The model or approach that combines behavioral skill training, cognitive intervention, and lifestyle coaching is which of the following?
   A. Relapse prevention
   B. The social cognitive model
   C. The TTM
   D. The socioecological model

DISCUSSION QUESTIONS FOR CASE STUDY EP-C.III

1. List a few cognitive and behavioral strategies you may help Mrs. Kelly with overcoming barriers with injuries, travel, and relapse prevention.

2. Looking at Mrs. Kelly's past exercise and medical history, list specific health metrics that increase her cardiometabolic risk. What is her BMI? How would you help her develop a goal to address her cardiometabolic profile?

DOMAIN IV: LEGAL AND PROFESSIONAL

CASE STUDY EP-C.IV

Author: **Matthew W. Parrot, PhD**
Author's Certifications: **ACSM EP-C**

Jimmy Strawn graduated with his Bachelor of Science in Exercise Physiology and attained the ACSM EP-C certification soon after. After researching his job options, Jimmy decided to start his own personal training studio and borrowed $100,000 with his parents cosigning the loan. In 2010, Westport Fitness Training became a reality. This small training studio was developed in the heart of an up-and-coming part of the city that appeared to mirror Jimmy's target market demographic. Jimmy started the facility with himself and one other employee along with 3,000 sq ft of commercial space filled with brand new fitness equipment. Shortly after the grand opening, another large commercial facility in the area closed its doors. As a result, Westport Fitness Training grew quickly from two employees to four, plus five contract personal trainers within the first 12 mo. Business was booming.

The influx of customers meant long hours for Jimmy and his staff. The trainers were busy with clients, and Jimmy could barely keep up with the increasing administrative demands and new business opportunities. Consequently, no preventive maintenance was performed on the exercise equipment in the first 5 yr of operation. The fact that the equipment was purchased brand new gave Jimmy the false impression that it would last for years without regular attention.

One summer day in July of 2015, a Westport Fitness Training client was working with Jimmy's top contract personal trainer when the unthinkable happened. The client was performing an exercise with the cable machine when a screw holding the pulley inexplicably fell out, causing the client to fall backward and hit his head on the other side of the machine. Jimmy was not on hand to witness the incident. Although embarrassed, the client claimed he felt fine and no other actions were taken by Jimmy's staff.

Consequences: A lawsuit was filed by the client claiming negligence on behalf of Jimmy Strawn and Westport Fitness Training. As Jimmy and his lawyer prepared their defense, a number of questions were posed.

MULTIPLE-CHOICE QUESTIONS FOR CASE STUDY EP-C.IV

1. Which of the following types of insurance coverage would be the *most* relevant in this case?
   A) General liability
   B) Professional liability
   C) Worker's compensation
   D) Property

2. Which of the following documents would be the *most* relevant in Jimmy's defense?
   A) Preactivity health screening
   B) Waiver of liability
   C) Membership agreement
   D) Personal training agreement

3. Although Jimmy and his staff took no action, which of the following actions would have been appropriate immediately following the incident, given the information we have?
   A) Call 911
   B) Holding an all-staff meeting
   C) Contacting his lawyer immediately
   D) Initiating first aid protocol and complete incident report

4. Which of the following activities is *most* likely to have prevented the injury from occurring?
   A) Completing and documenting preventive maintenance procedures according to manufacturer's recommendations
   B) Training staff on proper spotting techniques
   C) Ensuring all participants sign a liability waiver
   D) Developing and using a comprehensive emergency protocol according to ACSM standards

5. Which of the following first aid procedures would have been appropriate in this situation?
   A) Check scene for safety, complete initial assessment, and provide appropriate care.
   B) Check scene for safety, call 911, and complete initial assessment.
   C) Call 911, check scene for safety, and provide appropriate care.
   D) Provide appropriate care and apply ice and direct pressure to injury.

6. Which of the following actions would *not* have been appropriate according to HIPAA guidelines?
   A) Completing incident report and sending to insurance carrier
   B) Obtaining video surveillance of incident and sending to insurance carrier
   C) Sending the injured party's membership agreement to insurance carrier
   D) Distributing injured party's medical information to all facility members

7. Which of the following ethical responsibilities (under ACSM's Code of Ethics) did Jimmy and his staff *fail* to uphold?
   A) Members should treat or train athletes with the objective of maintaining the integrity of competition and fair play.
   B) The College, and its members, should safeguard the public and itself against members who are deficient in ethical conduct.
   C) Members should not advise, aid, or abet any athlete to use prohibited substances or methods of doping.
   D) None of the above

8. Which of the following knowledge areas did Jimmy *fail* to recognize prior to this incident?
    A) Knowledge of AED guidelines for implementation
    B) Knowledge of preventive maintenance schedules and audits
    C) Knowledge of preactivity screening, medical release, and waiver of liability for normal and at-risk participants
    D) Knowledge of employment verification requirements mandated by state and federal laws

9. Jimmy's employees failed to implement any type of emergency protocol as part of this incident. How can Jimmy prevent this from occurring in the future?
    A) Develop and distribute a policy and procedures manual
    B) Develop and distribute an emergency protocol

C) Hold regular emergency protocol training sessions with his staff
D) All of the above

10. Which if the following would not be part of an appropriate emergency protocol for this incident?
    A) Assessing injury
    B) Checking scene
    C) Activating EMS
    D) Contacting friends and family of injured party

DISCUSSION QUESTIONS FOR CASE STUDY EP-C.IV

1. Given the legal and professional job task analysis (JTA) associated with the EP-C, what areas should Jimmy have handled differently to better prepare himself and his business for this incident?

2. What are the requirements of an EP-C in terms of incident reporting?

3. What responsibilities does an EP-C have in terms of preventive maintenance, and how could those have reduced Jimmy's liability exposure in this incident?

4. What types of emergency procedures should have been implemented during this incident?

DOMAIN V: MANAGEMENT

CASE STUDY EP-C.V

Author: **Frederick Klinge, MBA**
Author's Certifications: **ACSM EP-C**

You are the personal training director for a large multipurpose health club that has been operating successfully in a competitive market for 19 yr. You oversee all fee-based personal training programs. For the past 4 yr, your department's year-end net profit has been slowly declining, starting at a high range of 24% and hitting a recent year-end low net profit of 11%. Budgeted net profit projections for your department always range from 25% to 30%.

You have recently decided to introduce a small group training program targeting competitive endurance sports athletes, called TriPower. This program is designed to compete against similar sports performance programs offered by other health clubs in the local market. The TriPower program is exclusively for club members, and the fees have been structured to be in line with the competition. Members will pay a program fee ranging from $65 to $100 per month, depending on the number of training sessions they wish to attend. Monthly membership dues at your club range from $80 for a single membership up to $120 for a family membership.

You report directly to the general manager of the club, who has asked you to focus on improving the overall net profit of your department.

EP-C

MULTIPLE-CHOICE QUESTIONS FOR CASE STUDY EP-C.V

1. Personnel: In order for a program to be successful, you need to hire competent, qualified trainers with strong educational backgrounds and defensible certifications. Before the hiring process starts, you must write the job description for TriPower Program Supervisor. This job description should include which of the following?
   A) Performance measures
   B) Qualifications and certification requirements
   C) Employee status
   D) Position overview
   E) All of the above

2. Program equipment: The TriPower program is going to involve different training modalities, including high-intensity interval training, strength training, plyometrics, and multiplanar functional movement training. You plan on using medicine balls, kettlebells, suspension training systems, dumbbells, and other similar types of equipment. As personal training director, you are responsible for inspecting and maintaining the equipment used in the TriPower program. Which of the following should be included on your equipment maintenance checklist?
   A) Store dumbbells in a safe position in the workout area when not in use
   B) Replace any equipment when a newer model becomes available
   C) Clean equipment once a week
   D) Equipment personally owned by the trainers delivering the program should never be used alongside the club-owned equipment.

3. Risk management: Proactive risk management can protect your club from costly legal proceedings. The TriPower program involves exercise modalities that require careful supervision and management. Which of the following should be included in the TriPower Risk Management Guidelines?
   A) Program participants should be strongly encouraged to wear athletic footwear, but the brand of footwear is to be chosen by the TriPower Manager.
   B) Because of the high-intensity nature of the TriPower program, participants over the age of 50 yr are not allowed to participate.
   C) All TriPower trainers should be familiar with the club's incident report system, which provides written documentation of all incidents that occur within the facility.
   D) Surveillance cameras should be installed in program workout areas to reduce liability exposure.

4. Fiscal management: You receive a monthly department income statement from your general manager that serves as a helpful department management tool. The department income statement lists operational revenues, expenses, and department net income and loss. Which of the following most accurately describes the term *net income*?
   A) A financial statement that projects revenues and expenses for a future period
   B) Gross income (revenue) less expenses representing the profit of a business (or department) for a specific period of time
   C) The movement of money in and out of a department through the collection of revenue and payment of expenses
   D) Gross income (revenue) less expenses representing the profit of a business (or department) at a specific point in time

5. Budgeting: Your management team relies heavily on budget analysis for evaluating program performance. Using previous years' financial data to develop a current and future year budget is referred to as a
   A) Zero-based budget
   B) Cash flow budget
   C) Financial budget
   D) Trend-line budget

6. Creating a budget: You have been asked by the general manager to create a budget projection for the TriPower program for the next year. Which of the following is important in creating an accurate budget?
   A) Make a list of all the current assets that will be used in the TriPower program
   B) Determine the operating costs for the program for the upcoming year, including percentage wage increases for program instructors and repairs to equipment used in the program
   C) Determine the wages and payroll taxes that will be payable for each of the 12 mo of the next fiscal year
   D) Calculate the approximate cost of issuing refunds to participants who get injured while participating in the program

EP-C

7. Budgeting: The TriPower program will be held in a 2,500 sq ft indoor performance center within your club and you've been charged with purchasing equipment for the program. One piece of equipment you have purchased is multistation strength training machine that costs $3,570, and it has an expected useful lifespan of 10 yr. This piece of equipment would be classified as what type of asset?
    A) Current asset
    B) Fixed asset
    C) Inventory asset
    D) Equity asset

8. Marketing: Determining the price of the TriPower program will be critical to the success and net profit of your department. Important issues to consider when determining the price of the TriPower program should include which of the following?
    A) Timing of the internal marketing program developed by in-house staff
    B) Feedback from member focus groups who were asked to discuss possible programs they would like to see the club offer
    C) The acceptable profitable profit margin predetermined by your management team
    D) The projected number of referrals to the program from other club departments

9. Marketing: The financial success of the TriPower program will be maximized by developing a successful advertising and marketing plan. This plan needs to target both internal and external markets and must be cost-effective. Which of the following is the most cost-effective marketing strategy?
    A) Add a new page to the club Web site featuring the TriPower program
    B) Contract with a local radio station affiliate to create a 30-s commercial plan that will run for 4 wk prior to the launch of the TriPower program
    C) Place an ad for the program in the local newspaper
    D) Develop an Internet marketing plan that focuses on promoting TriPower on the club's social media pages and sending an e-mail newsletter to all members who signed up to receive club e-mail correspondence

10. Program pricing: Determining the price of the TriPower program is multifaceted and important to the financial success of the program. Basic issues affecting price include which of the following?
    A) Profit margin
    B) Type of depreciation schedule for the equipment purchased for use in the program
    C) Real and perceived market value of the program
    D) Both A and C

DISCUSSION QUESTIONS FOR CASE STUDY EP-C.V

1. To ensure the ongoing success of any fitness program, it is important to evaluate both its qualitative and quantitative results. Considering the objectives of the TriPower program, list and describe some of the possible program evaluation techniques you might use as measures of its success.

2. It will be critical for you to generate member interest in your new TriPower program. What are some cost-effective, creative ways to increase the visibility of the program to your members and incentivize them to participate?

EP-C CASE STUDIES ANSWERS AND EXPLANATIONS

CASE STUDY EP-C.I

Multiple-Choice Answers for Case Study EP-C.I

1—C. $29.07 \text{ kg} \cdot \text{m}^{-2}$

Weight = 95.24 kg, height = 1.81 m

Therefore, $95.24 \text{ kg} / (1.81 \text{ m})^2 = 95.24 / 3.2761 = 29.07 \text{ kg} \cdot \text{m}^{-2}$

Resource: Swain D, senior editor. *ACSM'S Resource Manual for Guidelines for Exercise Testing and Prescription.* 7th ed. Philadelphia (PA): Wolters Kluwer; 2014. 896 p.

2—C. Overweight

Resource: Swain D, senior editor. *ACSM'S Resource Manual for Guidelines for Exercise Testing and Prescription.* 7th ed. Philadelphia (PA): Wolters Kluwer; 2014. 896 p.

3—D. $38.0 \text{ mL} \cdot \text{kg}^{-1} \cdot \text{min}^{-1}$

$\dot{V}O_{2\text{max}} (\text{mL} \cdot \text{kg}^{-1} \cdot \text{min}^{-1}) = 3.5 + 483/14 \text{ min}$

$= 3.5 + 34.5$

$= 38.0 \text{ mL} \cdot \text{kg}^{-1} \cdot \text{min}^{-1}$

Resource: Swain D, senior editor. *ACSM'S Resource Manual for Guidelines for Exercise Testing and Prescription.* 7th ed. Philadelphia (PA): Wolters Kluwer; 2014. 896 p.

4—D. Poor

Resources: Riebe D, senior editor. *ACSM'S Guidelines for Exercise Testing and Prescription.* 10th ed. Philadelphia (PA): Wolters Kluwer; 2018.

Swain D, senior editor. *ACSM'S Resource Manual for Guidelines for Exercise Testing and Prescription.* 7th ed. Philadelphia (PA): Wolters Kluwer; 2014. 896 p.

5—A. Excellent

Resources: Riebe D, senior editor. *ACSM'S Guidelines for Exercise Testing and Prescription.* 10th ed. Philadelphia (PA): Wolters Kluwer; 2018.

Swain D, senior editor. *ACSM'S Resource Manual for Guidelines for Exercise Testing and Prescription.* 7th ed. Philadelphia (PA): Wolters Kluwer; 2014. 896 p.

6—B. Average

Resources: Riebe D, senior editor. *ACSM'S Guidelines for Exercise Testing and Prescription.* 10th ed. Philadelphia (PA): Wolters Kluwer; 2018.

Swain D, senior editor. *ACSM'S Resource Manual for Guidelines for Exercise Testing and Prescription.* 7th ed. Philadelphia (PA): Wolters Kluwer; 2014. 896 p.

7—B. Excellent

Resources: Riebe D, senior editor. *ACSM'S Guidelines for Exercise Testing and Prescription.* 10th ed. Philadelphia (PA): Wolters Kluwer; 2018.

Swain D, senior editor. *ACSM'S Resource Manual for Guidelines for Exercise Testing and Prescription.* 7th ed. Philadelphia (PA): Wolters Kluwer; 2014. 896 p.

8—A. Well above average

Resources: Riebe D, senior editor. *ACSM'S Guidelines for Exercise Testing and Prescription.* 10th ed. Philadelphia (PA): Wolters Kluwer; 2018.

Swain D, senior editor. *ACSM'S Resource Manual for Guidelines for Exercise Testing and Prescription.* 7th ed. Philadelphia (PA): Wolters Kluwer; 2014. 896 p.

9—D. Fair

Resources: Riebe D, senior editor. *ACSM'S Guidelines for Exercise Testing and Prescription.* 10th ed. Philadelphia (PA): Wolters Kluwer; 2018.

Swain D, senior editor. *ACSM'S Resource Manual for Guidelines for Exercise Testing and Prescription.* 7th ed. Philadelphia (PA): Wolters Kluwer; 2014. 896 p.

Discussion Question Answers for Case Study EP-C.I

1. Testing should be completed only after Mike has participated in familiarization/practice sessions. Mike should warm up by completing a number of submaximal repetitions of the bench press that will be used to determine the 1-RM. Determine the 1-RM (or any multiple of 1-RM) within four trials with rest periods of 3–5 min between trials. Select an initial weight

that is within Mike's perceived capacity (~50%–70% of capacity). Resistance is progressively increased by 5%–10% for upper body exercise from previous successful attempts until Mike cannot complete the selected repetition(s); all repetitions should be performed at the same speed of movement and range of motion (ROM) to instill consistency between trials. The final weight lifted successfully is recorded as the absolute 1-RM or multiple-RM.

> **Resource**: Riebe D, senior editor. *ACSM'S Guidelines for Exercise Testing and Prescription.* 10th ed. Philadelphia (PA): Wolters Kluwer; 2018.

2. Ensure that the test area measures out to 1.5 mi. Inform Mike of the purpose of the test and the need to pace himself properly over 1.5 mi. Start the test and give Mike feedback on time to help him pace. Once the test is complete, record the total time to the nearest hundredth of a minute. Finally, calculate estimated $\dot{V}O_{2max}$ using the prediction equation for the 1.5-mi run test.

$\dot{V}O_{2max}$ (mL · kg^{-1} · min^{-1}) = 3.5 + 483/1.5 mi time (min)

For example:

If it takes Mike 11 min 15 s (11:15) to complete the 1.5-mi run, the time used in the given formula would be 11.25 (15 / 60 = 0.25)

$\dot{V}O_{2max}$ (mL · kg^{-1} · min^{-1}) = 3.5 + 483/1.5 mi time (min)

$\dot{V}O_{2max}$ (mL · kg^{-1} · min^{-1}) = 3.5 + 483/11.25 = 46.4 mL · kg^{-1} · min^{-1}

> **Resource**: Swain D, senior editor. *ACSM'S Resource Manual for Guidelines for Exercise Testing and Prescription.* 7th ed. Philadelphia (PA): Wolters Kluwer; 2014. 896 p.

CASE STUDY EP-C.II

Multiple-Choice Answers for Case Study EP-C.II

1—C. Stage I hypertension

Mr. McCain's resting BP was 140/84 mm Hg. Normal is <120 mm Hg (systolic) and <80 mm Hg (diastolic). Prehypertension is classified as 120–139 mm Hg (systolic) or 80–89 mm Hg (diastolic). Stage I hypertension is 140–159 mm Hg (systolic) or 90–99 mmHg (diastolic). Stage II hypertension is ≥160 mm Hg (systolic) or ≥100 mm Hg (diastolic). Thus, Mr. McCain's resting BP would place him in the category of stage I hypertension.

> **Resource**: Riebe D, senior editor. *ACSM'S Guidelines for Exercise Testing and Prescription.* 10th ed. Philadelphia (PA): Wolters Kluwer; 2018.

2—C. Good

Mr. McCain's $\dot{V}O_{2max}$ is 45.5 mL · kg^{-1} · min^{-1} and age is 36 yr. Using Table 4.7, the fitness category is "Good."

> **Resource**: Riebe D, senior editor. *ACSM'S Guidelines for Exercise Testing and Prescription.* 10th ed. Philadelphia (PA): Wolters Kluwer; 2018.

3—B. Very good

The chart in Table 4.14 is for a sit-and-reach box that has a zero point at 26 cm. Because the box used to test Mr. McCain is a 23-cm box, 3 cm must be subtracted from the score (40 − 3 = 37 cm).

Therefore, the score is 37 cm, and on the chart, for his age, the category is "Very Good."

> **Resource**: Riebe D, senior editor. *ACSM'S Guidelines for Exercise Testing and Prescription.* 10th ed. Philadelphia (PA): Wolters Kluwer; 2018.

4—C. 28.7 mL · kg^{-1} · min^{-1}

$\dot{V}O_2R$ = 45.5 mL · kg^{-1} · min^{-1} − 3.5 mL · kg^{-1} · min^{-1} = 42 mL · kg^{-1} · min^{-1}

60% of 42 mL · kg^{-1} · min^{-1} = 25.2 mL · kg^{-1} · min^{-1}

25.2 mL · kg^{-1} · min^{-1} + 3.5 mL · kg^{-1} · min^{-1} = 28.7 mL · kg^{-1} · min^{-1}

5—B. 396 kcal

Mr. McCain weighs 202 lb, which is 92 kg (202 lb / 2.205 = 92 kg). The intensity level is 28.7 mL · kg^{-1} · min^{-1} calculated in question 4.

(28.7 mL · kg^{-1} · min^{-1} × 92 kg) / 1,000 mL = 2.64 L/min

2.64 L/min × 5 kcal = 13.2 kcal/min

13.2 kcal/min × 30 min = 396 kcal

EP-C

Discussion Question Answers for Case Study EP-C.II

1. Mr. McCain should follow guidelines for hypertension, which include focusing weight reduction by increasing caloric expenditure coupled with reducing caloric intake.

   Frequency: Preferably aerobic exercise every day or most days of the week. Resistance training should be 2–3 d · wk^{-1}.

   Intensity: Moderate-intensity levels (40%–60% $\dot{V}O_2R$) is appropriate for aerobic activity; resistance training at 60%–80% of 1-RM

Time: Longer aerobic activities (>30 min) to increase caloric expenditure

Type: Choose activities that are enjoyable and use large muscle groups (e.g., walking, jogging, swimming) for aerobic; resistance training to include free weights or machine weights

2. Based on Mr. McCain, he should begin a low-intensity, long-duration exercise program. The goal is to lose weight and gradually increase muscle strength.

CASE STUDY EP-C.III

Multiple-Choice Answers for Case Study EP-C.III

1—D. Preparation

   Preparation, because she is currently trying to be active by walking her dog but is not meeting the guidelines. She is coming to you for help with a plan.

2—B. Health belief model

   The health belief model states that people are likely to change a behavior if that current behavior poses a perceived serious potential health problem, the threat is severe, and the person perceives themselves to be susceptible to the threat.

   Resource: Battista R, senior editor. *ACSM's Resources for the Personal Trainer*. 5th ed. Philadelphia (PA): Wolters Kluwer; 2017.

3—B. Client-centered approach

   Client-centered approach is a counseling style that "takes the client's perspective into account, features collaboration between the client and the practitioner, and includes genuine respect for the client's opinions."

   Resource: Battista R, senior editor. *ACSM's Resources for the Personal Trainer*. 5th ed. Philadelphia (PA): Wolters Kluwer; 2017.

4—A. Include Mrs. Kelly in a small group resistance training session with women of similar age and interests

   According to Bandura, providing vicarious experiences — watching others who are similar to you change their behavior — will increase a client's self-efficacy.

   Resources: Riebe D, senior editor. *ACSM'S Guidelines for Exercise Testing and Prescription*, 10th ed. Philadelphia (PA): Wolters Kluwer; 2018.

Swain D, senior editor. *ACSM'S Resource Manual for Guidelines for Exercise Testing and Prescription*. 7th ed. Philadelphia (PA): Wolters Kluwer; 2014. 896 p.

5—A. Enlist social support (e.g., working out with a friend)

   "Enlisting social support, i.e., walking with a neighbor" can help maintainers avoid boredom.

   Resource: Riebe D, senior editor. *ACSM'S Guidelines for Exercise Testing and Prescription*, 10th ed. Philadelphia (PA): Wolters Kluwer; 2018.

6—B. Increase total volume of cardiovascular exercise as tolerated until she meets the ACSM recommended amount of a minimum of 150 min of moderate-to-vigorous intensity activity each week

   She is currently walking, and increasing the time she is active in small increments will provide mastery experiences to increase her self-efficacy. Burning more calories will help her lose weight, and doing so slowly will aid in prevention of further injury to her knee. Small changes may also be more realistic and safe for her to achieve (small changes model).

   Resource: Battista R, senior editor. *ACSM's Resources for the Personal Trainer*. 5th ed. Philadelphia (PA): Wolters Kluwer; 2018.

7—A. Relapse prevention strategies

   The relapse prevention strategies are a combination of behavioral skill training, cognitive intervention, and lifestyle change

   Resource: Nigg C. *ACSM's Behavioral Aspects of Physical Activity and Exercise*. Philadelphia (PA): Lippincott Williams & Wilkins; 2014:107

Discussion Question Answers for Case Study EP-C.III

1. Provide guidance to Mrs. Kelly on overcoming specific barriers to physical activity. For example, provide her with workouts she can perform during travel, and encouraging her to fit in her activity when and where she can while taking care of her nephew will help keep her active until she can return to her normal life routine. Using a planning worksheet can help her think through (coping planning) and plan around her various barriers.

   Reducing her level of anxiety regarding committing to a regular exercise program is asking her to pay attention to her feelings about finally becoming more active (dramatic relief). It also addresses the cognitive portion of the RPM. To help her with the behavioral aspect of the RPM, you can develop activities she can participate in when traveling. To help her with her overall lifestyle change, she needs to see herself as an active person (social liberation).

   Resource: Nigg C. *ACSM's Behavioral Aspects of Physical Activity and Exercise*. Philadelphia (PA): Lippincott Williams & Wilkins; 2014:107.

2. Mrs. Kelly has elevated total cholesterol, borderline elevated LDL-C, decreased HDL-C, and elevated triglyceride and blood glucose levels. Although controlled by her medication, she also has high BP. Her BMI is 33.9 kg $\cdot$ m^{-2} placing her in the class I obesity category. By using motivational interviewing skills, she will understand the importance to lower her disease risk and BMI. Implementing goal setting principles that are specific, measurable, achievable, realistic, and time-oriented (SMART) will help her achieve her initial goal.

   Resources: Nigg C. *ACSM's Behavioral Aspects of Physical Activity and Exercise*. Philadelphia (PA): Lippincott Williams & Wilkins; 2014:76–77,137.

   Riebe D, senior editor. *ACSM's Guidelines for Exercise Testing and Prescription*. 10th ed. Philadelphia (PA): Wolters Kluwer; 2018.

CASE STUDY EP-C.IV

Multiple-Choice Answers for Case Study EP-C.IV

1—A. General liability

Resource: Swain D, senior editor. *ACSM'S Resource Manual for Guidelines for Exercise Testing and Prescription*. 7th ed. Philadelphia (PA): Wolters Kluwer; 2014. 896 p.

2—B. Waiver of liability

Resource: Riebe D, senior editor. *ACSM'S Guidelines for Exercise Testing and Prescription*, 10th ed. Philadelphia (PA): Wolters Kluwer; 2018.

3—D. Initiating first aid protocol and complete incident report

Resource: Swain D, senior editor. *ACSM'S Resource Manual for Guidelines for Exercise Testing and Prescription*. 7th ed. Philadelphia (PA): Wolters Kluwer; 2014. 896 p.

Tharrett SJ, Peterson JA. *ACSM's Health/Fitness Facilities Standards and Guidelines*. 4th ed. Champaign (IL): Human Kinetics; 2012. 256 p.

4—A. Completing and documenting preventive maintenance procedures according to manufacturer's recommendations

Tharrett SJ, Peterson JA. *ACSM's Health/Fitness Facilities Standards and Guidelines*. 4th ed. Champaign (IL): Human Kinetics; 2012. 256 p.

5—A. Check scene for safety, complete initial assessment, and provide appropriate care.

Resource: Swain D, senior editor. *ACSM'S Resource Manual for Guidelines for Exercise Testing and Prescription*. 7th ed. Philadelphia (PA): Wolters Kluwer; 2014. 896 p.

6—D. Distributing injured party's medical information to all facility members

Resource: Health Insurance Portability and Accountability Act of 1996 (HIPAA)

7—D. None of the above

Resource: Riebe D, senior editor. *ACSM'S Guidelines for Exercise Testing and Prescription*. 10th ed. Philadelphia (PA): Wolters Kluwer; 2018.

8—B. Knowledge of preventive maintenance schedules and audits

Resource: Tharrett SJ, Peterson JA. *ACSM's Health/Fitness Facilities Standards and Guidelines*. 4th ed. Champaign (IL): Human Kinetics; 2012. 256 p.

9—D. All of the above

Resource: Swain D, senior editor. *ACSM'S Resource Manual for Guidelines for Exercise Testing and Prescription*. 7th ed. Philadelphia (PA): Wolters Kluwer; 2014. 896 p.

10—D. Contacting friends and family of injured party

> *Resource*: Swain D, senior editor. *ACSM'S Resource Manual for Guidelines for Exercise Testing and Prescription.* 7th ed. Philadelphia (PA): Wolters Kluwer; 2014. 896 p.

Discussion Question Answers for Case Study EP-C.IV

1. The areas include policies and procedures manual, emergency procedure training, complete preventive maintenance as manufacturer's required, incident report training, safety procedures and supplies, understanding of insurance coverage differences for contractors versus employees, and installation of proper signage for equipment use.

   > Tharrett SJ, Peterson JA. *ACSM's Health/Fitness Facilities Standards and Guidelines,* 4th ed. Champaign (IL): Human Kinetics, 2012.

2. Develop a written incident report that includes name and contact information for injured party and witnesses, description of event and injuries, time and day of incident, and any actions taken by the staff. Complete this report for any injury, regardless of se-

verity and keep on file. To train all qualified subordinate staff on proper incident report completion.

> Tharrett, SJ and Peterson JA. *ACSM's Health/ Fitness Facilities Standards and Guidelines,* 4th ed. Champaign (IL): Human Kinetics, 2012.

3. An EP-C needs to be familiar with all preventive maintenance schedules as recommended by the manufacturer(s), to complete the preventive maintenance, and to document preventive maintenance procedures when completed.

   > Tharrett, SJ and Peterson JA. *ACSM's Health/ Fitness Facilities Standards and Guidelines.* 4th ed. Champaign (IL): Human Kinetics; 2012. 256 p.

4. Emergency procedures include incident report completion, first aid assessment by staff, first aid provided (if needed) by staff, and evaluation of emergency medical services (EMS) personnel involvement. Interview injured party and document all relevant information on the scene conditions, individuals present, extent of injury, and the incident itself.

   > Tharrett, SJ and Peterson, JA. *ACSM's Health/ Fitness Facilities Standards and Guidelines,* 4th ed. Champaign (IL): Human Kinetics, 2012.

CASE STUDY EP-C.V

Multiple-Choice Answers for Case Study EP-C.V

1—E. All of the above

> *Resource*: *ACSM's Resources for the Exercise Physiologist.* Revised Reprint Ed. Philadelphia (PA): Wolters Kluwer; 2015.

2—A. Store dumbbells in a safe position in the workout area when not in use

> *Resource*: *ACSM's Resources for the Exercise Physiologist.* Revised Reprint Ed. Philadelphia (PA): Wolters Kluwer; 2015.

3—C. All TriPower trainers should be familiar with the club's incident report system, which provides written documentation of all incidents that occur within the facility.

> *Resource*: *ACSM's Resources for the Exercise Physiologist.* Revised Reprint Ed. Philadelphia (PA): Wolters Kluwer; 2015.

4—B. Gross income (revenue) less expenses representing the profit of a business (or department) for a specific period of time

> *Resource*: *ACSM's Resources for the Exercise Physiologist.* Revised Reprint Ed. Philadelphia (PA): Wolters Kluwer; 2015.

5—D. Trend-line budget

> *Resource*: *ACSM's Resources for the Exercise Physiologist.* Revised Reprint Ed. Philadelphia (PA): Wolters Kluwer; 2015.

6—B. Determine the operating costs for the program for the upcoming year, including percentage wage increases for program instructors and repairs to equipment used in the program.

> *Resource*: *ACSM's Resources for the Exercise Physiologist.* Revised Reprint Ed. Philadelphia (PA): Wolters Kluwer; 2015.

7—B. Fixed asset

> *Resource*: *ACSM's Resources for the Exercise Physiologist.* Revised Reprint Ed. Philadelphia (PA): Wolters Kluwer; 2015.

8—C. The acceptable profitable profit margin predetermined by your management team

> *Resource*: *ACSM's Resources for the Exercise Physiologist.* Revised Reprint Ed. Philadelphia (PA): Wolters Kluwer; 2015.

9—D. Develop an Internet marketing plan that focuses on promoting TriPower on the club's social media pages and sending an e-mail newsletter to all

EP-C

members who signed up to receive club e-mail correspondence

Resource: *ACSM's Resources for the Exercise Physiologist*. Revised Reprint Ed. Philadelphia (PA): Wolters Kluwer; 2015.

10—D. Both A and C

Resource: *ACSM's Resources for the Exercise Physiologist*. Revised Reprint Ed. Philadelphia (PA): Wolters Kluwer; 2015.

Discussion Question Answers for Case Study EP-C.V

1. Possible program evaluation techniques include the following:

   - Performing a profit analysis would be an example of a quantitative evaluation method. A profit analysis would provide net income/loss performance information, taking into account the various sources of program revenue and expenses. Developing a monthly profit and loss statement would be an excellent example of an ongoing program evaluation method providing program management with profitability information.
   - A process evaluation might be a series of checklists used by the staff delivering the program that would provide management with information regarding program performance, for example, are the program staff members completing tasks involved in delivery the program services on a consistent basis and do these completed tasks help achieve program objectives.
   - Program participant surveys offer excellent feedback on participant satisfaction regarding the program services.
   - Outcome evaluation provide information that helps determine if program objectives were met. Outcome evaluations often consist of a program staff meeting following the conclusion of the

program and evaluating information gathered during the program as well as reviewing post-program financial results. This information is used to determine if the program met profitability goals.

Resource: *ACSM's Resources for the Exercise Physiologist*. Revised Reprint Ed. Philadelphia (PA): Wolters Kluwer; 2015.

2. Some cost-effective, creative ways include the following:

   - Harness the power of social media, for example, post-program TriPower class videos and participant photos on the club's Facebook page.
   - Use the club's management software system and send promotional e-mail blasts promoting the TriPower program to members who have expressed interest in receiving information regarding fitness programming. Offer a first-month 30% discount of the monthly program fee.
   - Use internal promotion methods, for example, signage, digital reach boards, newsletters, etc., to advertise an "Intro to TriPower" promotion. "Intro to TriPower" allows club members interested in trying the program to attend selected TriPower classes free of charge over a 2-wk period. TriPower staff members would design these specified "Intro to TriPower" classes to include beginner workouts and provide lots of information regarding the benefits to be gained from participating in the program.
   - TriPower participant referral promotion. Send an e-mail blast out to all current TriPower participants offering a $25 program credit for every new TriPower participant they refer to the program.

Resource: *ACSM's Resources for the Exercise Physiologist*. Revised Reprint Ed. Philadelphia (PA): Wolters Kluwer; 2015.

5 EP-C Job Task Analysis

Note: EP-C certification candidates may also review the knowledge and skills (KSs) found in Part 1, ACSM Certified Personal Trainer (CPT).

DOMAIN I: HEALTH AND FITNESS ASSESSMENT

A. Implement assessment protocols and preparticipation health screening procedures to maximize participant safety and minimize risk.		
Knowledge or Skill Statement	**Explanation/Examples**	**Resources**
Knowledge of preactivity screening procedures and tools that provide accurate information about the individual's health/medical history, current medical conditions, risk factors, sign/symptoms of disease, current physical activity habits, and medications	• American College of Sports and Medicine Exercise Preparticipation Health Screening Questionnaire for Exercise Professionals, Physical Activity Readiness Questionnaire (PAR-Q), informed consent, waiver	*ACSM's Guidelines for Exercise Testing and Prescription* (GETP), 10th edition (7) • Tables 2.1, 3.1 • Figures 2.1–2.3
Knowledge of the key components included in informed consent and health/medical history	• Content and extent may vary. • Participant should be familiar with the purpose and the risks of the procedures. • The form should be explained verbally.	*ACSM's Guidelines for Exercise Testing and Prescription* (GETP), 10th edition (7) • Figure 3.1 *ACSM'S Health-Related Physical Fitness Assessment Manual*, 5th edition (4) • Chapter 2
Knowledge of the limitations of informed consent and health/medical history	• The participant is playing a major role in the informed consent process. He or she must be liable and responsible for informing the certified exercise physiologist (EP-C) of any problems experienced (past, present, and during the assessment) that may increase the risk of the test or prohibit participation.	*ACSM's Health-Related Physical Fitness Assessment Manual*, 5th edition (4) • Chapter 2

B.	Determine participant's readiness to take part in a health-related physical fitness assessment and exercise program.	
Knowledge or Skill Statement	**Explanation/Examples**	**Resources**
Knowledge of preexercise readiness assessment as delineated in the current edition of *ACSM's Guidelines for Exercise Testing and Prescription*	• Consider positive and negative risk factors.	*ACSM's Guidelines for Exercise Testing and Prescription* (GETP), 10th edition (7) • Chapter 3
Knowledge of the major signs or symptoms suggestive of cardiovascular, pulmonary, renal, and metabolic disease	• Consider nine major signs and/or symptoms. • Be aware of clarifications/significance.	*ACSM's Guidelines for Exercise Testing and Prescription* (GETP), 10th edition (7) • Table 3.1
Knowledge of cardiovascular risk factors or conditions that may require consultation with medical personnel prior to exercise testing or training (*e.g.*, inappropriate changes in resting heart rate and/or blood pressure [BP]; new onset discomfort in chest, neck, shoulder, or arm; changes in the pattern of discomfort during rest or exercise, fainting, dizzy spells, claudication)	• Consider nine major signs and/or symptoms. • Be aware of clarifications/significance. • Be aware of the different termination criteria based on signs and symptoms.	*ACSM's Guidelines for Exercise Testing and Prescription* (GETP), 10th edition (7) • Chapters 3, 5, and 10 • Table 3.1
Knowledge of the pulmonary risk factors or conditions that may require consultation with medical personnel prior to exercise testing or training (*e.g.*, asthma, exercise-induced asthma/bronchospasm, extreme breathlessness at rest or during exercise, chronic bronchitis, emphysema)	• Nine major signs and/or symptoms. • Be aware of clarifications/significance. • Be aware of spirometry-related measures.	*ACSM's Guidelines for Exercise Testing and Prescription* (GETP), 10th edition (7) • Chapter 5
Knowledge of the metabolic risk factors or conditions that may require consultation with medical personnel prior to exercise testing or training (*e.g.*, obesity, metabolic syndrome, diabetes or glucose intolerance, hypoglycemia)	• Be aware of conditions that may postpone or terminate an exercise session.	*ACSM's Guidelines for Exercise Testing and Prescription* (GETP), 10th edition (7) • Chapter 10
Knowledge of the musculoskeletal risk factors or conditions that may require consultation with medical personnel prior to exercise testing or training (*e.g.*, acute or chronic pain, osteoarthritis, rheumatoid arthritis, osteoporosis, inflammation/pain, low back pain)	• Be aware of common signs and symptoms that are associated with these conditions.	*ACSM's Guidelines for Exercise Testing and Prescription* (GETP), 10th edition (7) • Chapters 10 and 11
Knowledge of ACSM preexercise readiness assessment and the implications for medical clearance before administration of an exercise test or participation in an exercise program	• Be aware of conditions that may require exercise testing in asymptomatic participants prior to the commencement of an exercise program.	*ACSM's Guidelines for Exercise Testing and Prescription* (GETP), 10th edition (7) • Chapter 3

EP-C

B. Determine participant's readiness to take part in a health-related physical fitness assessment and exercise program. (cont.)		
Knowledge or Skill Statement	**Explanation/Examples**	**Resources**
Knowledge of risk factors that may be favorably modified by physical activity habits	• Consider the benefits of regular physical activity and/or exercise.	*ACSM's Guidelines for Exercise Testing and Prescription* (GETP), 10th edition (7)
Knowledge of medical terminology including but not limited to total cholesterol (TC), high-density lipoprotein cholesterol (HDL-C), low-density lipoprotein cholesterol (LDL-C), triglycerides, impaired fasting glucose, impaired glucose tolerance, hypertension, atherosclerosis, myocardial infarction, dyspnea, tachycardia, claudication, syncope, and ischemia	• Consider key medical terms that influence health and may affect exercise prescription and outcome.	*ACSM's Guidelines for Exercise Testing and Prescription* (GETP), 10th edition (7)
Knowledge of recommended plasma cholesterol levels for adults based on National Cholesterol Education Program (NCEP)/Adult Treatment Panel (ATP) Guidelines	• Adapted from the "Third Report of the Expert Panel on Detection, Evaluation, and Treatment of High Blood Cholesterol in Adults," ATP IV outlines the NCEP's recommendations for cholesterol testing and management. • Guideline may be adjusted periodically.	*ACSM's Guidelines for Exercise Testing and Prescription* (GETP), 10th edition (7)
Knowledge of recommended BP levels for adults based on National High Blood Pressure Education Program Guidelines	• Adapted from "The Seventh Report of the Joint National Committee on Prevention, Detection, Evaluation, and Treatment of High Blood Pressure (JNC8)." • Guideline may be adjusted periodically.	*ACSM's Guidelines for Exercise Testing and Prescription* (GETP), 10th edition (7) • Table 3.2
Knowledge of medical supervision recommendations for cardiorespiratory fitness testing	• When recommended to have a medical doctor (MD) supervision during a test, one should be in close proximity and readily available.	*ACSM's Guidelines for Exercise Testing and Prescription* (GETP), 10th edition (7) • Chapters 2 and 3
Knowledge of the components of a health history questionnaire (*e.g.,* past and current medical history, family history of cardiac disease, orthopedic limitations, prescribed medications, activity patterns for exercise and work, nutritional habits, stress and anxiety levels, and smoking and alcohol use)	• This process should be thorough and include past and present items.	*ACSM's Guidelines for Exercise Testing and Prescription* (GETP), 10th edition (7) • Figure 2.3
Skill in the administration of a preexercise readiness assessment and recognition of major signs or symptoms suggestive of cardiovascular, pulmonary, or metabolic disease and/or the presence of known cardiovascular, pulmonary, and metabolic disease status	• Review health/medical history for known disease, signs/symptoms, using the American College of Sports Medicine (ACSM) Preparticipation Screening Algorithm.	*ACSM's Guidelines for Exercise Testing and Prescription* (GETP), 10th edition (7) • Figures 2.2 and 2.3

EP-C

B. Determine participant's readiness to take part in a health-related physical fitness assessment and exercise program. (cont.)

Knowledge or Skill Statement	Explanation/Examples	Resources
Skill in the administration of a preexercise readiness assessment to determine the need for medical clearance prior to exercise and to select appropriate physical fitness assessment protocols	• Review, when applied, self-guided or professionally guided screening forms. • Consider various physical fitness assessment protocols such as body composition, cardiorespiratory fitness, muscular strength and muscular endurance, and flexibility.	*ACSM's Guidelines for Exercise Testing and Prescription* (GETP), 10th edition (7) • Chapters 2–4

C. Select and prepare physical fitness assessments for healthy participants and those with controlled disease.

Knowledge or Skill Statement	Explanation/Examples	Resources
Knowledge of the physiological basis of the major components of physical fitness — cardiorespiratory fitness, body composition, flexibility, muscular strength, and muscular endurance	• If detailed exercise physiology review is warranted, review *ACSM's Exercise Management for Persons with Chronic Diseases and Disabilities*, 4th edition (2).	*ACSM's Guidelines for Exercise Testing and Prescription* (GETP), 10th edition (7) • Chapter 4 *ACSM's Exercise Management for Persons with Chronic Diseases and Disabilities*, 4th edition (2)
Knowledge of selecting the most appropriate testing protocols for each participant based on preliminary screening data	• Consider specific fitness goals. • Consider injury history. • Consider if risks of health-related physical fitness testing may outweigh potential benefits.	*ACSM's Guidelines for Exercise Testing and Prescription* (GETP), 10th edition (7) • Chapter 4
Knowledge of calibration techniques and proper use of fitness testing equipment	• To ensure the accuracy of the collected data, devices and related equipment (stationary bikes, treadmills, etc.) must be calibrated prior to the testing session. • Review equipment manuals for specifics.	*ACSM's Guidelines for Exercise Testing and Prescription* (GETP), 10th edition (7) • Chapter 4 *ACSM's Health-Related Physical Fitness Assessment Manual*, 5th edition (4) • Chapter 1
Knowledge of the purpose and procedures of fitness testing protocols for the components of health-related fitness	• Review pretest instruction and follow appropriate test order. • Be aware of different modes to measure the components of health-related physical fitness.	*ACSM's Guidelines for Exercise Testing and Prescription* (GETP), 10th edition (7) • Chapter 4
Knowledge of test termination criteria and proper procedures to be followed after discontinuing health fitness tests	• These indications apply for exercise tests but could also be applied for any health-related physical fitness components tests.	*ACSM's Guidelines for Exercise Testing and Prescription* (GETP), 10th edition (7) • Chapter 4 • Box 4.4
Knowledge of fitness assessment sequencing	• These may apply to related forms, equipment to be used, and environmental conditions.	*ACSM's Guidelines for Exercise Testing and Prescription* (GETP), 10th edition (7) • Chapter 4

EP-C

C. Select and prepare physical fitness assessments for healthy participants and those with controlled disease. (cont.)

Knowledge or Skill Statement	Explanation/Examples	Resources
Knowledge of the effects of common medications and substances on exercise testing (*e.g.*, antianginals, antihypertensives, antiarrhythmics, bronchodilators, hypoglycemics, psychotropics, alcohol, diet pills, cold tablets, caffeine, nicotine)	• For each class of common medication and substances, recognize drug name and related brand and effect on heart rate, blood pressure, electrocardiogram (ECG), and exercise capacity.	*ACSM's Guidelines for Exercise Testing and Prescription* (GETP), 10th edition (7) • Appendix A
Knowledge of the physiologic and metabolic responses to exercise testing associated with each chronic diseases and conditions (*e.g.*, heart disease, hypertension, diabetes mellitus, obesity, pulmonary disease)	• Review pathophysiology, exercise responses, and the effects of exercise training for each chronic condition.	*ACSM's Exercise Management for Persons with Chronic Diseases and Disabilities*, 4th edition (2)
Skill in analyzing and interpreting information obtained from assessment of the components of health-related fitness	• Use appropriate criterion-referenced and normative standard tables to analyze and interpret data.	*ACSM's Guidelines for Exercise Testing and Prescription* (GETP), 10th edition (7) • Chapter 4
Skill in modifying protocols and procedures for testing children, adolescents, older adults, and individuals with special considerations	• Be aware of the differences between testing an apparently healthy population and healthy population with special considerations.	*ACSM's Guidelines for Exercise Testing and Prescription* (GETP), 10th edition (7) • Chapters 2, 3, and 7

D. Conduct and interpret cardiorespiratory fitness assessments.

Knowledge or Skill Statement	Explanation/Examples	Resources
Knowledge of common submaximal and maximal cardiorespiratory assessment protocols	• Be aware of the pros and cons of using different modes of exercise and different protocols to determine cardiorespiratory performance.	*ACSM's Guidelines for Exercise Testing and Prescription* (GETP), 10th edition (7) • Chapter 4 *ACSM's Health-Related Physical Fitness Assessment Manual*, 5th edition (4) • Chapters 7 and 8
Knowledge of blood pressure (BP) measurement techniques	• Be aware of different conditions and considerations that may affect resting BP measurements such as body posture, appropriate cuff size, etc.	*ACSM's Guidelines for Exercise Testing and Prescription* (GETP), 10th edition (7) • Chapter 3 • Boxes 3.5 and 3.6 *ACSM's Health-Related Physical Fitness Assessment Manual*, 5th edition (4) • Chapter 3
Knowledge of Korotkoff sounds for determining systolic BP (SBP) and diastolic BP (DBP)	• Be aware of the significance and the difference between the fourth (true DBP) and the fifth (clinical DBP) Korotkoff sounds in respect to resting and exercise measurements.	*ACSM's Guidelines for Exercise Testing and Prescription* (GETP), 10th edition (7) • Chapter 3 • Boxes 3.5 and 3.6 *ACSM's Health-Related Physical Fitness Assessment Manual*, 5th edition (4) • Box 3.1

EP-C

D. Conduct and interpret cardiorespiratory fitness assessments. (cont.)

Knowledge or Skill Statement	Explanation/Examples	Resources
Knowledge of the BP response to exercise	• Be aware of abnormal responses to exercise such as a drop in SBP and substantial increase in DBP. • Be aware of the significance of rate-pressure product.	*ACSM's Guidelines for Exercise Testing and Prescription* (GETP), 10th edition (7) • Chapter 3
Knowledge of techniques of measuring heart rate (HR) and HR response to exercise	• Be aware of the two common anatomical palpation sites. • Be aware of the wide interindividual variability with respect to HR responses during exercise and therefore the potential inaccuracy in predicting maximal heart rate (HR_{max}).	*ACSM's Guidelines for Exercise Testing and Prescription* (GETP), 10th edition (7) • Chapter 4
Knowledge of the rating of perceived exertion (RPE)	• Be aware of the limitation of the RPE scale. • Similar to HR responses to exercise, the RPE scale presents a wide interindividual variability and therefore should be used with caution.	*ACSM's Guidelines for Exercise Testing and Prescription* (GETP), 10th edition (7) • Chapter 4 • Table 4.6
Knowledge of HR, BP, and RPE monitoring techniques before, during, and after cardiorespiratory fitness testing	• Be aware that there are several techniques to measure HR. • BP should be measured at the horizontal level of the heart. • The subjective measure of perceived exertion may be influenced by many factors and therefore should be used with caution.	*ACSM's Guidelines for Exercise Testing and Prescription* (GETP), 10th edition (7) • Chapter 4
Knowledge of the anatomy and physiology of the cardiovascular and pulmonary systems	• This information could also be found in any undergraduate- or graduate-level exercise physiology textbook.	
Knowledge of cardiorespiratory terminology including angina pectoris, tachycardia, bradycardia, arrhythmia, and hyperventilation	• These terms could be found in any other reputable clinical exercise physiology textbook.	*Clinical Exercise Physiology*, 2nd edition (11) • Glossary, pp. 593–610
Knowledge of the pathophysiology of myocardial ischemia, myocardial infarction (MI), stroke, hypertension, and hyperlipidemia	• Be familiar with the different stages (significance) and progression of atherosclerosis. • Be aware of the intimate relationship that each condition often has with one another.	
Knowledge of the effects of myocardial ischemia, MI, hypertension, claudication, and dyspnea on cardiorespiratory responses during exercise	• Be aware of the multifaceted relationship between atherosclerosis and these conditions.	*ACSM's Exercise Management for Persons with Chronic Diseases and Disabilities*, 4th edition (2)
Knowledge of oxygen consumption dynamics during exercise (*e.g.*, HR, stroke volume, cardiac output, ventilation, ventilatory threshold)	• This information could also be found in any undergraduate or graduate level exercise physiology textbook	*ACSM's Guidelines for Exercise Testing and Prescription* (GETP), 10th edition (7) • Chapters 4 and 6

EP-C

D. Conduct and interpret cardiorespiratory fitness assessments. (cont.)

Knowledge or Skill Statement	Explanation/Examples	Resources
Knowledge of methods of calculating maximal volume of oxygen consumed per unit of time (VO_{2max})	• Be aware that there are several methods of calculating $\dot{V}O_{2max}$. Each of the methods provides some pros and cons in respect to the level of difficulty and accuracy of performing the test.	*ACSM's Guidelines for Exercise Testing and Prescription* (GETP), 10th edition (7) • Chapters 4 and 5 *ACSM's Health-Related Physical Fitness Assessment Manual*, 5th edition (4) • Chapters 7 and 8
Knowledge of cardiorespiratory responses to acute graded exercise of conditioned and unconditioned participants	• This information could be found in any other reputable exercise physiology textbook.	*Exercise Physiology: Integrating Theory and Application* (18) • Chapter 5
Skill in interpreting cardiorespiratory fitness test results	• Consider the pros and cons of each method in respect to the level of difficulty and accuracy of the results.	*ACSM's Guidelines for Exercise Testing and Prescription* (GETP), 10th edition (7) • Chapters 4 and 5 *ACSM's Health-Related Physical Fitness Assessment Manual*, 5th edition (4) • Chapters 7 and 8
Skill in locating anatomic landmarks for palpation of peripheral pulses and BP	• Palpate for the brachial artery prior to attempting to measure BP.	
Skill in measuring HR, BP, and RPE at rest and during exercise and conducting submaximal exercise tests (*e.g.*, cycle ergometer, treadmill, field testing, step test)	• Consider the order of measurements during a submaximal or maximal graded exercise test.	*ACSM's Guidelines for Exercise Testing and Prescription* (GETP), 10th edition (7) • Chapter 4 • Table 4.6
Skill in determining cardiorespiratory fitness based on submaximal exercise test results	• Consider the pros and cons of using different modes of exercise and different protocols to determine cardiorespiratory fitness.	*ACSM's Health-Related Physical Fitness Assessment Manual*, 5th edition (4) • Chapter 7

E. Conduct assessments of muscular strength, muscular endurance, and flexibility.

Knowledge or Skill Statement	Explanation/Examples	Resources
Knowledge of common muscular strength, muscular endurance, and flexibility assessment protocols	• Be aware of the pros and cons of using different common muscular strength, muscular endurance, and flexibility assessment protocols.	*ACSM's Health-Related Physical Fitness Assessment Manual*, 5th edition (4) • Chapters 5 and 6
Knowledge of interpreting muscular strength, muscular endurance, and flexibility assessments	• Use appropriate criterion-referenced and normative standard tables to analyze and interpret data.	*ACSM's Health-Related Physical Fitness Assessment Manual*, 5th edition (4) • Chapters 5 and 6
Knowledge of relative strength, absolute strength, and one repetition maximum (1-RM) estimation	• Be aware that there are other methods of measuring strength using both static and isokinetic assessments.	
Knowledge of the anatomy of bone, skeletal muscle, and connective tissues	• Be aware of the relationship these different systems have in respect to human movement.	*ACSM's Health-Related Physical Fitness Assessment Manual*, 5th edition (4) • Chapter 5

EP-C

E.   Conduct assessments of muscular strength, muscular endurance, and flexibility. (cont.)

Knowledge or Skill Statement	Explanation/Examples	Resources
Knowledge of muscle action terms including anterior, posterior, inferior, superior, medial, lateral, supination, pronation, flexion, extension, adduction, abduction, hyperextension, rotation, circumduction, agonist, antagonist, and stabilizer	• Be aware of the different joints in the body in respect to planes and axes of rotation and associated movements. • Be aware of the different roles performed by each muscle.	*Basic Biomechanics*, 6th edition (15) • Chapter 6
Knowledge of the planes and axes in which movement action occurs	• Be aware that the starting position for recognizing planes and axis of all movements in the human body is the anatomical position.	
Knowledge of the interrelationships among center of gravity, base of support, balance, stability, posture, and proper spinal alignment	• This information could be found in any other reputable biomechanics textbook.	*Basic Biomechanics*, 6th edition (15) • Chapters 9 and 13
Knowledge of the normal curvatures of the spine and common assessments of postural alignment	• Be aware of the difference between primary and secondary spinal curves. • This information could be found in any other reputable biomechanics textbook.	*Basic Biomechanics*, 6th edition (15) • pp. 283–284
Knowledge of the location and function of the major muscles (*e.g.*, pectoralis major, trapezius, latissimus dorsi, biceps, triceps, rectus abdominis, internal and external obliques, erector spinae, gluteus maximus, quadriceps, hamstrings, adductors, abductors, and gastrocnemius)	• Be aware of the relationship between muscles location, line of pull, and specific movements.	
Knowledge of the major joints and their associated movement	• Be aware of each joint's classification and the relationship to planes and axes.	
Skill in identifying the major bones, muscles, and joints	• Be aware of the adjacent bones, muscles, and joints.	
Skill in conducting assessments of muscular strength, muscular endurance and flexibility (*e.g.*, 1-RM, hand grip dynamometer, push-ups, sit-and-reach)	• Be aware of the pros and cons of using different common muscular strength, muscular endurance, and flexibility tests.	*ACSM's Health-Related Physical Fitness Assessment Manual*, 5th edition (4) • Chapters 5 and 6
Skill in estimating 1-RM using lower resistance (2–10 RM)	• Consider the advantages and disadvantages of using an estimation rather than measuring 1-RM.	*Designing Resistance Training Programs*, 3rd edition (12) • Chapter 5
Skill in interpreting results of muscular strength, muscular endurance, and flexibility assessments	• Use appropriate criterion-referenced and normative standard tables to analyze and interpret data.	*ACSM's Health-Related Physical Fitness Assessment Manual*, 5th edition (4) • Chapters 5 and 6

EP-C

F. Conduct anthropometric and body composition assessments.

Knowledge or Skill Statement	Explanation/Examples	Resources
Knowledge of the advantages, disadvantages, and limitations of body composition techniques (*e.g.*, air displacement plethysmography [BOD POD], dual-energy X-ray absorptiometry [DEXA], hydrostatic weighing, skinfolds, and bioelectrical impedance)	• Be aware of the pros and cons of each method in respect to the level of difficulty and accuracy of the results.	*ACSM's Health-Related Physical Fitness Assessment Manual*, 5th edition (4) • Chapter 4
Knowledge of the standardized descriptions of circumference and skinfold sites	• Be familiar with the differences between circumference and skinfold measurement in respect to accuracy, significance, and use.	*ACSM's Health-Related Physical Fitness Assessment Manual*, 5th edition (4) • Chapter 4 *ACSM's Guidelines for Exercise Testing and Prescription* (GETP), 10th edition (7) • Chapter 4
Knowledge of procedures for determining body mass index (BMI) and taking skinfold and circumference measurements	• Be aware of the pros and cons of each method in respect to the level of difficulty and accuracy of the results.	*ACSM's Health-Related Physical Fitness Assessment Manual*, 5th edition (4) • Chapter 4 *ACSM's Guidelines for Exercise Testing and Prescription* (GETP), 10th edition (7) • Chapter 4
Knowledge of the health implications of variation in body fat distribution patterns and the significance of BMI, waist circumference, and waist-to-hip ratio	• Be aware of the relationship between BMI, waist circumference, and the related disease risk.	*ACSM's Guidelines for Exercise Testing and Prescription* (GETP), 10th edition (7) • Chapter 4
Skill in locating anatomic landmarks for skinfold and circumference measurements	• Consider the anatomic landmarks differences between skinfold and circumference sites.	*ACSM's Guidelines for Exercise Testing and Prescription* (GETP), 10th edition (7) • Chapter 4 • Boxes 4.2 and 4.3
Skill in interpreting the results of anthropometric and body composition assessments	• Consider the process of calculating skinfold measurement, specifically, body density conversion to body fat percentage.	*ACSM's Guidelines for Exercise Testing and Prescription* (GETP), 10th edition (7) • Chapter 4 • Tables 4.3–4.5

EP-C

DOMAIN II: EXERCISE PRESCRIPTION, IMPLEMENTATION, AND ONGOING SUPPORT

A. Review preparticipation readiness assessments including self-guided health questionnaires and appraisals, exercise history, and fitness assessments.

Knowledge or Skill Statement	Explanation/Examples	Resources
Knowledge of preexercise readiness assessment as delineated in the current edition of *ACSM's Guidelines for Exercise Testing and Prescription* **Knowledge** of the frequency (how often), intensity, (how hard), time (duration or how long), type (mode or what kind), total volume (amount), and progression (advancement) or the FITT-VP principle of exercise prescription and of the provision of recommendations on exercise pattern to be consistent with the ACSM recommendations made in its companion evidence-based position stand **Skill** in synthesizing prescreening results and reviewing them with participants	• Be aware of the major changes to the preparticipation procedures in this edition of *Guidelines for Exercise Testing and Prescription* (GETP) when compared to previous publications of American College of Sports Medicine (ACSM).	*ACSM's Guidelines for Exercise Testing and Prescription* (GETP), 10th edition (7) • Chapters 2 and 3

B. Determine safe and effective exercise programs to achieve desired outcomes and goals and translate assessment results into appropriate exercise prescriptions.

Knowledge or Skill Statement	Explanation/Examples	Resources
Knowledge of strength, cardiovascular, and flexibility-based exercise	• Be aware of the basic components of an exercise training session; quantity of exercise; and frequency, intensity, time, type, volume, and progression (FITT-VP) principles.	*ACSM's Guidelines for Exercise Testing and Prescription* (GETP), 10th edition (7) • Chapter 6
Knowledge of the benefits and precautions associated with exercise training in apparently healthy participants and those with controlled disease	• Be familiar with the benefits of regular physical activity and/or exercise. • Be familiar with the risk that is associated with physical activity and/or exercise.	*ACSM's Guidelines for Exercise Testing and Prescription* (GETP), 10th edition (7) • Chapter 1 • Box 1.2 • Tables 1.2–1.5
Knowledge of program development for specific client needs (*e.g.*, sport-specific training, performance, health, lifestyle, functional ability, balance, agility, aerobic, anaerobic)	• Consider client-specific fitness goals (health and performance related). • Collect baseline and follow-up data in order to provide individualized and appropriate exercise prescription.	*ACSM's Guidelines for Exercise Testing and Prescription* (GETP), 10th edition (7) • Chapter 4
Knowledge of the six motor skill–related physical fitness components: agility, balance, coordination, reaction time, speed, and power	• Be aware of the fundamental differences between health-related physical fitness components and skill-related physical fitness components.	*ACSM's Guidelines for Exercise Testing and Prescription* (GETP), 10th edition (7) • Chapter 1 • Box 1.1

B. Determine safe and effective exercise programs to achieve desired outcomes and goals, and translate assessment results into appropriate exercise prescriptions. (cont.)

Knowledge or Skill Statement	Explanation/Examples	Resources
Knowledge of the physiologic changes associated with an acute bout of exercise	• Be familiar with changes in heart rate (HR), stroke volume (SV), cardiac output (CO [Q̇]), blood flow, blood pressure, arteriovenous oxygen difference (a-vO2 DIFF), and ventilation. • This information could also be found in any undergraduate- or graduate-level exercise physiology textbook.	*ACSM's Guidelines for Exercise Testing and Prescription* (GETP), 10th edition (7) • Chapters 4 and 6
Knowledge of the physiologic adaptations following chronic exercise training	• This information could be found in any reputable exercise physiology textbook. • The adaptations that are associated with chronic exercise training improve physiological function, reduce coronary artery disease (CAD) risk factors, decrease morbidity and mortality rates, and provide other health-related benefits.	*ACSM's Guidelines for Exercise Testing and Prescription* (GETP), 10th edition (7) • Chapter 1
Knowledge of American College of Sports Medicine (ACSM) exercise prescription guidelines for strength, cardiovascular, and flexibility-based exercise for apparently healthy clients, clients with increased risk, and clients with controlled disease	• Be familiar with FITT-VP principles. • The information may apply to apparently healthy population, healthy population with special consideration, and inpatient and outpatient rehabilitation programs.	*ACSM's Guidelines for Exercise Testing and Prescription* (GETP), 10th edition (7) • Chapters 6–9
Knowledge of the components and sequencing incorporated into an exercise session (*e.g.*, warm-up, conditioning or sports-related exercise, cool-down, stretching)	• Be aware that these components should be incorporated in some form with aerobic exercise as well as muscular fitness exercise.	*ACSM's Guidelines for Exercise Testing and Prescription* (GETP), 10th edition (7) • Chapter 6
Knowledge of the physiological principles related to warm-up and cool-down	• Although both the warm-up and cool-down are often overlooked by many professionals, the physiological principles are important and valid.	
Knowledge of the principles of reversibility, progressive overload, individual differences and specificity of training, and how they relate to exercise prescription	• When determining an appropriate exercise prescription, be aware of client/patient goals. Prescribe appropriate exercise and be mindful of attainable goals.	
Knowledge of the role of aerobic and anaerobic energy systems in the performance of various physical activities	• Be very familiar with the intricate relationship between the aerobic and anaerobic systems as they relate to the intensity and duration of different physical activities.	
Knowledge of the basic biomechanical principles of human movement	• Be familiar with biomechanics and the relationship to activities of daily living (ADL) as well as to sport performance. • This information could also be found in any reputable undergraduate- or graduate-level biomechanics textbook.	

B.   Determine safe and effective exercise programs to achieve desired outcomes and goals, and translate assessment results into appropriate exercise prescriptions. (cont.)

Knowledge or Skill Statement	Explanation/Examples	Resources
Knowledge of the psychological and physiological signs and symptoms of overtraining	• Be familiar with differences between overtraining from aerobic exercise and overtaining from resistance exercise.	
Knowledge of the signs and symptoms of common musculoskeletal injuries associated with exercise (*e.g.*, sprain, strain, bursitis, tendonitis)	• Be aware of the differences between musculature and joint-related injuries. • This information could also be found in any reputable undergraduate or graduate athletic training textbook.	*Basic Biomechanics*, 6th edition (15) • Chapter 5
Knowledge of the advantages and disadvantages of exercise equipment (*e.g.*, free weights, selectorized machines, cardiovascular equipment)	• Both free weights and exercise machines can be beneficial if used appropriately and when following published guidelines.	
Skill in teaching and demonstrating exercises	• The certified exercise physiologist (EP-C) is expected to be able to properly instruct aerobic, resistance, and flexibility exercises.	*ACSM's Guidelines for Exercise Testing and Prescription* (GETP), 10th edition (7) • Chapters 6–9
Skill in designing safe and effective training programs	• EP-C is expected to be able to take raw data that is collected during exercise tests, interpret the results, and design safe and effective training programs.	*ACSM's Guidelines for Exercise Testing and Prescription* (GETP), 10th edition (7) • Chapters 6–9
Skill in implementing exercise prescription guidelines for apparently healthy clients, clients with increased risk, and clients with controlled disease	• EP-C is expected to be able to take raw data that is collected during exercise tests, interpret the results, and provide a population-specific exercise prescription.	*ACSM's Guidelines for Exercise Testing and Prescription* (GETP), 10th edition (7) • Chapters 6–9

C.   Implement cardiorespiratory exercise prescriptions using the frequency, intensity, time, and type (FITT) principle for apparently healthy participants based on current health status, fitness goals, and availability of time.

Knowledge or Skill Statement	Explanation/Examples	Resources
Knowledge of the recommended FITT framework for the development of cardiorespiratory fitness	• The certified exercise physiologist (EP-C) should be very familiar with the FITT-VP framework, more specifically, the intricate relationship between frequency, intensity, time, and type of exercise.	*ACSM's Guidelines for Exercise Testing and Prescription* (GETP), 10th edition (7) • Chapter 6
Knowledge of the benefits, risks, and contraindications of a wide variety of cardiovascular training exercises based on client experience, skill level, current fitness level, and goals	• Consider appropriate risk classification. • Consider individualized and appropriate exercise prescription.	*ACSM's Guidelines for Exercise Testing and Prescription* (GETP), 10th edition (7) • Chapter 1
Knowledge of the minimal threshold of physical activity required for health benefits and/or fitness development	• EP-C should be aware that FITT principles applies to aerobic, resistance, and flexibility exercises.	*ACSM's Guidelines for Exercise Testing and Prescription* (GETP), 10th edition (7) • Chapter 6

EP-C

C. Implement cardiorespiratory exercise prescriptions using the frequency, intensity, time, and type (FITT) principle for apparently healthy participants based on current health status, fitness goals, and availability of time. (cont.)

Knowledge or Skill Statement	Explanation/Examples	Resources
Knowledge of determining exercise intensity using heart rate reserve (HRR), oxygen uptake reserve ($\dot{V}O_2R$), peak heart rate (HR_{peak}) method, peak volume of oxygen consumed per unit of time (VO_{2peak}) method, peak metabolic equivalents (MET) method, and the rating of perceived exertion (RPE) scale.	• Be aware that the RPE scale and other measures of perceived effort and/or affective variability should not be used as primary method of prescribing exercise intensity.	*ACSM's Guidelines for Exercise Testing and Prescription* (GETP), 10th edition (7) • Chapters 6 and 12 • Box 6.2 • Table 6.1
Knowledge of the accuracy of HRR, $\dot{V}O_2R$, HR_{peak} method, $\dot{V}O_{2peak}$ method, peak MET method, and the RPE scale	• Be aware of different prediction equation for maximal heart rate (HR_{max}). • The HRR or $\dot{V}O_2R$ methods may be preferable when compared to $\%HR$ and $\%\dot{V}O_2$.	*ACSM's Guidelines for Exercise Testing and Prescription* (GETP), 10th edition (7) • Chapter 6 • Table 6.2
Knowledge of abnormal responses to exercise (*e.g.*, hemodynamic, cardiac, ventilatory)	• Be aware that these variables play a major role when assessing the therapeutic, diagnostic, and prognostic application of a test.	*ACSM's Guidelines for Exercise Testing and Prescription* (GETP), 10th edition (7) • Chapter 5
Knowledge of metabolic calculations (*e.g.*, unit conversions, deriving energy cost of exercise, caloric expenditure)	• Be aware of the different unit conversions. • These formulas are most accurate during a steady-state exercise.	*ACSM's Guidelines for Exercise Testing and Prescription* (GETP), 10th edition (7) • Chapter 6
Knowledge of calculating the caloric expenditure of an exercise session (kilocalories per session)	• 1 lb (0.45 kg) of fat = 3,500 kcal • Be aware of the MET level equation of calculating caloric expenditure per minute.	
Knowledge of methods for establishing and monitoring levels of exercise intensity including heart rate (HR), RPE, and MET.	• Be aware that the RPE scale and other measures of perceived effort and/or affective valence should not be used as primary method of prescribing exercise intensity.	*ACSM's Guidelines for Exercise Testing and Prescription* (GETP), 10th edition (7) • Chapters 6 and 12 • Box 6.2 • Table 6.1
Knowledge of the applications of anaerobic training principles	• Be aware that plyometric training is also considered as a method of anaerobic training.	
Knowledge of the anatomy and physiology of the cardiovascular and pulmonary systems including the basic properties of cardiac muscle	• Be aware of the relationship between these two systems in respect to normal function at rest and during exercise. • Be aware of the relationship between these two systems in respect to upper limitation of aerobic performance. • This information could be found in any other reputable exercise physiology textbook.	*Exercise Physiology: Integrating Theory and Application* (18) • Chapters 5 and 6

C. Implement cardiorespiratory exercise prescriptions using the frequency, intensity, time, and type (FITT) principle for apparently healthy participants based on current health status, fitness goals, and availability of time. (cont.)

Knowledge or Skill Statement	Explanation/Examples	Resources
Knowledge of the basic principles of gas exchange	• Be familiar with the concept of open-circuit spirometry. • Be familiar with the significance of respiratory exchange ratio (RER) and the relationship to respiratory quotient (RQ).	*ACSM's Guidelines for Exercise Testing and Prescription* (GETP), 10th edition (7) • Chapter 4
Skill in determining appropriate exercise FITT for clients with various fitness levels	• Be familiar with the interaction between the different components of FITT-VP principles, specifically, intensity and time (duration) of the activity. • Be aware of different prediction equation for HR_{max}. • The HRR or $\dot{V}O_2R$ methods may be preferable when compared to %HR and %$\dot{V}O_2$. • Be aware that the RPE scale and other measures of perceived effort and/or affective valence should not be used as primary method of prescribing exercise intensity.	*ACSM's Guidelines for Exercise Testing and Prescription* (GETP), 10th edition (7) • Chapters 6 to 9
Skill in determining the energy cost, absolute and relative oxygen costs ($\dot{V}O_2$), and MET levels of various activities and apply the information to an exercise prescription	• Consider the conversions between relative and absolute O_2 (mL $\cdot$ kg^{-1} $\cdot$ min^{-1} $\rightarrow$ L $\cdot$ min^{-1} $\rightarrow$ /1,000 $\times$ body mass), relative $\dot{V}O_2$, and MET (mL $\cdot$ kg^{-1} $\cdot$ min^{-1} $\rightarrow$ MET$\rightarrow$ /3.5) and vice versa.	*ACSM's Guidelines for Exercise Testing and Prescription* (GETP), 10th edition (7) • Chapter 6 • Figure 6.1 • Table 6.3
Skill in identifying improper technique in the use of cardiovascular equipment	• Consider the client-specific FITT-VP principles. • If needed, consider consulting the specific manual of the cardiovascular exercise equipment.	*ACSM's Guidelines for Exercise Testing and Prescription* (GETP), 10th edition (7) • Chapter 6
Skill in teaching and demonstrating the use of various cardiovascular exercise equipment	• Consider the client-specific FITT-VP principles. • If needed, consider consulting the specific manual of the cardiovascular exercise equipment.	*ACSM's Guidelines for Exercise Testing and Prescription* (GETP), 10th edition (7) • Chapters 4 and 6

D. Implement exercise prescriptions using the frequency, intensity, time, type, volume, and progression (FITT-VP) principle for flexibility, muscular strength, muscular endurance, balance, agility, and reaction time for apparently healthy participants and those with controlled disease based on current health status, fitness goals, and availability of time.

Knowledge or Skill Statement	Explanation/Examples	Resources
Knowledge of the recommended FITT framework for the development of muscular strength, muscular endurance, and flexibility	• Be aware of the differences between prescribing muscular strength and endurance in respect to the number of repetitions and the intensity (percentage of one repetition maximum [1-RM]). • Be aware of the different types of flexibility exercises.	*ACSM's Guidelines for Exercise Testing and Prescription* (GETP), 10th edition (7) • Chapter 6
Knowledge of the minimal threshold of physical activity required for health benefits and/or fitness development	• Be aware of the interaction between the intensity and the time of the exercise. • Minimal threshold intensity may vary and be affected by individual's corticotropin-releasing factor level, age, health status, physiologic differences, genetics, habitual physical activity, and social and psychological factors.	*ACSM's Guidelines for Exercise Testing and Prescription* (GETP), 10th edition (7) • Chapter 6
Knowledge of safe and effective exercises designed to enhance muscular strength and/or endurance of major muscle groups	• When determining an appropriate exercise prescription, be aware of client/patient goals. • Prescribe appropriate exercise and be mindful of attainable goals.	
Knowledge of safe and effective stretches that enhance flexibility	• There are many effective stretching exercises that may involve major muscle groups and/or individual muscles. • Be aware of the differences between static, dynamic, ballistic stretches, and proprioceptive neuromuscular facilitation (PNF).	*Stretching for Functional Flexibility* (8) • Chapter 5
Knowledge of indications for water-based exercise (*e.g.*, arthritis, obesity)	• Although aquatic exercise may be appropriate for some populations, there are some notable disadvantages (*i.e.*, non–weight-bearing exercise).	*Therapeutic Exercise: From Theory to Practice* (17) • Table 12.1
Knowledge of the types of resistance training programs (*e.g.*, total body, split routine) and modalities (*e.g.*, free weights, variable resistance equipment, pneumatic machines, bands)	• When choosing total body or a variation of a split routine, be mindful of other variables such as number of training sessions per week and frequency of training. • Be aware of the pros and cons of both free weights and variable resistance equipment.	
Knowledge of acute (*e.g.*, load, volume, sets, repetitions, rest periods, order of exercises) and chronic training variables (*e.g.*, periodization)	• Be aware of the interaction between the number of repetitions and the load. • Be aware of the variation in volume of the training and periodization schedule.	

EP-C

D. Implement exercise prescriptions using the frequency, intensity, time, type, volume, and progression (FITT-VP) principle for flexibility, muscular strength, muscular endurance, balance, agility, and reaction time for apparently healthy participants and those with controlled disease based on current health status, fitness goals, and availability of time. (cont.)

Knowledge or Skill Statement	Explanation/Examples	Resources
Knowledge of the types of muscle contractions (*e.g.*, eccentric, concentric, isometric)	• Be aware of the pros and cons of using each of the types of muscle contractions.	
Knowledge of joint movements (*e.g.*, flexion, extension, adduction, abduction) and the muscles responsible for them	• This information could be found in any other reputable kinesiology or biomechanics textbook.	*Basic Biomechanics*, 6th edition (15) • Chapters 7–9 • Tables 7.1–7.3, 8.1, 8.2, and 9.1
Knowledge of acute and delayed onset muscle soreness (DOMS)	• DOMS is related to microtears of myocytes rather than lactate accumulation. • This information could be found in any other reputable exercise physiology textbook.	*Exercise Physiology: Integrating Theory and Application* (18) • Chapter 3
Knowledge of the anatomy and physiology of skeletal muscle fiber, the characteristics of fast- and slow-twitch muscle fibers, and the sliding-filament theory of muscle contraction	• This information is fairly extensive and should be covered thoroughly. • This information could be found in any other reputable exercise physiology textbook.	*Exercise Physiology: Integrating Theory and Application* (18) • Chapter 3
Knowledge of the stretch reflex, proprioceptors, Golgi tendon organ (GTO), muscle spindles, and how they relate to flexibility	• Be aware of the positive and negative effects that these sensory organs have on the different modes of flexibility training such as static, ballistic and dynamic flexibility, and PNF. • This information could be found in any other reputable exercise physiology, kinesiology, or biomechanics textbook.	*Exercise Physiology: Integrating Theory and Application* (18) • Chapter 3 *Basic Biomechanics*, 6th edition (15) • Chapter 5
Knowledge of muscle-related terminology including atrophy, hyperplasia, and hypertrophy	• Be aware of the differences between those terms and the prevalence among humans in response to exercise or lack of it. • This information could be found in any other reputable exercise physiology, kinesiology, or biomechanics textbook.	*Exercise Physiology: Integrating Theory and Application* (18) • Chapter 3
Knowledge of the Valsalva maneuver and its implications during exercise	• This maneuver should not be overlooked. In both apparently healthy and diseased populations, this maneuver could lead to significant and dangerous hemodynamic-related alterations.	
Knowledge of the physiology underlying plyometric training and common plyometric exercises (*e.g.*, box jumps, leaps, bounds)	• Plyometric exercises are considered as a form of anaerobic training and can be prescribed as a form of resistance training exercises. • Intensity may be adjusted by varying different components of the same exercise (*i.e.*, the height of the box, one vs. two leg exercise)	*Exercise Physiology: Integrating Theory and Application* (18) • Chapter 3

D. Implement exercise prescriptions using the frequency, intensity, time, type, volume, and progression (FITT-VP) principle for flexibility, muscular strength, muscular endurance, balance, agility, and reaction time for apparently healthy participants and those with controlled disease based on current health status, fitness goals, and availability of time. (cont.)

Knowledge or Skill Statement	Explanation/Examples	Resources
Knowledge of the contraindications and potential risks associated with muscular conditioning activities (*e.g.*, straight-leg sit-ups, double-leg raises, squats, hurdler's stretch, yoga plough, forceful back hyperextension, and standing bent-over toe touch, behind neck press/lat pull-down)	• Consider appropriate exercise techniques.	*Advanced Fitness Assessment and Exercise Prescription*, 4th edition (16) • Appendices C and F
Knowledge of prescribing exercise using the calculated %1-RM	• This knowledge is vital when there is a need to vary the intensity of the exercise such as between different periodization cycles.	
Knowledge of spotting positions and techniques for injury prevention and exercise assistance	• Spotter should be very familiar with the given the exercise. • Spotting is paramount for proper and safe exercise.	
Knowledge of periodization (*e.g.*, macrocycles, microcycles, mesocycles) and associated theories	• Be aware of the differences between linear and nonlinear periodization methods. • Be aware of the differences between microcycle, mesocycle, and macrocycle. • Be aware of the relationship between volume, intensity, and the specificity of exercises in relationship to different periodization cycles.	
Knowledge of safe and effective Olympic weightlifting exercises	• Consider if these exercises are appropriate for the client. • This information is fairly extensive and should be covered thoroughly.	*Explosive Lifting for Sports—Enhanced Edition* (22) • Chapters 4–9
Knowledge of safe and effective core stability exercises (*e.g.*, planks, crunch, bridges, cable twists)	• Consider the use of different aids (*i.e.*, stability and medicine balls).	*Strength Ball Training*, 2nd edition (14) • Chapters 3 and 4
Skill in identifying improper technique in the use of resistive equipment (*e.g.*, stability balls, weights, bands, resistance bars, and water exercise equipment)	• Lead and demonstrate the correct technique of using different resistive equipment.	*Advanced Fitness Assessment and Exercise Prescription*, 4th edition (16) • Appendices C and F *Strength Ball Training*, 2nd edition (14) • Chapters 3 and 4 *Therapeutic Exercise: From Theory to Practice* (17) • Table 12.1
Skill in teaching and demonstrating appropriate exercises for enhancing musculoskeletal flexibility	• Differentiate between static, dynamic, ballistic stretches, and PNF.	*Stretching for Functional Flexibility* (8) • Chapter 5

EP-C

D. Implement exercise prescriptions using the frequency, intensity, time, type, volume, and progression (FITT-VP) principle for flexibility, muscular strength, muscular endurance, balance, agility, and reaction time for apparently healthy participants and those with controlled disease based on current health status, fitness goals, and availability of time. (cont.)

Knowledge or Skill Statement	Explanation/Examples	Resources
Skill in teaching and demonstrating safe and effective muscular strength and endurance exercises (*e.g.*, free weights, weight machines, resistive bands, Swiss balls, body weight, and all other major fitness equipment)	• This information is fairly extensive and should be covered thoroughly. • Lead by example!	*Advanced Fitness Assessment and Exercise Prescription*, 4th edition (16) • Appendices C and F *Strength Ball Training*, 2nd edition (14) • Chapters 3 and 4

E. Establish exercise progression guidelines for resistance, aerobic, and flexibility activity to achieve the goals of apparently healthy participants.

Knowledge or Skill Statement	Explanation/Examples	Resources
Knowledge of the basic principles of exercise progression	• Regarding cardiovascular exercise prescription, be aware of the different progression stages. • Be aware of different methods to progress resistance exercises (*i.e.*, periodization).	*ACSM's Guidelines for Exercise Testing and Prescription* (GETP), 10th edition (7) • Chapter 6
Knowledge of adjusting the frequency, intensity, time, and type (FITT) framework in response to individual changes in conditioning	• Be familiar with the interaction between the different components of FITT-VP principles.	*ACSM's Guidelines for Exercise Testing and Prescription* (GETP), 10th edition (7) • Chapter 6
Knowledge of the importance of performing periodic reevaluations to assess changes in fitness status	• This information is vital to the adjustment and development of sound exercise prescription as well as short- and long-term goals.	*ACSM's Guidelines for Exercise Testing and Prescription* (GETP), 10th edition (7) • Chapter 4
Knowledge of the training principles that promote improvements in muscular strength, muscular endurance, cardiorespiratory fitness, and flexibility	• Be aware of the underlying physiological differences between muscular strength, muscular endurance, and cardiorespiratory fitness. • Be familiar with the interaction between the different components of FITT-VP principles in respect to both resistance and cardiorespiratory exercises.	*ACSM's Guidelines for Exercise Testing and Prescription* (GETP), 10th edition (7) • Chapters 4 and 6
Skill in recognizing the need for progression and communicating updates to exercise prescriptions	• Gradual progression may reduce the risk of cardiovascular disease (CVD) and musculoskeletal injury. • Client goals may be more achievable.	"American College of Sports Medicine Position Stand. Quantity and Quality of Exercise for Developing and Maintaining Cardiorespiratory, Musculoskeletal, and Neuromotor Fitness in Apparently Healthy Adults: Guidance for Prescribing Exercise" (13)

EP-C

F.	Implement a weight management program as indicated by personal goals that are supported by preparticipation health screening, health history, and body composition/anthropometrics.	
Knowledge or Skill Statement	**Explanation/Examples**	**Resources**
Knowledge of exercise prescriptions for achieving weight management, including weight loss, weight maintenance, and weight gain goals	• Consider different weight loss programs/approaches. • Consider client's caloric intake, expenditure, and current body fat percentage.	*ACSM's Guidelines for Exercise Testing and Prescription* (GETP), 10th edition (7)
Knowledge of energy balance and basic nutritional guidelines (*e.g.*, MyPyramid, United States Department of Agriculture [USDA] Dietary Guidelines for Americans)	• Be aware of various diet assessments and their advantages and disadvantages. • The assessment of nutritional status may serve as an important secondary tool to exercise prescription.	
Knowledge of weight management terminology including but not limited to obesity, overweight, body fat percentage, body mass index (BMI), lean body mass (LBM), anorexia nervosa, bulimia, binge eating, metabolic syndrome, body fat distribution, adipocyte, bariatrics, ergogenic aid, fat-free mass (FFM), resting metabolic rate (RMR), and thermogenesis	• Be aware of the differences between the different terms in respect to a description of a disease condition, anthropometric assessment, and/or physiological descriptor.	*ACSM's Guidelines for Exercise Testing and Prescription* (GETP), 10th edition (7) • Chapter 10 *Exercise Physiology: Integrating Theory and Application* (18) • Chapter 11
Knowledge of the relationship between body composition and health	• Be aware of the link between overweight and obesity and other debilitating chronic conditions such as cardiovascular disease (CVD) and diabetes. • Be aware of the link between overweight and obesity and other risk factors such as hypertension.	*ACSM's Guidelines for Exercise Testing and Prescription* (GETP), 10th edition (7) • Chapter 11
Knowledge of the unique dietary needs of participant populations (*e.g.*, women, children, older adults, pregnant women)	• In order to fully comprehend this information, the certified exercise physiologist (EP-C) needs to be fully aware of dietary needs of the general population.	"USDA Center for Nutrition Policy and Promotion" (26)
Knowledge of common nutritional ergogenic aids, their purported mechanisms of action, and associated risks and benefits (*e.g.*, protein/amino acids, vitamins, minerals, herbal products, creatine, steroids, caffeine)	• Many ergogenic aids are effective in improving performance, but many are barred from use in official competition.	*Exercise Physiology: Integrating Theory and Application* (18) • Chapter 14
Knowledge of methods for modifying body composition including diet, exercise, and behavior modification	• In many cases and in order to achieve lasting results, modifying body composition requires simultaneous use of diet, exercise, and behavior modification.	*ACSM's Guidelines for Exercise Testing and Prescription* (GETP), 10th edition (7) • Chapter 11
Knowledge of fuel sources for aerobic and anaerobic metabolism including carbohydrates, fats, and proteins	• Be aware of the interaction between the different fuel sources in respect to both aerobic and anaerobic exercises. • This information could be found in any other reputable exercise physiology textbook.	*Exercise Physiology: Integrating Theory and Application* (18) • Chapter 2

EP-C

F. Implement a weight management program as indicated by personal goals that are supported by preparticipation health screening, health history, and body composition/anthropometrics. (cont.)		
Knowledge or Skill Statement	**Explanation/Examples**	**Resources**
Knowledge of the effects of overall dietary composition on healthy weight management	• The application of "proper diet" may vary based on such factors as age, gender, and activity level (sedentary lifestyle vs. active lifestyle). • This information is fairly extensive and should be covered thoroughly.	
Knowledge of the importance of maintaining normal hydration before, during, and after exercise	• There are several ways to assess hydration (*i.e.,* urine color and osmolality). • Be aware of hyponatremia and its association with overhydration.	*Exercise Physiology: Integrating Theory and Application* (18) • Chapter 9
Knowledge of the consequences of inappropriate weight loss methods (*e.g.,* saunas, dietary supplements, vibrating belts, body wraps, overexercising, very low calorie diets, electric stimulators, sweat suits, fad diets)	• Proper and substantial weight loss is a long-term process.	
Knowledge of the kilocalorie levels of carbohydrate, fat, protein, and alcohol	• Energy content of different nutrients is not equal.	
Knowledge of the relationship between kilocalorie expenditures and weight loss	• Deficit of 3,500 kcal = loss of 1 lb of body mass. • This is common knowledge among exercise scientists.	*Exercise Physiology: Integrating Theory and Application* (18) • Chapter 11
Knowledge of published position statements on obesity and the risks associated with it (*e.g.,* National Institutes of Health, American Dietetic Association, American College of Sports Medicine [ACSM])	• Be aware of the difference between overweight and obesity in respect to the definition of these terms.	*ACSM's Guidelines for Exercise Testing and Prescription* (GETP), 10th edition (7) • Chapter 11
Knowledge of the relationship between body fat distribution patterns and health	• Android obesity ("apple shape") vs. gynoid ("pear shape") • Visceral vs. subcutaneous fat distribution	
Knowledge of the physiology and pathophysiology of overweight and obese participants	• Individuals who are overweight and/ or obese are often present with comorbidities and/or debilitating orthopedic conditions.	*ACSM's Exercise Management for Persons with Chronic Diseases and Disabilities*, 4th edition (2) • Chapter 21
Knowledge of the recommended frequency, intensity, time, and type (FITT) framework for participants who are overweight or obese	• The amount of physical activity may need to be greater than recommended for apparently healthy individuals. • Exercise should be coupled with sound nutritional and behavior change interventions.	*ACSM's Guidelines for Exercise Testing and Prescription* (GETP), 10th edition (7) • Chapter 11

EP-C

F. Implement a weight management program as indicated by personal goals that are supported by preparticipation health screening, health history, and body composition/anthropometrics. (cont.)

Knowledge or Skill Statement	Explanation/Examples	Resources
Knowledge of comorbidities and musculoskeletal conditions associated with overweight and obesity that may require medical clearance and/or modifications to exercise testing and prescription	• Due to the potential existence of other chronic and orthopedic issues, additional medical intervention may be warranted.	*ACSM's Guidelines for Exercise Testing and Prescription* (GETP), 10th edition (7) • Chapter 11
Skill in applying behavioral strategies (*e.g.,* exercise, diet, behavioral modification strategies) for weight management	• Be aware that the appropriate way to lose weight may require some time and may involve additional exercise and/or diet, exercise, and/or behavior modification.	*ACSM's Guidelines for Exercise Testing and Prescription* (GETP), 10th edition (7) • Chapter 11
Skill in modifying exercises for individuals limited by body size	• Exercise prescription may need to be individualized and modified based on abilities and the presence or absence of comorbidities and/or preexisting orthopedic limitations.	
Skill in calculating the volume of exercise in terms of kilocalories per session	• Be aware of all the conversions that are at the bottom of the table (Table 6.3).	*ACSM's Guidelines for Exercise Testing and Prescription* (GETP), 10th edition (7) • Table 6.3

G. Prescribe and implement exercise programs for participants with controlled cardiovascular, pulmonary, and metabolic diseases and other clinical populations and work closely with clients' health care providers as needed.

Knowledge or Skill Statement	Explanation/Examples	Resources
Knowledge of American College of Sports Medicine (ACSM) risk stratification and exercise prescription guidelines for participants with cardiovascular, pulmonary, and metabolic diseases and other clinical populations	• This information is fairly extensive and should be covered thoroughly.	*ACSM's Guidelines for Exercise Testing and Prescription* (GETP), 10th edition (7) • Chapters 3, 10, and 11 • Table 3.1 • Box 3.1
Knowledge of ACSM relative and absolute contraindications for initiating exercise sessions or exercise testing and indications for terminating exercise sessions and exercise testing	• Be aware of the difference between relative and absolute contraindications in respect to the benefits vs. risks that are associated with exercise/testing.	*ACSM's Guidelines for Exercise Testing and Prescription* (GETP), 10th edition (7)
Knowledge of physiology and pathophysiology of cardiac disease, arthritis, diabetes mellitus, dyslipidemia, hypertension, metabolic syndrome, musculoskeletal injuries, overweight and obesity, osteoporosis, peripheral artery disease, and pulmonary disease	• Extensive prior knowledge of cardiopulmonary physiology is highly recommended.	*ACSM's Guidelines for Exercise Testing and Prescription* (GETP), 10th edition (7) • Chapters 10 and 11
Knowledge of the effects of diet and exercise on blood glucose levels in diabetics	• Be aware of special considerations that may affect exercise such as hypoglycemia; blood glucose before, during, and immediately following exercise; hyperglycemia; polyurea; neuropathy; nephropathy; and retinopathy.	*ACSM's Guidelines for Exercise Testing and Prescription* (GETP), 10th edition (7) • Chapters 10 and 11

EP-C

G. Prescribe and implement exercise programs for participants with controlled cardiovascular, pulmonary, and metabolic diseases and other clinical populations and work closely with clients' health care providers as needed. (cont.)

Knowledge or Skill Statement	Explanation/Examples	Resources
Knowledge of the recommended frequency, intensity, time, and type (FITT) principle for the development of cardiorespiratory fitness, muscular fitness, and flexibility for participants with cardiac disease, arthritis, diabetes mellitus, dyslipidemia, hypertension, metabolic syndrome, musculoskeletal injuries, overweight and obesity, osteoporosis, peripheral artery disease, and pulmonary disease	• In order to fully comprehend this information, the certified exercise physiologist (EP-C) needs to be fully aware of FITT-VP principles because they apply to apparently healthy individuals. • This information is fairly extensive and should be covered thoroughly.	*ACSM's Guidelines for Exercise Testing and Prescription* (GETP), 10th edition (7) • Chapters 10 and 11
Skill in progressing exercise programs, according to the FITT principle, in a safe and effective manner	• Rate of progression in both aerobic and strength exercises should be individualized.	*ACSM's Guidelines for Exercise Testing and Prescription* (GETP), 10th edition (7) • Chapter 6
Skill in modifying the exercise prescription and/or exercise choice for individuals with cardiac disease, arthritis, diabetes mellitus, dyslipidemia, hypertension, metabolic syndrome, musculoskeletal injuries, overweight and obesity, osteoporosis, peripheral artery disease, and pulmonary disease	• To make appropriate modifications, the EP-C needs to be fully aware of FITT-VP principles because they apply to apparently healthy individuals. • To make appropriate modifications, one needs to fully comprehend the physiology and pathophysiology of these conditions.	*ACSM's Guidelines for Exercise Testing and Prescription* (GETP), 10th edition (7) • Chapters 10 and 11
Skill in identifying improper exercise techniques and modifying exercise programs for participants with low back, neck, shoulder, elbow, wrist, hip, knee, and/or ankle pain	• To make appropriate modifications, one needs to fully comprehend the physiology and pathophysiology of these conditions. • If warranted, consult with appropriate professional (*i.e.*, physical therapist [PT])	

H. Prescribe and implement exercise programs for healthy special populations (*i.e.*, older adults, youth, pregnant women).

Knowledge or Skill Statement	Explanation/Examples	Resources
Knowledge of normal maturational changes from childhood to old age and their effects on the skeletal muscle, bone, reaction time, coordination, posture, heat and cold tolerance, maximal oxygen consumption, strength, flexibility, body composition, resting and maximal heart rate, and resting and maximal blood pressure	• Knowledge of related exercise physiology is critical. • This information is fairly extensive and should be covered thoroughly.	*ACSM's Guidelines for Exercise Testing and Prescription* (GETP), 10th edition (7) • Chapters 7 and 8 *ACSM's Exercise Management for Persons with Chronic Diseases and Disabilities*, 4th edition (2)

H. Prescribe and implement exercise programs for healthy special populations (*i.e.,* older adults, youth, pregnant women). (cont.)

Knowledge or Skill Statement	Explanation/Examples	Resources
Knowledge of techniques for the modification of cardiovascular, flexibility, and resistance exercises based on age, functional capacity, and physical condition	• To make appropriate modifications, the certified exercise physiologist (EP-C) needs to be fully aware of FITT-VP principles because they apply to apparently healthy individuals. • To make appropriate modifications, the EP-C needs to fully comprehend the anatomical and physiological differences between apparently healthy and healthy special populations.	*ACSM's Guidelines for Exercise Testing and Prescription* (GETP), 10th edition (7) • Chapters 4, 7, and 8
Knowledge of techniques for the development of exercise prescriptions for children, adolescents, and older adults regarding strength, functional capacity, and motor skills	• To make appropriate exercise prescription, the EP-C needs to fully comprehend the anatomical and physiological differences between these populations.	*ACSM's Guidelines for Exercise Testing and Prescription* (GETP), 10th edition (7) • Chapters 4 and 7
Knowledge of the unique adaptations to exercise training in children, adolescents, and older participants regarding strength, functional capacity, and motor skills	• Extensive prior knowledge of related exercise physiology is critical. • This information is fairly extensive and should be covered thoroughly.	*ACSM's Guidelines for Exercise Testing and Prescription* (GETP), 10th edition (7) • Chapters 4 and 7 *ACSM's Exercise Management for Persons with Chronic Diseases and Disabilities*, 4th edition (2) • Chapter 5
Knowledge of the benefits and precautions associated with exercise training across the lifespan	• The risk of a cardiovascular event during exercise is very low in apparently healthy individuals. • The risk of a cardiovascular event during exercise is directly related to the intensity of the exercise and the severity of diagnosed or undiagnosed occlusion cardiovascular disease (CVD).	*ACSM's Guidelines for Exercise Testing and Prescription* (GETP), 10th edition (7) • Chapter 1
Knowledge of the recommended frequency, intensity, time, type, volume, and progression (FITT-VP) framework for the development of cardiorespiratory fitness, muscular fitness, and flexibility in apparently healthy children and adolescents	• To make appropriate modifications, the EP-C needs to be fully aware of FITT-VP principles because they apply to apparently healthy populations. • Children are not miniature adults, and therefore, exercise prescription should be modified accordingly.	*ACSM's Guidelines for Exercise Testing and Prescription* (GETP), 10th edition (7) • Chapters 6 and 7
Knowledge of the effects of the aging process on the musculoskeletal and cardiovascular structures and functions during rest, exercise, and recovery	• Be aware of the effects of the aging process as well as the effects of physical activity or sedentary lifestyle on the musculoskeletal and cardiovascular structures.	*Physiology of Exercise and Healthy Aging* (25) • Chapters 1 and 2
Knowledge of the recommended FITT-VP framework necessary for the development of cardiorespiratory fitness, muscular fitness, balance, and flexibility in apparently healthy older adults	• Be aware of any aging-related conditions that may affect exercise prescription.	*ACSM's Guidelines for Exercise Testing and Prescription* (GETP), 10th edition (7) • Chapter 7

EP-C

H. Prescribe and implement exercise programs for healthy special populations (*i.e.*, older adults, youth, pregnant women). (cont.)

Knowledge or Skill Statement	Explanation/Examples	Resources
Knowledge of common orthopedic and cardiovascular exercise considerations for older adults	• When prescribing exercise to older adults, one needs to be aware of all existing mental, physical, and medical conditions and respond accordingly.	
Knowledge of the relationship between regular physical activity and the successful performance of activities of daily living (ADL) for older adults	• The physical fitness components that may improve with regular physical activity are muscular strength and endurance, cardiovascular endurance, balance, and flexibility.	
Knowledge of the recommended frequency, intensity, type, and duration of physical activity necessary for the development of cardiorespiratory fitness, muscular fitness, and flexibility in apparently healthy pregnant women	• To make appropriate modifications, the EP-C needs to be fully aware of FITT-VP principles because they apply to apparently healthy individuals. • Prior to prescribing exercise in this population, the EP-C needs to be aware of the physiological responses to exercise, contraindications for exercising, and other special considerations because they relate to this population.	*ACSM's Guidelines for Exercise Testing and Prescription* (GETP), 10th edition (7) • Chapter 7
Skill in teaching and demonstrating appropriate exercises for healthy populations with special considerations	• The EP-C must be aware of the anatomical and physiological differences between these populations. • The EP-C must modify the exercise accordingly. • Lead by example!	*ACSM's Guidelines for Exercise Testing and Prescription* (GETP), 10th edition (7) • Chapters 6 and 7
Skill in modifying exercises based on age, physical condition, and current health status	• To make appropriate modifications, the EP-C needs to fully comprehend the physiological differences between apparently healthy populations and healthy populations with special considerations.	*ACSM's Guidelines for Exercise Testing and Prescription* (GETP), 10th edition (7) • Chapter 7

I. Modify exercise prescriptions based on environmental conditions.

Knowledge or Skill Statement	Explanation/Examples	Resources
Knowledge of the effects of a hot, cold, or high-altitude environment on the physiologic response to exercise	• This information is fairly extensive and should be covered thoroughly. • This information could be found in any reputable exercise physiology textbook.	*ACSM's Guidelines for Exercise Testing and Prescription* (GETP), 10th edition (7) • Chapter 8 *Exercise Physiology: Integrating Theory and Application* (18) • Chapter 10

I. Modify exercise prescriptions based on environmental conditions. (cont.)

Knowledge or Skill Statement	Explanation/Examples	Resources
Knowledge of special precautions and program modifications for exercise in a hot, cold, or high-altitude environment	• By knowing the physiology as it relates to these conditions, one may develop and implement some prevention strategies.	*ACSM's Guidelines for Exercise Testing and Prescription* (GETP), 10th edition (7) • Chapter 8 *Exercise Physiology: Integrating Theory and Application* (18) • Chapter 10
Knowledge of the role of acclimatization when exercising in a hot or high-altitude environment	• By knowing the physiology as it relates to these conditions, one may develop an individualized exercise prescription using acclimatization protocols to achieve optimal physical and cognitive (in altitude) performances.	*ACSM's Guidelines for Exercise Testing and Prescription* (GETP), 10th edition (7) • Chapter 8 *Exercise Physiology: Integrating Theory and Application* (18) • Chapter 10
Knowledge of appropriate fluid intake during exercise in a hot, humid environments as well as cold, and high-altitude	• Be aware of techniques to assess hydration (*i.e.*, urine color and osmolality). • Be aware of hydration needs prior to, during, and after exercise.	*Exercise Physiology: Integrating Theory and Application* (18) • Chapter 9

DOMAIN III: EXERCISE COUNSELING AND BEHAVIORAL STRATEGIES

A. Optimize adoption and adherence to exercise programs and other healthy behaviors by applying effective communication techniques.

Knowledge or Skill Statement	Explanation/Examples	Resources
Knowledge of the effective and timely uses of communication modes (*e.g.*, e-mail, telephone, Web site, newsletters)	• The use of the mode of communication may be related to factors such as age, gender, ethnicity, locality, and other subjective preferences.	
Knowledge of verbal and nonverbal behaviors that communicate positive reinforcement and encouragement (*e.g.*, eye contact, targeted praise, empathy)	• Because the behavioral aspect needs to be addressed early in the intervention, it is critical that positive reinforcement and encouragement are communicated to your client.	
Knowledge of group leadership techniques for working with participants of all ages	• The information and the tools that are being used to motivate and educate participants need to be adjusted to fit the group population.	
Knowledge of active listening techniques	• Consider more advanced consoling skills. • Consider both listening and making reflective statements.	
Knowledge of learning modes (auditory, visual, kinesthetic)	• Using different modes to enhance task completion.	*The Kinesthetic Classroom: Teaching and Learning through Movement* (19) • Chapter 1
Knowledge of types of feedback (*e.g.*, evaluative, supportive, descriptive)	• Feedback is vital to behavior modification in an environment that supports a client-centered approach.	

A. Optimize adoption and adherence to exercise programs and other healthy behaviors by applying effective communication techniques. (cont.)

Knowledge or Skill Statement	Explanation/Examples	Resources
Skill in using active listening techniques	• Consider more advanced consoling skills. • The ability to listen, analyze, and communicate is critical.	
Skill in applying teaching and training techniques to optimize participant training sessions	• Extensive knowledge of related behavioral strategies to enhance physical activity participation is critical. • Program should be client-centered.	
Skill in using feedback to optimize participant training sessions	• Must be familiar with motivational and behavior modification techniques such as client-centered approach and active listening. • Must be familiar with basic motivational and behavior modification terms such empathy and rapport.	
Skill in applying verbal and nonverbal communications with diverse participant populations	• Vary the mode of communication based on age, gender, ethnicity, locality, and other subjective preferences.	

B. Optimize adoption of and adherence to exercise programs and other healthy behaviors by applying effective behavioral and motivational strategies.

Knowledge or Skill Statement	Explanation/Examples	Resources
Knowledge of behavior change models and theories (*e.g.*, health belief model, theory of planned behavior, socioecological model, transtheoretical model, social cognitive theory, cognitive evaluation theory)	• This information is fairly extensive and should be covered thoroughly. • These behavior change models and theories play a key role in the overall process of moving from sedentary to physically active lifestyle.	
Knowledge of the basic principles involved in motivational interviewing	• Have a client-centered approach. • May involve various counseling skills	
Knowledge of intervention strategies and stress management techniques	• The intervention strategy that may be used should depend on the individual stage of change.	
Knowledge of the stages of motivational readiness (*e.g.*, transtheoretical model)	• Be aware of the following: precontemplation, contemplation, preparation, action, and maintenance.	
Knowledge of behavioral strategies for enhancing exercise and health behavior change (*e.g.*, reinforcement; specific, measurable, attainable, realistic and relevant, and time-bound [SMART] goal setting; social support)	• This information is fairly extensive and should be covered thoroughly. • Using sound and effective behavioral strategies is key for enhancing exercise and health behavior change.	

B. Optimize adoption of and adherence to exercise programs and other healthy behaviors by applying effective behavioral and motivational strategies. (cont.)

Knowledge or Skill Statement	Explanation/Examples	Resources
Knowledge of behavior modification terminology including but not limited to self-esteem, self-efficacy, antecedents, cues to action, behavioral beliefs, behavioral intentions, and reinforcing factors	• Understanding these concepts play a major role in the overall process of behavior modification and moving from a sedentary to physically active lifestyle.	*Behavior Modification: What It Is And How to Do It*, 9th edition (20) • Part II
Knowledge of behavioral strategies (*e.g.*, exercise, diet, behavioral modification strategies) for weight management	• A successful weight loss program is a lengthy and ongoing process that should include exercise, diet, and behavior modification.	
Knowledge of the role that affect, mood, and emotion play in exercise adherence	• Many factors affect exercise adherence (*i.e.*, personal, behavioral).	
Knowledge of common barriers to exercise initiation and compliance (*e.g.*, time management, injury, fear, lack of knowledge, weather)	• Recognizing and overcoming barriers to exercise is a vital step in the development of viable behavior change program.	
Knowledge of techniques that facilitate motivation (*e.g.*, goal setting, incentive programs, achievement recognition, social support)	• Many aspects are involved in facilitating motivation. • The form of motivation could be described as either extrinsic or intrinsic.	
Knowledge of the role extrinsic and intrinsic motivation plays in the adoption and maintenance of behavior change	• Program-based incentive is an example of a form of extrinsic motivation. • A personal reward for behavior is an example of a form of intrinsic motivation.	
Knowledge of relapse prevention strategies and plans of action	• Relapse in exercising is usually due to an inevitable event (illness or injury, professional engagements, etc.). • Relapse prevention may involve developing a restart plan, the use of reinforcement or rewards system, etc.	
Knowledge of applying health coaching principles and lifestyle management techniques related to behavior change	• This topic is fairly extensive and may include strategies to enhance physical activity participation, diet modification, stress reduction techniques, etc.	
Knowledge of strategies that increase nonstructured physical activity levels (*e.g.*, stair walking, parking farther away, bike to work)	• May involve making a conscious decision to become more active • Related to behavior change	
Skill in explaining the purpose and value of understanding perceived exertion	• A valuable secondary tool to monitor exercise tolerance • Scale must be explained prior to the commencement of the test.	*ACSM's Guidelines for Exercise Testing and Prescription* (GETP), 10th edition (7) • Chapter 4 • Table 4.6

EP-C

B. Optimize adoption of and adherence to exercise programs and other healthy behaviors by applying effective behavioral and motivational strategies. (cont.)

Knowledge or Skill Statement	Explanation/Examples	Resources
Skill in using imagery as a motivational tool	• The use of images for reinforcing and promoting physical activity	
Skill in evaluating behavioral readiness to optimize exercise adherence	• Use tools such as the self-motivation assessment scale and physical activity stages of change.	
Skill in applying the theories related to behavior change to diverse populations	• This theoretical knowledge is fairly extensive and should be covered thoroughly. • Consider decision-making theory, social cognitive theory, etc.	
Skill in developing intervention strategies to increase self-efficacy and self-confidence	• Applied to different health behavior change theories • Skill to recognize the degree of self-efficacy and self-confidence	
Skill in developing reward systems that support and maintain program adherence	• The information is fairly extensive because it applies to different aspects of behavioral strategies to enhance physical activity participation.	
Skill in setting effective behavioral goals	• Goal setting should be realistic, target-specific behaviors, measurable, and time frame specific (long term vs. short term).	

C. Provide educational resources to support clients in the adoption and maintenance of healthy lifestyle behaviors.

Knowledge or Skill Statement	Explanation/Examples	Resources
Knowledge of the relationship between physical inactivity and common chronic diseases (*e.g.,* atherosclerosis, Type 2 diabetes, obesity, dyslipidemia, arthritis, low back pain, hypertension)	• There is an inverse relationship between physical activity and the severity and the number of common chronic diseases. • Dose response related	*ACSM's Guidelines for Exercise Testing and Prescription* (GETP), 10th edition (7) • Chapter 1
Knowledge of the dynamic interrelationship between fitness level, body composition, stress, and overall health	• The benefits of regular physical activity may include but not limited to improvement in cardiovascular and respiratory functions, reduction in coronary artery disease (CAD) risk factors, and decreased in overall morbidity and mortality.	*ACSM's Guidelines for Exercise Testing and Prescription* (GETP), 10th edition (7) • Chapter 1

C. Provide educational resources to support clients in the adoption and maintenance of healthy lifestyle behaviors. (cont.)		
Knowledge or Skill Statement	**Explanation/Examples**	**Resources**
Knowledge of modifications necessary to promote healthy lifestyle behaviors for diverse populations	• To make appropriate modifications, the certified exercise physiologist (EP-C) needs to be fully aware of FITT-VP principles because they apply to apparently healthy populations. • To make appropriate modifications, the EP-C needs to fully comprehend the physiology and pathophysiology of common chronic diseases conditions. • To make appropriate modifications, the EP-C needs to fully comprehend the anatomical and physiological differences between apparently healthy and healthy special populations.	*ACSM's Guidelines for Exercise Testing and Prescription* (GETP), 10th edition (7) • Chapters 7–11
Knowledge of stress management techniques and relaxation techniques (*e.g.,* progressive relaxation, guided imagery, massage therapy)	• Each of these techniques may be useful for stress reduction and may be used individually or in conjunction with one another.	*The Relaxation and Stress Reduction Workbook*, 6th edition (10) • Chapters 4–7
Knowledge of the activities of daily living (ADL) and how they relate to overall health	• ADL may be affected negatively by many chronic conditions and may be affected positively by endurance and strength-based exercises.	
Knowledge of accessing and disseminating scientifically based, relevant health, exercise, nutrition, and wellness-related resources and information	• Be aware of the concept and importance of research. • Have the ability to "translate" scientific literature to practical use.	*Exercise Physiology: Integrating Theory and Application* (18) • Chapter 1
Knowledge of specific, age-appropriate leadership techniques and educational methods to increase client engagement	• The selection of an appropriate program to increase client engagement should be individualized and client-centered.	
Knowledge of community-based exercise programs that provide social support and structured activities (*e.g.,* walking clubs, intramural sports, golf leagues, cycling clubs)	• These programs could be supported and organized by schools, work sites, religious institutions, etc.	
Skill in accessing and delivering health, exercise, and wellness-related information	• The EP-C must be able to make use of technology to locate, assess, and use relevant health-related information.	*Exercise Physiology: Integrating Theory and Application* (18) • Chapter 1
Skill in educating clients about benefits and risks of exercise and the risks of sedentary behavior	• The EP-C must have the skill to access, disseminate, and simplify scientifically based, health-related information. • Be able to explain complex information in layman's terms.	*Exercise Physiology: Integrating Theory and Application* (18) • Chapter 1

EP-C

D. Provide support within the scope of practice of a certified exercise physiologist (EP-C) and refer to other health professionals as indicated.

Knowledge or Skill Statement	Explanation/Examples	Resources
Knowledge of the side effects of common over-the-counter and prescription drugs that may impact a client's ability to exercise	• Be aware of the effects of these medications on heart rate (HR), blood pressure (BP), electrocardiogram (ECG), and exercise capacity.	*ACSM's Guidelines for Exercise Testing and Prescription* (GETP), 10th edition (7) • Appendix A
Knowledge of signs and symptoms of mental health states (*e.g.,* anxiety, depression, eating disorders) that may necessitate referral to a medical or mental health professional	• Affect wide range of populations • Proper treatment will allow a substantial improvement in psychological functioning and quality of life.	
Knowledge of symptoms and causal factors of test anxiety (*i.e.,* performance, appraisal threat during exercise testing) and how they may affect physiological responses to testing	• Exercise has a positive effect on symptoms of anxiety. • Consider the relationship between anxiety and exercise adherence.	
Knowledge of client needs and learning styles that may impact exercise sessions and exercise testing procedures	• A client-centered approach should be adopted for all aspects that are related to exercise. • Exercise prescription should be individualized.	
Knowledge of conflict resolution techniques that facilitate communication among exercise cohorts	• Be aware of conflict resolution techniques that may be used to resolve a conflict, argument, or disagreement.	"Conflict Resolution Skills" (24)
Skill in communicating the need for medical, nutritional, or mental health intervention	• One should be able to evaluate and assess physical activity, nutritional, and psychological statuses and provide and communicate appropriate and sound responses.	

DOMAIN IV: LEGAL AND PROFESSIONAL

A. Create and disseminate risk management guidelines (with the assistance of the human resources and/or legal departments) for a health/fitness facility department or organization to reduce member, employee, and business risk.

Knowledge or Skill Statement	Explanation/Examples	Resources
Knowledge of employee criminal background checks, child abuse clearances, and drug and alcohol screenings	• Laws may vary between states.	"Performing Pre-Employment Background Checks" (30)
Knowledge of employment verification requirements mandated by state and federal laws	• Laws may vary between states.	"Performing Pre-Employment Background Checks" (30)

EP-C

A. Create and disseminate risk management guidelines (with the assistance of the human resources and/or legal departments) for a health/fitness facility department or organization to reduce member, employee, and business risk. (cont.)

Knowledge or Skill Statement	Explanation/Examples	Resources
Knowledge of safe handling and disposal of body fluids and employee safety (Occupational Safety and Health Administration [OSHA] guidelines)	• Applies to occupational exposure to blood/body fluids or other potentially infectious materials	OSHA Standards (29 CFR) 1910.1030(d)(4)(iii)(C) (23)
Knowledge of insurance coverage common to the health/fitness industry including general liability, professional liability, workers' compensation, property, and business interruption	• Be aware of insurance reimbursement and the role of Medicaid and Medicare. • Be aware of the following topics: malpractice, negligence, and standards of practice.	
Knowledge of sexual harassment policies and procedures	• Must understand the federal law prohibiting sexual harassment in the workplace • Most states have some additional laws that relates to sexual harassment and discrimination.	"Title VII of the Civil Rights Act of 1964" (29)
Knowledge of interviewing techniques	• Avoid questions that may violate discrimination laws (what is your sexual orientation, religion, etc.).	"Title VII of the Civil Rights Act of 1964" (29)
Knowledge of basic precautions taken in an exercise setting to ensure participant safety	• Safety is always first. • Proper screening and emergency policy standards are paramount.	*ACSM's Guidelines for Exercise Testing and Prescription* (GETP), 10th edition (7) • Chapters 2 and 3 • Tables 2.1 and 3.1–3.4 • Figures 2.1–2.3 and 3.1 *ACSM's Health/Fitness Facility Standards and Guidelines*, 4th edition (3) • Chapter 3 • Table 3.1
Knowledge of preactivity screening, medical release, and waiver of liability for normal and at-risk participants	• This information is fairly extensive and should be covered thoroughly.	*ACSM's Guidelines for Exercise Testing and Prescription* (GETP), 10th edition (7) • Chapters 2 and 3
Knowledge of emergency response systems and procedures employee assistance program	• The procedures should be clearly stated, reviewed regularly, and known to all employees.	*ACSM's Health/Fitness Facility Standards and Guidelines*, 4th edition (3) • Chapter 3
Knowledge of the use of signage	• Be aware of the differences between cautionary signage, danger signage, and warning signage.	*ACSM's Health/Fitness Facility Standards and Guidelines*, 4th edition (3) • Chapter 8
Knowledge of preventive maintenance schedules and audits	• Be aware of the differences between daily, weekly, and monthly care.	*ACSM's Health/Fitness Facility Standards and Guidelines*, 4th edition (3) • Chapter 7 • Tables 7.3 and 7.4
Knowledge of techniques and methods of evaluating the condition of exercise equipment to reduce the potential risk of injury	• Be aware of the differences between daily, weekly, and monthly care.	*ACSM's Health/Fitness Facility Standards and Guidelines*, 4th edition (3) • Chapter 7 • Tables 7.3 and 7.4

A. Create and disseminate risk management guidelines (with the assistance of the human resources and/or legal departments) for a health/fitness facility department or organization to reduce member, employee, and business risk. (cont.)

Knowledge or Skill Statement	Explanation/Examples	Resources
Knowledge of the legal implications of documented safety procedures, the use of incident documents, and ongoing safety training documentation for the purpose of safety and risk management	• Be aware of tort and contract principles because they relate to physical activity legal issues. • Regardless of severity, every incident (injury) should be documented.	*ACSM's Health/Fitness Facility Standards and Guidelines*, 4th edition (3) • Chapter 3
Knowledge of documentation procedures for cardiopulmonary resuscitation (CPR) and automated external defibrillator (AED) certification for employees	• CPR and AED certification is critical and required for the certified exercise physiologist (EP-C).	*ACSM's Health/Fitness Facility Standards and Guidelines*, 4th edition (3) • Chapter 3
Knowledge of AED guidelines for implementation	• AED plays a major role in the resuscitative process in ventricular fibrillation–related cardiac arrest. • In some states, a legislation was passed that requires health/fitness facilities to carry AED. • The procedures should be reviewed regularly and known to all AED-certified employees.	*ACSM's Health/Fitness Facility Standards and Guidelines*, 4th edition (3) • Chapter 3
Knowledge of the components of the American College of Sports Medicine (ACSM) Code of Ethics and the ACSM Certified EP-C scope of practice	• The ACSM Code of Ethics has five components. • In recent years, the scope of practice was adjusted and based on the Job Task Analysis (JTA).	ACSM's Code of Ethics (5)
Skill in developing and disseminating a policy and procedures manual	• Chapter 1 provides a good introduction to what a policies and procedures manual should include. • This information is fairly extensive and should be covered thoroughly.	*ACSM's Health/Fitness Facility Standards and Guidelines*, 4th edition (3) • Chapters 1–8
Skill in developing and implementing confidentiality policies	• Because personnel in health/fitness facilities are exposed to confidential health-related information, HIPAA regulations should be used as a guide when developing such a policy.	Health Insurance Portability and Accountability Act of 1996 (HIPAA) (27)
Skill in maintenance of a safe exercise environment (*e.g.*, equipment operation, proper sanitation, safety and maintenance of exercise areas, and overall facility maintenance)	• Follow the recommended daily, weekly, and/or monthly equipment and facility cleaning and maintenance.	*ACSM's Health/Fitness Facility Standards and Guidelines*, 4th edition (3) • Chapters 5 and 7 • Tables 5.4–5.6, 7.3, and 7.4
Skill in the organization, communication, and human resource management required to implement risk management policies and procedures.	• Be aware of both standards and guidelines for risk management and emergency policies.	*ACSM's Health/Fitness Facility Standards and Guidelines*, 4th edition (3) • Chapter 3
Skill in training employees to identify high-risk situations	• Employees should have the appropriate education, certification, and experience to identify high-risk situations. • Employees should be familiar with emergency response protocols.	*ACSM's Health/Fitness Facility Standards and Guidelines*, 4th edition (3) • Chapter 4

EP-C

B. Create an effective injury prevention program and ensure that emergency policies and procedures are in place.

Knowledge or Skill Statement	Explanation/Examples	Resources
Knowledge of emergency procedures (*i.e.*, telephone procedures, written emergency procedures, personnel responsibilities) in a health and fitness setting	• Staff should be familiar with and have access to all written emergency guidelines and procedures. • Emergency plan should be current and documented.	*ACSM's Health/Fitness Facility Standards and Guidelines,* 4th edition (3)
Knowledge of basic first aid procedures for exercise-related injuries, such as bleeding, strains/sprains, fractures, and exercise intolerance (dizziness, syncope, heat and cold injuries)	• This information is fairly extensive, and the certified exercise physiologist (EP-C) should have the knowledge to appropriately recognize and treat the emergency.	
Knowledge of the EP-C responsibilities and limitations and the legal implications of carrying out emergency procedures	• To protect participants/clients and to minimize the risk of legal ramifications, the EP-C must be familiar with each facility's policies and procedures (place of employment).	"ACSM's Certified Health Fitness Specialist Scope of Practice" (1)
Knowledge of safety plans, emergency procedures, and first aid techniques needed during fitness evaluations, exercise testing, and exercise training	• Be aware of the facility's policies and procedures. • Be aware of different medical conditions/emergencies and the proper acute and emergency (if applicable) response.	*ACSM's Health/Fitness Facility Standards and Guidelines,* 4th edition (3)
Knowledge of potential musculoskeletal injuries (*e.g.*, contusions, sprains, strains, fractures), cardiovascular/pulmonary complications (*e.g.*, tachycardia, bradycardia, hypotension/hypertension, dyspnea) and metabolic abnormalities (*e.g.*, fainting/syncope, hypoglycemia/hyperglycemia, hypothermia/hyperthermia)	• The knowledge of these conditions is fairly extensive. • Be aware of the conditions, signs, and symptoms as well as acute responses.	
Knowledge of the initial management and first aid techniques associated with open wounds, musculoskeletal injuries, cardiovascular/pulmonary complications, and metabolic disorders	• The EP-C should recognize and be able to provide acute care for each of these conditions.	
Knowledge of emergency documentation and appropriate document use	• Regardless of severity, every incident (injury) should be documented.	*ACSM's Health/Fitness Facility Standards and Guidelines,* 4th edition (3) • Chapter 3
Skill in applying basic first aid procedures for exercise-related injuries, such as bleeding, strains/sprains, fractures, and exercise intolerance (dizziness, syncope, heat and cold injuries)	• The EP-C should have the knowledge, recognize, and be able to provide acute yet skillful care to each of these conditions.	

EP-C

B. Create an effective injury prevention program and ensure that emergency policies and procedures are in place. (cont.)

Knowledge or Skill Statement	Explanation/Examples	Resources
Skill in applying basic life support, first aid, cardiopulmonary resuscitation (CPR), and automated external defibrillator (AED) techniques	• The EP-C must have a current adult CPR/AED certification with a practical skills component.	*ACSM's Health/Fitness Facility Standards and Guidelines*, 4th edition (3) • Chapter 4
Skill in designing an evacuation plan	• The plan should be developed as part of the exercise program safety and emergencies procedures.	*ACSM's Health/Fitness Facility Standards and Guidelines*, 4th edition (3) • Appendix J
Skill in demonstrating emergency procedures during exercise testing and/or training	• The EP-C must be familiar with each facility's emergency policies and procedures. • The EP-C must have a current adult CPR/AED certification with a practical skills component.	*ACSM's Health/Fitness Facility Standards and Guidelines*, 4th edition (3) • Chapter 4

DOMAIN V: MANAGEMENT

A. Manage human resources in accordance with leadership, organization, and management techniques.

Knowledge or Skill Statement	Explanation/Examples	Resources
Knowledge of industry benchmark compensation and employee benefit guidelines	• The information that is presented by the BLS regarding compensation may vary from year to year. • Employee benefits will vary widely from one employer to another.	Bureau of Labor Statistics (BLS) (9)
Knowledge of federal, state, and local laws pertaining to staff qualifications and credentialing requirements	• Staff qualifications and credentialing requirements will vary from state to state.	*ACSM's Health/Fitness Facility Standards and Guidelines*, 4th edition (3) • Chapter 4
Knowledge of techniques for tracking and evaluating member retention	• Consider using focus groups, surveys, in-depth interviews, and feedback systems.	
Skill in applying policies, practices, and guidelines to efficiently hire, train, supervise, schedule, and evaluate employees	• Be very familiar with the facility policies and procedures. • Be very familiar with federal, state, and local laws pertaining to staff qualifications and credentialing requirements.	*ACSM's Health/Fitness Facility Standards and Guidelines*, 4th edition (3) • Chapter 4
Skill in applying conflict resolution techniques	• Negotiate and mediate in the interpersonal level (between employees and/or members) in order to resolve a conflict, argument, or disagreement.	"Conflict Resolution Skills" (24)

EP-C

B. Manage fiscal resources in accordance with leadership, organization, and management techniques.

Knowledge or Skill Statement	Explanation/Examples	Resources
Knowledge of fiduciary roles and responsibilities inherent in managing an exercise and health promotion program	• Be aware of Employee Retirement Income Security Act (ERISA).	"Meeting Your Fiduciary Responsibilities" (28)
Knowledge of principles of financial planning and goal setting, institutional budgeting processes, forecasting, and allocation of resources	• This information is fairly extensive and requires understanding of the basic principles, rules, and regulations of business administration.	"Understanding the Basics" (31)
Knowledge of basic software systems that facilitate accounting (*e.g.*, Microsoft Excel)	• This spreadsheet application is being updated periodically. • There are other basic software systems that may assist facility accounting such as Quicken.	Microsoft Excel (21)
Knowledge of industry benchmarks for budgeting and finance	• This information is fairly extensive and requires understanding of the basic principles, rules, and regulations of business administration.	"Understanding the Basics" (31)
Knowledge of basic sales techniques that promote health, fitness, and wellness services	• Be aware of common techniques such as cold calling, drop box leads, etc.	
Skill in efficiently managing financial resources and performing related tasks (*e.g.*, planning, budgeting, resource allocation, revenue generation)	• Be very familiar with finance and accounting management because it relates to business administration. • Be very familiar with federal, state, and local laws pertaining to business administration.	"Understanding the Basics" (31)
Skill in administering fitness- and wellness-related programs within established budgetary guidelines	• Be very familiar with the rules and regulations of business administration.	"Understanding the Basics" (31)

C. Establish policies and procedures for the management of health/fitness facilities based on accepted safety and legal guidelines, standards, and regulations.

Knowledge or Skill Statement	Explanation/Examples	Resources
Knowledge of accepted guidelines, standards, and regulations used to establish policies and procedures for the management of health/fitness facilities	• Chapter 1 provides a good introduction to what a policy and procedures manual should include. • This information is fairly extensive and should be covered thoroughly.	*ACSM's Health/Fitness Facility Standards and Guidelines*, 4th edition (3) • Chapters 1–8
Knowledge of facility design and operation principles	• This information is fairly extensive and should be covered thoroughly. • Be aware of the differences between fitness only and multipurpose facilities in respect to design and overall operations.	*ACSM's Health/Fitness Facility Standards and Guidelines*, 4th edition (3) • Chapters 5 and 16

EP-C

C. Establish policies and procedures for the management of health/fitness facilities based on accepted safety and legal guidelines, standards, and regulations. (cont.)

Knowledge or Skill Statement	Explanation/Examples	Resources
Knowledge of facility and equipment maintenance guidelines	• Be aware of the differences between daily, weekly, and monthly equipment maintenance.	*ACSM's Health/Fitness Facility Standards and Guidelines*, 4th edition (3) • Chapters 5 and 7
Knowledge of documentation techniques for health/fitness facility management	• Facilities should have written policies and procedures. • Be aware that policies and procedures will vary from state to state.	*ACSM's Health/Fitness Facility Standards and Guidelines*, 4th edition (3) • Chapter 5
Knowledge of federal, state, and local laws as they relate to health/fitness facility management	• Check federal, state, and local laws because facility management rules and regulation will vary from state to state.	*ACSM's Health/Fitness Facility Standards and Guidelines*, 4th edition (3) • Chapter 5

D. Develop and execute a marketing plan to promote programs, services, and facilities.

Knowledge or Skill Statement	Explanation/Examples	Resources
Knowledge of lead generation techniques	• Use membership referral, lead boxes, cold calling, etc.	*ACSM's Resources for the Exercise Physiologist*, 2nd edition (6) • Chapters 15 and 17
Knowledge of the four *P*'s of marketing: product, price, placement, and promotion	• Marketing plays a major role in the viability of health/fitness facilities. • The management team should consider an array of marketing tools to promote the facility and fitness-related programs.	*ACSM's Resources for the Exercise Physiologist*, 2nd edition (6) • Chapters 15 and 17
Knowledge of public relations, community awareness, and sponsorship and their relationship to branding initiatives	• Use tools such as developing alliances with Home Owners Association's (HOA) and realtors, initiate community involvement, etc.	*ACSM's Resources for the Exercise Physiologist*, 2nd edition (6) • Chapters 15 and 17
Knowledge of advertising techniques	• Consider scatter gun approach, sharp shooter method, promotional massages, etc.	*ACSM's Resources for the Exercise Physiologist*, 2nd edition (6) • Chapters 15 and 17
Knowledge of target market (internal) assessment techniques	• Assess internal factors that may provide advantages or disadvantages in meeting the needs of the target market (clients). • Consider market trends, conduct regular evaluations, etc.	*ACSM's Resources for the Exercise Physiologist*, 2nd edition (6) • Chapters 15 and 17
Knowledge of target market (external) assessment techniques	• Assess external factors such as offering by competitors, the state of the economy, etc.	*ACSM's Resources for the Exercise Physiologist*, 2nd edition (6) • Chapters 15 and 17
Skill in applying marketing techniques that promote client retention	• Use tools such as focus groups, surveys, in-depth interviews, and feedback systems.	*ACSM's Resources for the Exercise Physiologist*, 2nd edition (6) • Chapters 15 and 17

D. Develop and execute a marketing plan to promote programs, services, and facilities. (cont.)

Knowledge or Skill Statement	Explanation/Examples	Resources
Skill in applying marketing techniques that attract new clients	• Must be very familiar with marketing techniques such as lead boxes, direct mail, cold calling, etc.	*ACSM's Resources for the Exercise Physiologist*, 2nd edition (6) • Chapters 15 and 17
Skill in designing and writing promotional materials	• Must be very familiar with developing materials that will positively and aggressively market the facility	*ACSM's Resources for the Exercise Physiologist*, 2nd edition (6) • Chapters 15 and 17
Skill in collaborating with community and governmental agencies and organizations	• Must be very familiar with strategic alliance strategies	*ACSM's Resources for the Exercise Physiologist*, 2nd edition (6) • Chapters 15 and 17
Skill in providing customer service	• Pivotal factor in health/fitness facilities • Some ways to improve customer service relate to providing superior service, maintain exercise equipment, etc.	*ACSM's Resources for the Exercise Physiologist*, 2nd edition (6) • Chapters 15 and 17

E. Use effective communication techniques to develop professional relationships with other allied health professionals (*e.g.*, nutritionists, physical therapists, physicians, nurses).

Knowledge or Skill Statement	Explanation/Examples	Resources
Knowledge of communication styles and techniques	• In addition to face-to-face communications (meetings, conferences, etc.), it is common today to use a wide range of electronic communications such as e-mails, tweets, etc.	*ACSM's Resources for the Exercise Physiologist*, 2nd edition (6) • Chapters 15 and 17
Knowledge of networking techniques	• Meet and maintain a relationship with other allied health professionals (conferences, webinars, etc.). • Maintain communications (keep in touch). • Consider developing strategic alliances.	*ACSM's Resources for the Exercise Physiologist*, 2nd edition (6) • Chapters 15 and 17
Skill in planning meetings	• Requires experience in advertising, the use of other promotional materials, direct mail, etc.	*ACSM's Resources for the Exercise Physiologist*, 2nd edition (6) • Chapters 15 and 17

EP-C

REFERENCES

ACSM REFERENCES:

1. American College of Sports Medicine. ACSM's certified health fitness specialist scope of practice. American College of Sports Medicine [Internet]. [cited 2016 December]. Available from: http://www.acsm.org/AM/Template.cfm?Section=HealthFitness_Instructor1&Template=/CM/ContentDisplay.cfm&ContentID=10829#HFI_Scope_of_Practice2011

2. American College of Sports Medicine. *ACSM's Exercise Management for Persons with Chronic Diseases and Disabilities*. 4th ed. Champaign (IL): Human Kinetics; 2016. 416 p.

3. American College of Sports Medicine. *ACSM's Health/Fitness Facility Standards and Guidelines*. 4th ed. Champaign (IL): Human Kinetics; 2012. 203 p.

4. American College of Sports Medicine. *ACSM's Health-Related Physical Fitness Assessment Manual*. 5th ed. Philadelphia (PA): Wolters Kluwer; 2018. 172 p.

5. American College of Sports Medicine. Code of ethics of American College of Sports Medicine. American College of Sports Medicine [Internet]. [cited 2016 December]. Available from: http://www.acsm.org/Content/NavigationMenu/MemberServices/MemberResources/CodeofEthics/Code_of_Ethics.htm

6. Magyari P, editor. *ACSM's Resources for the Exercise Physiologist*. 2nd ed. Philadelphia (PA): Wolters Kluwer; 2018. p.

7. Riebe D, senior editor. *ACSM's Guidelines for Exercise Testing and Prescription*. 10th ed. Philadelphia (PA): Wolters Kluwer; 2018. p.

NON-ACSM REFERENCES:

8. Armiger P, Martyn MA. *Stretching for Functional Flexibility*. Philadelphia (PA): Lippincott Williams & Wilkins; 2010. 263 p.

9. Bureau of Labor Statistics. Occupational outlook handbook, 2010–2011 edition, fitness workers. United States Department of Labor [Internet]. [cited 2016 December]. Available from: http://www.bls.gov/oco/ocos296.htm

10. Davis M, Eshelman ER, McKay M. *The Relaxation and Stress Reduction Workbook*. 6th ed. Oakland (CA): New Harbinger Publications; 2008. 371 p.

11. Ehrman JK. *Clinical Exercise Physiology*. 2nd ed. Champaign (IL): Human Kinetics; 2009. 691 p.

12. Fleck SJ, Kraemer WJ. *Designing Resistance Training Programs*. 3rd ed. Champaign (IL): Human Kinetics; 2004. 377 p.

13. Garber CE, Blissmer B, Deschenes MR, et al. American College of Sports Medicine position stand. Quantity and quality of exercise for developing and maintaining cardiorespiratory, musculoskeletal, and neuromotor fitness in apparently healthy adults: guidance for prescribing exercise. *Med Sci Sports Exerc*. 2011;43(7):1334–59.

14. Goldenberg L, Twist P. *Strength Ball Training*. 2nd ed. Champaign (IL): Human Kinetics; 2007. 285 p.

15. Hall SJ. *Basic Biomechanics*. 6th ed. Boston (MA): WCB/McGraw-Hill; 2011. 577 p.

16. Heyward VH. *Advanced Fitness Assessment and Exercise Prescription*. 4th ed. Champaign (IL): Human Kinetics; 2002. 369 p.

17. Higgins M. *Therapeutic Exercise: From Theory to Practice*. Philadelphia (PA): F. A. Davis Company; 2011. 807 p.

18. Kraemer WJ, Fleck SJ, Deschenes MR. *Exercise Physiology: Integrating Theory and Application*. Philadelphia (PA): Lippincott Williams & Wilkins; 2012. 488 p.

19. Lengel T, Kuczala M. *The Kinesthetic Classroom: Teaching and Learning through Movement*. Thousand Oaks (CA): Corwin Press; 2010. 156 p.

20. Martin G, Pear J. *Behavior Modification: What It Is and How to Do It*. 9th ed. Boston (CA): Pearson Education/Allyn & Bacon; 2011. 462 p.

21. Microsoft Corporation. Excel. Microsoft Corporation [Internet]. [cited 2016 December]. Available from: http://office.microsoft.com/en-us/excel/

22. Newton H. *Explosive Lifting for Sports—Enhanced Edition*. Champaign (IL): Human Kinetics; 2006. 191 p.

23. Occupational Safety and Health Administration. Occupational safety and health standards: toxic and hazardous substances (standard number 1910.1030). United States Department Labor [Internet]. [cited 2016 December]. Available from: http://www.osha.gov/pls/oshaweb/owadisp.show_document?p_table=standards&p_id=10051

24. Segal J, Smith M. Conflict resolution skills. Helpguide [Internet]. [cited 2011 Sep 22]. Available from: http://helpguide.org/mental/eq8_conflict_resolution.htm

25. Taylor AW, Johnson MJ. *Physiology of Exercise and Healthy Aging*. Champaign (IL): Human Kinetics; 2008. 274 p.

26. U.S. Department of Agriculture. USDA center for nutrition policy and promotion. United States Department of Agriculture [Internet]. [cited 2016 December]. Available from: http://www.choosemyplate.gov/index.html

27. U.S. Department of Health and Human Services. Summary of the HIPAA privacy rule. U.S. Department of Health and Human Services [Internet]. [cited 2016 December]. Available from: http://www.hhs.gov/ocr/privacy/hipaa/understanding/summary/privacysummary.pdf

28. U.S. Department of Labor. Meeting your fiduciary responsibilities. United States Department of Labor [Internet]. [cited 2016 December]. Available from: http://www.dol.gov/ebsa/publications/fiduciary-responsibility.html

29. U.S. Equal Employment Opportunity Commission. Title VII of the Civil Rights Act of 1964. U.S. Equal Employment Opportunity Commission [Internet]. [cited 2016 December]. Available from: http://www.eeoc.gov/laws/statutes/titlevii.cfm

30. U.S. Small Business Administration. Performing pre-employment background checks. U.S. Small Business Administration [Internet]. [cited 2016 December]. Available from: http://www.sba.gov/content/performing-pre-employment-background-Checks

31. U.S. Small Business Administration. Understanding the basics. U.S. Small Business Administration [Internet]. [cited 2016 December]. Available from: http://www.sba.gov/category/navigation-structure/starting-managing-business/starting-business/preparing-your-finances/understanding-basics

EP-C

Note: EP-C certification candidates may also review the practice examination found in Part 1, ACSM Certified Personal Trainer (CPT).

DIRECTIONS: Each of the numbered items or incomplete statements in this section is followed by answers or by completions of the statement. Select the ONE lettered answer or completion that is BEST in each case.

1. Underweight is classified as a body mass index (BMI) of _____.
   A) $<19.9 \text{ kg} \cdot \text{m}^{-2}$
   B) $<18.5 \text{ kg} \cdot \text{m}^{-2}$
   C) $<24.9 \text{ kg} \cdot \text{m}^{-2}$
   D) $<20.5 \text{ kg} \cdot \text{m}^{-2}$

2. When measuring regional body circumferences, an average of duplicate measures is used provided that those measurements do not differ by more than _____.
   A) 3 mm
   B) 10 mm
   C) 5 mm
   D) 12 mm

3. Which of the following represents the demarcation point of a *very high* health risk for young women when using waist-to-hip ratio (WHR)?
   A) >0.86
   B) >0.95
   C) >1.00
   D) >1.03

4. Which of the following is accepted as the criterion measure of cardiorespiratory fitness?
   A) Field test performance
   B) Maximal volume of oxygen consumed per unit time ($\dot{V}O_{2max}$)
   C) Body fat percentage
   D) Maximal heart rate (HR_{max})

5. When estimating $\dot{V}O_{2max}$ using the YMCA cycle ergometer protocol, which of the following best describes the relationship between heart rate (HR) >110 bpm and 85% age-predicted HR_{max} or 70% heart rate reserve (HRR)?
   A) Logarithmic
   B) Inverse
   C) Curvilinear
   D) Linear

6. Which of the following variables is unique to the Rockport One-Mile Fitness Walking Test's regression equation to estimate $\dot{V}O_{2max}$?
   A) Age
   B) HR
   C) Gender
   D) Body mass

7. What is the suggested work rate for a deconditioned, female individual performing the Astrand-Rhyming cycle ergometer protocol?
   A) 150 or 300 $\text{kg} \cdot \text{m} \cdot \text{min}^{-1}$ (25 or 50 W)
   B) 300 or 450 $\text{kg} \cdot \text{m} \cdot \text{min}^{-1}$ (50 or 75 W)
   C) 450 or 600 $\text{kg} \cdot \text{m} \cdot \text{min}^{-1}$ (75 or 100 W)
   D) 600 or 900 $\text{kg} \cdot \text{m} \cdot \text{min}^{-1}$ (100 or 150 W)

8. The Queens College Step Test (also known as McArdle Step Test) is performed for how long?
   A) 45 s
   B) 90 s
   C) 3 min
   D) 5 min

9. Which of the following is not a general category for clinical exercise testing?
   A) Prognosis
   B) Implementation
   C) Evaluation
   D) Diagnosis

10. Which of the following is considered the "gold standard" to objectively measure exercise capacity?
    A) Maximal exercise test using indirect calorimetry
    B) Submaximal exercise test using hemodynamic responses
    C) Physician exam
    D) Walk/run field test

11. Whose legal responsibility is it to supervise the clinical exercise laboratory and interpret all clinical exercise testing results in a diagnostic setting?
    A) The test administrator
    B) The clinical exercise physiologist
    C) The on-call physician assistant
    D) The supervising physician

12. Which of the following graded exercise protocols is most widely used in the United States in a clinical setting?
   A) Bruce treadmill protocol
   B) Queens College Step Test
   C) Astrand-Rhyming cycle ergometer test
   D) All are used equally.

13. HR, blood pressure (BP), and electrocardiogram (ECG) should be recorded regularly during the clinical exercise test and through at least _____ of recovery.
   A) 90 s
   B) 3 min
   C) 6 min
   D) 10 min

14. The normal HR response to incremental exercise is to increase workloads at an HR of _____ per 1 metabolic equivalent (MET).
   A) 10 bpm
   B) 5 bpm
   C) 20 bpm
   D) 15 bpm

15. The purpose of the cool-down period following an exercise session includes all of the following except _____.
   A) Gradual recovery of HR
   B) Gradual recovery of BP
   C) Improvement in range of motion (ROM)
   D) Removal of metabolic end products

16. What is the frequency of combined aerobic exercise recommended for most adults?
   A) 5–7 d · wk^{-1}
   B) 4–6 d · wk^{-1}
   C) 3–5 d · wk^{-1}
   D) 1–3 d · wk^{-1}

17. Which of the following percentages of HRR would classify as "moderate" aerobic exercise intensity?
   A) 34%
   B) 52%
   C) 65%
   D) 91%

18. Which of the following methods is *not* recommended for estimating exercise intensity for exercise prescription (Ex R$_x$)?
   A) HRR
   B) Oxygen uptake reserve ($\dot{V}O_2R$)
   C) Ventilatory threshold (VT)
   D) Maximum heart rate percentage (%HR$_{max}$)

19. What is the minimum recommended target volume for energy expenditure (EE) to promote overall health and well-being in an Ex R$_x$?
   A) 500–1,000 MET-min · wk^{-1}
   B) 250–500 MET-min · wk^{-1}
   C) 150–250 MET-min · wk^{-1}
   D) 1,000–1,500 MET-min · wk^{-1}

20. What is the minimum recovery time recommended for a muscle group following a resistance training bout?
   A) 12 h
   B) 24 h
   C) 48 h
   D) 72 h

21. Which of the following is *not* a purpose of physical fitness testing?
   A) To bring in extra income to pay off other major expenses of the testing company
   B) To educate participants about their present health and fitness status relative to health-related standards and age- and sex-matched norms
   C) To motivate participants by establishing reasonable and attainable health/fitness goals
   D) To allow evaluation of progress following an exercise program and long-term monitoring of participants

22. When performing a battery of tests in a single testing session, which of the following orders is most optimal for testing multiple health-related components of fitness?
   A) Sit-and-reach test, resting heart rate (HR$_{rest}$), Queens College Step Test, ACSM push-up test
   B) Queens College Step Test, HR$_{rest}$, ACSM push-up test, sit-and-reach test
   C) ACSM push-up test, Queens College Step Test, sit-and-reach test, HR$_{rest}$
   D) HR$_{rest}$, Queens College Step Test, ACSM push-up test, sit-and-reach test

23. The degenerative loss of muscle mass and, thus, strength due to reduced physical activity and aging is known as _____.
   A) Rheumatoid arthritis
   B) Sarcopenia
   C) Hypertension
   D) Osteoporosis

24. Which of the following is *not* a valid test for muscular strength?
   A) Grip strength test
   B) YMCA bench press test
   C) 3-repetition maximum (RM) bench press test
   D) 10-RM shoulder press test

EP-C

25. The _____ skinfold site is performed using a diagonal fold method.
    A) Thigh
    B) Medial calf
    C) Suprailiac
    D) Abdominal

26. _____ is not a contraindication of maximal exercise testing in the clinical setting.
    A) Acute myocarditis or pericarditis
    B) Ongoing unstable angina
    C) Recent stroke or transient ischemia attack
    D) Resting systolic blood pressure (SBP) between 125 and 140 mm Hg or diastolic blood pressure (DBP) between 60 and 75 mm Hg

27. Clinical exercise testing among adult patients with chronic heart failure (HF) should observe the following recommendations *except* _____.
    A) Maximal exercise testing is reasonable to help determine whether HF is the cause of exercise limitation when the contribution of HF is uncertain.
    B) Maximal exercise testing is not a realistic way to identify candidates for cardiac transplantation or other advanced treatments due to inherent risk of heart stress.
    C) Exercise testing should be considered to detect reversible myocardial ischemia.
    D) Exercise testing should be considered to aid in the prescription of exercise training.

28. _____ pertains to the ability to correctly identify patients who do not have a given condition.
    A) Sensitivity
    B) Specificity
    C) Positive percent value
    D) Negative predictive value

29. All of the following are among the ACSM guidelines to determine "maximal" effort during a graded exercise test (GXT) *except* _____.
    A) Achievement of age-predicted HR_{max}
    B) A postexercise venous lactate concentration greater than 8 mmol $\cdot$ L^{-1}
    C) A rating of perceived exertion (RPE) at peak exercise greater than 17 on the 6–20 scale or greater than 7 on the 0–10 scale
    D) A peak respiratory exchange ratio (RER) greater than or equal to 1.10

30. Which of the following BP readings would be characterized as hypertension in an adult?
    A) 100/60 mm Hg
    B) 110/70 mm Hg
    C) 140/90 mm Hg
    D) 120/80 mm Hg

31. The informed consent document _____.
    A) Is a legal document
    B) Provides immunity from prosecution
    C) Provides an explanation of the test to the client
    D) Legally protects the rights of the client

32. At minimum, professionals performing fitness assessments on others should possess which combination of the following?
    A) Cardiopulmonary resuscitation (CPR) and ACSM Certified Exercise Physiologist (EP-C)
    B) Advanced cardiac life support and ACSM Certified Clinical Exercise Physiologist
    C) Advanced cardiac life support and ACSM Registered Clinical Exercise Physiologist
    D) Only physicians can perform fitness assessments.

33. The optimal Ex R_x should address which of the following?
    A) Cardiorespiratory (aerobic) fitness
    B) Body composition
    C) Neuromotor fitness
    D) All of the above

34. _____ involves holding the stretched position using the strength of the agonist muscle as is common in many forms of yoga.
    A) Passive static stretching
    B) Active static stretching
    C) Proprioceptive neuromuscular facilitation (PNF)
    D) Dynamic stretching

35. The ACSM recommends a frequency of at least _____ d of moderate exercise or at least _____ d of vigorous exercise per week for aerobic exercise training.
    A) 5; 3
    B) 4; 4
    C) 3; 5
    D) 4; 2

36. If a 175-lb man jogged for 30-min treadmill at an intensity of 26 mL $\cdot$ kg^{-1} $\cdot$ min^{-1}, what would his approximate caloric expenditure be for the entire 30-min session?
    A) 10 kcal
    B) 80 kcal
    C) 310.5 kcal
    D) 3,900 kcal

37. _____ is not recommended because of the significant chance of injury, severe muscle soreness, and serious complications such as rhabdomyolysis that can ensue.
    A) Resistance training composed exclusively of eccentric contractions conducted at very high intensities
    B) The Valsalva maneuver
    C) Resistance training composed exclusively of static contractions for periods longer than 60 s
    D) The use of a weight belt during power lifting

EP-C

38. Which of the following is *not* true regarding the psychological benefits of regular exercise in the elderly?
    A) Self-concept
    B) Life satisfaction
    C) Stimulate appetite
    D) Self-efficacy

39. Which statement is true regarding physical activity for children?
    A) Children should participate in several bouts of physical activity lasting more than 120 min each day.
    B) Children should perform 30 min of moderate-intensity and 30 min of vigorous-intensity physical activity on most days of the week.
    C) Children should focus on just one or two modes of physical activity to develop exceptional skills in those areas.
    D) Children need to have several periods of 2 h or more of inactivity during the day in order to have adequate rest.

40. What does the acronym FITT-VP stand for?
    A) Fast, intense, time, type, volume, and progression
    B) Frequency, independent, time, type, volume, and persistence
    C) Frequency, intensity, time, type, volume, and progression
    D) Force, impulse, torque, time, volume, and progression

41. Optimal Ex R_x should contain which of the following?
    A) Cardiorespiratory fitness, muscular strength, muscular endurance, flexibility, body composition, and neuromotor fitness
    B) Cardiorespiratory fitness, muscular power, muscular force, flexibility, body composition, and neuromotor fitness
    C) Cardiorespiratory fitness, muscular strength, muscular force, body composition, and neuromotor fitness
    D) Cardiorespiratory fitness, muscular power, muscular endurance, flexibility, and body composition

42. According to the most recent ACSM guidelines, in order to gain health benefits, it is recommended that moderate physical activity should be performed how many days per week?
    A) $2 \, d \cdot wk^{-1}$
    B) $7 \, d \cdot wk^{-1}$
    C) $5 \, d \cdot wk^{-1}$
    D) $3 \, d \cdot wk^{-1}$

43. For health benefits, it is recommended that vigorous physical activity should be performed how many days per week?
    A) $2 \, d \cdot wk^{-1}$
    B) $7 \, d \cdot wk^{-1}$
    C) $5 \, d \cdot wk^{-1}$
    D) $3 \, d \cdot wk^{-1}$

44. Moderate exercise is considered to be _____.
    A) 59%–79% HRR or $\dot{V}O_2R$
    B) 40%–59% HRR or $\dot{V}O_2R$
    C) 30%–45% HRR or $\dot{V}O_2R$
    D) 60%–89% HRR or $\dot{V}O_2R$

45. Vigorous exercise is considered to be _____.
    A) 59%–79% HRR or $\dot{V}O_2R$
    B) 40%–59% HRR or $\dot{V}O_2R$
    C) 30%–45% HRR or $\dot{V}O_2R$
    D) 60%–89% HRR or $\dot{V}O_2R$

46. The recommended exercise duration for moderate exercise is _____.
    A) 30–$60 \, min \cdot d^{-1}$
    B) 20–$50 \, min \cdot d^{-1}$
    C) 20–$30 \, min \cdot d^{-1}$
    D) 30–$40 \, min \cdot d^{-1}$

47. When using a pedometer, how many steps should most individuals achieve?
    A) $5,000 \, steps \cdot d^{-1}$
    B) $9,000 \, steps \cdot d^{-1}$
    C) $7,000 \, steps \cdot d^{-1}$
    D) $11,000 \, steps \cdot d^{-1}$

48. Muscular fitness refers to _____.
    A) Muscular endurance, muscular force, muscular strength
    B) Muscular endurance, muscular power, and muscular strength
    C) Muscular power, muscular force, and muscle soreness
    D) Muscular strength, anaerobic power, and muscular power

49. Ideal resistance training volume for most adults should be _____.
    A) 2–4 sets with 8–12 repetitions
    B) 1–2 sets with 8–12 repetitions
    C) 2–4 sets with 12–15 repetitions
    D) 3–5 sets with 8–12 repetitions

50. Which of the following medications is designed to modify blood cholesterol levels?
    A) Nitrates
    B) β–Blockers
    C) Antihyperlipidemics
    D) Aspirin

51. Which of the following represents more than 90% of the fat stored in the body and is composed of a glycerol molecule connected to three fatty acids?
    A) Phospholipids
    B) Cholesterol
    C) Triglycerides
    D) Free fatty acids

52. Which of the following BP readings represents the prehypertension category in adults?
    A) 100/60 mm Hg
    B) 110/70 mm Hg
    C) 160/90 mm Hg
    D) 118/84 mm Hg

53. For every 1 MET increase in exercise intensity during submaximal exercise, SBP should increase _____.
    A) Approximately 10 mm Hg
    B) 15–20 mm Hg
    C) 25–30 mm Hg
    D) 30–35 mm Hg

54. Which of the following would not terminate a maximal or submaximal exercise test in a low-risk adult?
    A) Subject requests to stop
    B) Shortness of breath
    C) A slight decrease in diastolic pressure
    D) Failure of HR to increase with increased intensity

55. The ACSM recommends that, in apparently healthy individuals, aerobic exercise intensity be prescribed within what percentage of HR_{max} range?
    A) 40% and 60%
    B) 50% and 80%
    C) 60% and 90%
    D) 70% and 100%

56. The ACSM recommends how many reps of each exercise for muscular endurance?
    A) 5–6
    B) 15–25
    C) 12–20
    D) More than 25

57. For higher intensity activities, _____.
    A) The benefit outweighs any potential risk.
    B) The risk of orthopedic and cardiovascular complications is increased.
    C) The risk of orthopedic and cardiovascular complications is minimal.
    D) There is no increased risk of orthopedic and cardiovascular complications.

58. What is the recommended repetition range when resistance training adults for general muscular fitness?
    A) 1–5
    B) 6–10
    C) 8–12
    D) 15–20

59. Feeling good about being able to perform an activity or skill, such as finally being able to run a mile or to increase the speed of walking a mile, is an example of an _____.
    A) Extrinsic reward
    B) Intrinsic reward
    C) External stimulus
    D) Internal stimulus

60. In the *2015–2020 Dietary Guidelines for Americans*, it is recommended that adults need at least _____ min of moderate-intensity physical activity and should perform muscle strengthening exercises on _____ or more days per week.
    A) 90, 1
    B) 120, 2
    C) 150, 2
    D) 180, 1

61. The health belief model assumes that people will engage in a behavior, such as exercise, when _____.
    A) There is a perceived threat of disease.
    B) External motivation is provided.
    C) Optimal environmental conditions are met.
    D) Internal motivation outweighs external circumstances.

62. If a client exercises too much without rest days or develops a minor injury and does not allow time for the injury to heal, what can occur?
    A) An overuse injury
    B) Shin splints
    C) Sleep deprivation
    D) Decreased physical conditioning

63. Which of the following is a *false* statement regarding an informed consent?
    A) The informed consent is not a legal document.
    B) The informed consent does not provide legal immunity to a facility or individual in the event of injury to an individual.
    C) Negligence, improper test administration, inadequate personnel qualifications, and insufficient safety procedures are all items that are expressly covered by the informed consent.
    D) The consent form does not relieve the facility or individual of the responsibility to do everything possible to ensure the safety of the individual.

64. To determine program effectiveness, psychological theories provide a conceptual framework for assessment and _____.
    A) Management of programs or interventions
    B) Application of cognitive-behavioral or motivational principles
    C) Measurement
    D) All of the above

65. An important safety consideration for exercise equipment in a fitness center includes _____.
    A) Flexibility of equipment to allow for different body sizes
    B) Affordability of equipment to allow for changing out equipment periodically
    C) Mobility of equipment to allow for easy rearrangement
    D) None of the above

66. Which of the following personnel is responsible for overall facility management and is often responsible for assisting the development of programs?
    A) Administrative assistant
    B) Front desk staff
    C) Facility operator or program director
    D) CPT

67. What is the purpose of agreements, releases, and consent forms?
    A) To inform the client of participation risks as well as the rights of the client and the facility
    B) To inform the client what he or she can and cannot do in the facility
    C) To define the relationship between the facility operator and the EP-C
    D) To detail the rights and responsibilities of the club owner to reject an application by a prospective client

68. Which of the following is a possible medical emergency that a client can experience during an exercise session?
    A) Hypoglycemia
    B) Hypotension
    C) Hyperglycemia
    D) All of the above

69. Which of the following muscle actions occurs when muscle tension increases but the length of the muscle does not change?
    A) Concentric isotonic
    B) Eccentric isotonic
    C) Isokinetic
    D) Isometric

70. Which of the following activities provides the greatest improvement in aerobic fitness for someone who is beginning an exercise program?
    A) Weight training
    B) Downhill snow skiing
    C) Stretching
    D) Walking

71. A source of intimal injury thought to initiate the process of atherogenesis is _____.
    A) Dyslipidemia
    B) Hypertension
    C) Turbulence of blood flow within the vessel
    D) All of the above

72. According to the ACSM, at what level is high-density lipoprotein (HDL) considered a risk factor in the development of cardiovascular disease (CVD)?
    A) $<200 \text{ mg} \cdot \text{dL}^{-1}$
    B) $<110 \text{ mg} \cdot \text{dL}^{-1}$
    C) $<60 \text{ mg} \cdot \text{dL}^{-1}$
    D) $<40 \text{ mg} \cdot \text{dL}^{-1}$

73. From rest to maximal exercise, the SBP should _____ progressively with an increasing workload.
    A) Increase
    B) Decrease
    C) Stay the same
    D) Decrease with isometric or increase with isotonic contractions

74. Fitness assessment is an important aspect of the training program because it provides information for which of the following?
    A) Developing the Ex R_x
    B) Evaluating proper nutritional choices
    C) Diagnosing musculoskeletal injury
    D) Developing appropriate billing categories

75. Which of the following is an example of how to progressively overload the muscular system via resistance training?
    A) Increasing amount of resistance lifted
    B) Performing more sets per muscle group
    C) Increasing days per week the muscle groups are trained
    D) All of the above are examples of progressive overload.

76. Exercise adherence is increased when _____.
    A) There is social and health care provider support for the individual.
    B) A regular schedule of exercise is established.
    C) Muscle soreness and injury are minimal.
    D) Individualized, attainable goals and objectives are identified.
    E) All of the above

77. Which of the following is a change seen as a result of regular aerobic exercise?
    A) Decreased HR at rest
    B) Increased stroke volume at rest
    C) No change for cardiac output at rest
    D) All of the above

78. While assessing the behavioral changes associated with an exercise program, which of the following would be categorized under the cognitive process of the transtheoretical model?
    A) Stimulus control
    B) Reinforcement management
    C) Self-reevaluation
    D) Self-liberation

79. A measure of muscular endurance is _____.
    A) 1-RM
    B) 3-RM
    C) Number of curl-ups in 1 min
    D) Number of curl-ups in 3 min

80. Following an acute musculoskeletal injury, the appropriate action calls for stabilization of the area and incorporating the RICES treatment method. RICES is the acronym for which of the following?
    A) Recovery, ibuprofen, compression, education, stabilization
    B) Rest and ice, care for injury, support
    C) Rest, ice, compression, elevation, and stabilization
    D) Rotate, ice, care, evaluate, support

81. Implementation of emergency procedures must include the fitness center's _____.
    A) Management
    B) Staff
    C) Clients
    D) Management and staff

82. Which of the following will increase stability?
    A) Lowering the center of gravity
    B) Raising the center of gravity
    C) Decreasing the base of support
    D) Moving the center of gravity farther from the edge of the base of support

83. During aerobic exercise, which of the following responses would *not* be considered normal in individuals without CVD?
    A) Increased SBP
    B) Increased pulse pressure
    C) Increased mean arterial pressure
    D) Increased DBP

84. An exercise program for elderly persons generally should emphasize increased _____.
    A) Frequency
    B) Intensity
    C) Duration
    D) Intensity and frequency

85. The loss of elasticity (or "hardening") of the arteries is known as _____.
    A) Atherosclerosis
    B) Arteriosclerosis
    C) Atheroma
    D) Adventitia

86. Which of the following assumes that a person will adopt appropriate health behaviors if he or she feels the consequences are severe and feel personally vulnerable?
    A) Learning theories
    B) Health belief model
    C) Transtheoretical model
    D) Stages of motivational readiness

87. Generally, low-fit or sedentary persons may benefit from _____.
    A) Shorter duration, higher intensity, and higher frequency of exercise
    B) Longer duration, higher intensity, and higher frequency of exercise
    C) Shorter duration, lower intensity, and higher frequency of exercise
    D) Shorter duration, higher intensity, and lower frequency of exercise

88. In commercial settings, clients should be more extensively screened for potential health risks. The information solicited should include which of the following?
    A) Personal medical history
    B) Present medical status
    C) Medication
    D) All of the above

89. What is the planning tool that addresses the organization's short- and long-term goals; identifies the steps needed to achieve the goals; and gives the time line, priority, and allocation of resources to each goal?
    A) Financial plan
    B) Strategic plan
    C) Risk management plan
    D) Marketing plan

90. When periodizing training for a marathon runner (26.2 mi) who is doing a long run each Sunday, which is appropriate? Each Sunday run should _____.
    A) Be the same distance at about 20–22 mi
    B) Gradually increase in distance weekly with a slightly lower distance Sunday every fourth week or so
    C) Gradually increase in distance every week by about 10%
    D) Rapidly increase distance weekly then avoid all long runs the last 2 months

91. In prevention of osteoporosis, it is important to regularly perform what kind of exercise?
    A) Only chair exercises
    B) Aquatic exercise only
    C) Stationary cycling only
    D) All modes of weight-bearing exercise

92. Both the Karvonen (HRR) and the direct HR_{max} formulas of calculating target heart rate (THR) begin subtracting variables from a set number. What is this first number used in both formulas?
    A) Estimated HR_{max}
    B) Maximal SBP
    C) Body weight
    D) Gender

93. Which grouping lists the three training principles that you need to consider when prescribing exercise for individuals?
    A) Overload, intensity, progression
    B) Frequency, intensity, duration
    C) Specificity, overload, redundancy
    D) Overload, specificity, progression

94. If you want your client to exercise at 55%–70% of her HR_{max} in today's workout and she is 24 yr old and does not know her observed HR_{max}, what HR should she be using today?
    A) 97–123 bpm
    B) 108–137 bpm
    C) 110–140 bpm
    D) 121–154 bpm

95. Which of the following types of muscle stretching can cause residual muscle soreness, is time-consuming, and typically requires a partner?
    A) Static
    B) Ballistic
    C) PNF
    D) All of the above

96. Identify the appropriate subjective self-evaluation tool used as a quick health screening before beginning any exercise program.
    A) Physical Activity Readiness Questionnaire + (PAR-Q+)
    B) Health Status Questionnaire (HSQ)
    C) Exercise electrocardiogram (E-ECG)
    D) RPE-Borg scale (RPE)

97. After completing an examination of your client's health screening documents and the prior physiological resting measurements that were recorded, you decide to proceed with a single session of fitness assessments. Identify the recommended order of administration.
    A) Body composition, flexibility, cardiorespiratory fitness, and muscular fitness
    B) Flexibility, body composition, muscular fitness, and cardiorespiratory fitness
    C) Flexibility, cardiorespiratory fitness, body composition, and muscular fitness
    D) Body composition, cardiorespiratory fitness, muscular fitness, and flexibility

98. When participating in exercise at high altitudes, HR will _____ at the same RPE as compared to when exercising at sea level.
    A) Be lower
    B) Have no relation and cannot be monitored
    C) Be higher
    D) Remain the same

99. Considering the following list of activities, which are considered activities of daily living (ADL)?
    A) Walking (transferring)
    B) Singing
    C) Lifting extremely heavy items
    D) Reading and writing

100. Which of the following exercises should be avoided after the first trimester for a pregnant woman?
    A) Upright exercises such as walking on an outdoor track
    B) Sitting exercises such as semirecumbent cycling
    C) Prone position exercises
    D) Supine position exercises

EP-C EXAMINATION ANSWERS AND EXPLANATIONS

1—B. $<18.5 \text{ kg} \cdot \text{m}^{-2}$

BMI, a calculation of body weight in kilograms divided by height in squared meters, is generally used to establish a relationship between the height of an individual and the amount of mass on that frame. BMI norms have been established by the ACSM and the Expert Panel on the Identification, Evaluation, and Treatment of Overweight and Obesity in Adults. "Normal" BMI is defined as a number between 18.5 and 24.9 $\text{kg} \cdot \text{m}^{-2}$. Therefore, a BMI below 18.5 $\text{kg} \cdot \text{m}^{-2}$ would classify as "underweight," meaning that there is too little mass on the body given its height.

2—C.   5 mm

When recording regional body circumferences, it is recommended that two measurements be recorded (in rotational order) and then averaged together. This helps ensure reliability and accuracy of the measurement. Acceptable error is ±5 mm between measurements. In the event that the two measurements exceed 5 mm in difference, the administrator should remeasure to ensure accurate results.

3—A. >0.86

Due to the different distribution of fat between males and females, risk stratification using WHR is different between men and women. Males tend to carry more visceral fat around the abdomen and subsequently have higher WHR than females. A *very high* risk value is set at >0.95 for young men and >1.03 for men between the ages of 60 and 69 yr. Women carry excess adipose tissue around the hips and buttocks; therefore, the risk of cardiovascular and other diseases is higher at lower ratios compared to males.

4—B.   Maximal volume of oxygen consumed per unit time ($\dot{V}O_{2max}$)

$\dot{V}O_{2max}$ is the best (only) direct measure of cardiorespiratory fitness. $\dot{V}O_{2max}$ is less subject to overestimations and is a far more stable and valid indicator of cardiorespiratory fitness. This is in large part due to the close relation $\dot{V}O_{2max}$ has to the functional capacity of the heart (stroke volume, HR, arteriovenous O_2 difference).

5—D.   Linear

As work rate on a submaximal test increases, HR will respond in a linear manner once it surpasses 110 bpm. HR increases and reaches a steady state at each exercise work rate and will rise incrementally with each stage of exercise. This response will continue at each stage as long as the physiological limits of that individual are not reached.

6—C.   Gender

Males have approximately 15% higher relative $\dot{V}O_{2max}$ than females across different ages and physical activity levels. The Rockport One-Mile Fitness Walking Test formula is $\dot{V}O_{2max}$ (mL · $\text{kg}^{-1} \cdot \text{min}^{-1}$) = 132.853 − (0.1692 × body mass in kg) − (0.3877 × age in years) + (6.315 × gender) − (3.2649 × time in minutes) − (0.1565 × HR), where gender = 0 for female, 1 for male. The Rockport regression equation adjusts for the physiological advantage males have over females.

7—B.   300 or 450 $\text{kg} \cdot \text{m} \cdot \text{min}^{-1}$ (50 or 75 W)

The Astrand-Rhyming protocol provides varying work rates depending on gender and fitness level. For untrained, female individuals, the minimum recommendation protocol is 50 revolutions per minute (RPM) with a load of 1 kg (on a Monark cycle ergometer with 6 m flywheel circumference). 1 kg · 6 m · 50 RPM = 300 $\text{kg} \cdot \text{m} \cdot \text{min}^{-1}$. The range of up to 450 $\text{kg} \cdot \text{m} \cdot \text{min}^{-1}$ allows for some physical fitness variation within the population.

8—C.   3 min

The Queens College Step Test lasts 3 min in order to provide steady-state HR as a result of aerobic exercise. Then, to estimate $\dot{V}O_{2max}$, early recovery HR is measured for 15 s (multiplied by 4). Exercise less than 3 min runs the risk of not establishing steady-state HR, and exercise greater than 5 min is redundant, as HR has plateaued and continued exercise introduces the potential of local muscular fatigue.

9—B.   Implementation

Clinical exercise testing generally consists of three components: prognosis (determining the risk for an adverse event), evaluation (determining the physiological response to exercise), and diagnosis (determining the presence of a disease/disorder).

10—A.   Maximal exercise test using indirect calorimetry

Maximal exercise testing, usually conducted as a graded exercise or exercise tolerance test, provides the truest measure of exercise capacity (*e.g.*, peak oxygen uptake [$\dot{V}O_{2peak}$]) for each individual. All other forms of testing/examination rely on estimations, which, although beneficial, often over- or undercompensate and can therefore be misleading.

11—D. The supervising physician

In a diagnostic clinical setting, exercise testing should be conducted under the auspices of a physician. However, recent trends have moved many exercise testing laboratories away from the physician and toward allied health paraprofessionals (*e.g.*, clinical exercise physiologists, physician assistants). This has been done in large part as a cost-cutting move as well as to free up time for physicians. The use of these paraprofessionals to administer exercise testing can be done legally as long as the supervising physician is "in the immediate vicinity . . . and available for emergencies." However, it is important to note that the safety of the client is still the priority of the supervising physician.

12—A. Bruce treadmill protocol

Treadmill protocols remain the most popular form of clinical exercise testing in the United States. Cycle ergometry has become increasingly popular in Europe; however, it has been shown that cycle ergometry can underestimate peak exercise capacity by 5%–20%. The Bruce protocol continues to be the most commonly used protocol for exercise testing due to its familiarity among physicians, amount of research supporting the protocol, and ability to be modified to meet the needs of low functional capacity clients.

13—C. 6 min

Following completion of peak exercise during a clinical exercise test, the test administrator should continue to monitor the vital signs of the client regularly (*e.g.*, every 1–2 min) through at least 6 min of recovery. This timeframe is used to help determine the rate of return of vital signs as well as to ensure the health and safety of the client following exhaustive work. This is particularly true in cases where low functional capacity exists or the risk of a sudden cardiac event is elevated.

14—A. 10 bpm

Research has suggested that for every MET increase, the subsequent HR response should be approximately 10 bpm. This rise is sufficient to challenge the heart to appropriately respond to the increased metabolic demand.

15—C. Improvement in range of motion (ROM)

Improvements in ROM are a benefit of the stretching phase of an exercise session. Although oftentimes included as part of the cool-down, the stretching phase is distinct and should follow the cool-down phase. This is to promote improved flexibility and ROM in the muscles, as they will still be warm from the increased blood flow during the exercise session.

16—C. $3\text{–}5 \text{ d} \cdot \text{wk}^{-1}$

It is recommended that individuals perform a minimum of $5 \text{ d} \cdot \text{wk}^{-1}$, or vigorous-intensity aerobic exercise done at least $3 \text{ d} \cdot \text{wk}^{-1}$, or a weekly combination of $3\text{–}5 \text{ d} \cdot \text{wk}^{-1}$ of moderate- and vigorous-intensity exercise to promote and maintain health and fitness benefits. Aerobic exercise performed less than $3 \text{ d} \cdot \text{wk}^{-1}$ does not provide the body with enough stimulus to maximize improvements in cardiorespiratory fitness. Benefits from aerobic exercise performed in excess of $5 \text{ d} \cdot \text{wk}^{-1}$ have been suggested to plateau as well as increase the risk of musculoskeletal injury and burnout.

17—B. 52%

Moderate-intensity aerobic exercise is considered to fall in the range of 40%–59% of an individual's HRR ($HR_{max} - HR_{rest}$). Vigorous exercise includes an HRR range of 60%–89%.

18—D. Maximum heart rate percentage (%HR_{max})

It is not recommended to use HR-dependent methods when prescribing exercise intensities because of the over/underestimation that can occur. Additionally, HR can vary depending on the method used to establish HR (*e.g.*, palpation, HR monitor). Direct measurements of physiological responses (HRR, $\dot{V}O_2R$, VT, etc.) are preferred because these tend to be less subject to variation and provide a truer indication of fitness.

19—A. $500\text{–}1,000 \text{ MET-min} \cdot \text{wk}^{-1}$

This volume of EE is considered adequate for most adults. An exercise volume between 500 and $1,000 \text{ MET-min} \cdot \text{wk}^{-1}$ is roughly equivalent to (a) $1,000 \text{ kcal} \cdot \text{wk}^{-1}$ of moderate-intensity physical activity (or about 150 min wk^{-1}); (b) an exercise intensity of 3–5.9 METs (for individuals weighing ~68–91 kg [~150–200 lb]); and (c) $10 \text{ MET-h} \cdot \text{wk}^{-1}$. These have all been associated with improved physical health and well-being as well as significantly lower rates of CVD and premature mortality.

20—C. 48 h

Exercising muscle requires time to recover/repair in between bouts. If inadequate recovery time is given to muscle prior to exercising again, the muscle will continue to damage and subsequent performance will be compromised. The general consensus is a minimum of 48 h of recovery to ensure the body has time to repair the damage to the muscle fiber. Some individuals may require longer (upward of 96 h). It is important to note that split routines and other variations of resistance training can allow for individuals to continue to work within that 48 h window as long as care is given to not engage the previously exercised muscle group(s) during succeeding bouts.

21—A. To bring in extra income to pay off other major expenses of the testing company

The purpose of physical fitness testing is not and should not be for any reason other than to benefit the participant. Even research studies involving physical fitness testing should offer beneficial data for the study's participants. Educating, motivating, and evaluating the progress of participants are all effective purposes of physical fitness testing.

22—D. HR_{rest}, Queens College Step Test, ACSM push-up test, sit-and-reach test

To get the most accurate and appropriate information, the following order of testing is recommended: resting measurements (*e.g.*, HR, BP, blood analysis), body composition, cardiorespiratory fitness (*e.g.*, Queens College Step Test), muscular fitness (*e.g.*, ACSM push-up test), and flexibility (*e.g.*, sit-and-reach test). Often, several methods of body composition assessment are sensitive to hydration status, and some tests of cardiorespiratory and muscular fitness may affect hydration. Therefore, it is inappropriate to administer those specific tests before the body composition assessment. Assessing cardiorespiratory fitness often uses measures of HR. Some tests of muscular fitness and flexibility affect HR. Hence, they are inappropriate to administer before cardiorespiratory fitness testing since the elevated HR from those assessments may have a negative impact on the cardiorespiratory fitness testing results.

23—B. Sarcopenia

Similar to osteoporosis (loss of bone mass due to aging and reduced physical activity), sarcopenia is associated with a reduced ability to perform ADL and increases the risk of musculoskeletal injury. Muscular strength and endurance may improve or maintain bone mass and muscle mass, thus reducing the risk of osteoporosis and sarcopenia.

24—B. YMCA bench press test

The YMCA bench press test is a valid test for upper body muscular endurance because the test is conducted with a set resistance and the goal is to successfully complete as many repetitions as possible.

25—C. Suprailiac

The suprailiac skinfold site should be a diagonal fold in line with the natural angle of the iliac crest taken in the anterior axillary line immediately superior to the iliac crest.

26—D. Resting systolic blood pressure (SBP) between 125 and 140 mm Hg or diastolic blood pressure (DBP) between 60 and 75 mm Hg

A contraindication is any situation in which the risk associated with undergoing the exercise test is likely to exceed the information to be gained from it. Box 5.2: Contraindications to Symptom-Limited Maximal Exercise Testing outlines the contraindications of clinical exercise testing. Resting SBP above 200 mm Hg or DBP above 110 mm Hg are the appropriate contraindications.

Resource: Riebe D, senior editor. *ACSM's Guidelines for Exercise Testing and Prescription.* 10th ed. Philadelphia (PA): Wolters Kluwer; 2018.

27—B. Maximal exercise testing is not a realistic way to identify candidates for cardiac transplantation or other advanced treatments due to inherent risk of heart stress.

Maximal exercise testing with measurement of respiratory gas exchange is reasonable to identify high-risk patients presenting with HF who are candidates for cardiac transplantation or other advanced treatments according to Box 5.1: Select Evidence-Based Recommendations Regarding the Utility of Clinical Exercise Testing among Patients with Heart Disease.

Resource: Riebe D, senior editor. *ACSM's Guidelines for Exercise Testing and Prescription.* 10th ed. Philadelphia (PA): Wolters Kluwer; 2018.

28—B. Specificity

As indicated in Box 5.6 in regard to ischemic heart disease (IHD), specificity is the percentage of patients without IHD who have a negative test for IHD. So, specificity represents the true negative cases among the test sample.

Resource: Riebe D, senior editor. *ACSM's Guidelines for Exercise Testing and Prescription.* 10th ed. Philadelphia (PA): Wolters Kluwer; 2018.

29—A. Achievement of age-predicted HR_{max}

ACSM considers "failure of HR to increase with increases in workload" as the criterion used to confirm that a maximal effort has been elicited.

30—C. 140/90 mm Hg

To be classified as hypertensive, the SBP must equal or exceed 140 mm Hg or the DBP must equal or exceed 90 mm Hg as measured on two separate occasions, preferably days apart. An elevation of either the systolic or diastolic pressure is classified as hypertension.

31—C.   Provides an explanation of the test to the client.

Informed consent is not a legal document. It does not provide legal immunity to a facility or individual in the event of injury to a client nor does it legally protect the rights of the client. It simply provides evidence that the client was made aware of the purposes, procedures, and risks associated with the test or exercise program. The consent form does not relieve the facility or individual of the responsibility to do everything possible to ensure the safety of the client. Negligence, improper test administration, inadequate personnel qualifications, and insufficient safety procedures all are items that are not expressly covered by informed consent. Because of the limitations associated with informed consent documents, legal counsel should be sought during the development of the document.

32—A.   Cardiopulmonary resuscitation (CPR) and ACSM Certified Exercise Physiologist (EP-C)

At minimum, professionals performing fitness assessments on others should possess CPR and ACSM EP-C certification.

33—D.   All of the above

In addition to cardiorespiratory fitness, body composition, and neuromotor fitness, the ideal exercise training program should also address muscular strength, muscular endurance, and flexibility in most adults who are seeking to maintain or improve their all-around fitness.

34—B.   Active static stretching

Static stretching is characteristic of a lack of movement during the stretch, where the stretch is held for a period of time (*i.e.*, 10–30 s). The primary difference between active and passive static stretching is the source of assistance. In passive static stretching, the muscle/tendon group being stretched is held by a partner or device such as an elastic band.

35—A.   5; 3

The ACSM provides evidence-based recommendations (Table 6.5) of at least 5 d · wk^{-1} of moderate exercise, or at least 3 d · wk^{-1} of vigorous exercise, or a combination of moderate and vigorous exercise on at least 3–5 · wk^{-1}.

Resource: Riebe D, senior editor. *ACSM's Guidelines for Exercise Testing and Prescription*. 10th ed. Philadelphia (PA): Wolters Kluwer; 2018.

36—C.   310.5 kcal

Caloric expenditure = Absolute O_2 consumed × Caloric equivalent

The steps are as follows:
- Convert 175 lb to 79.55 kg (divide by 2.2)
- Convert relative $\dot{V}O_2$ of 26 mL · kg^{-1} · min^{-1} to absolute $\dot{V}O_2$ of 2.07 L · min^{-1}
- With an absolute O_2 consumption of 2.07 L · min^{-1}, you can then multiply by 5 kcal · min^{-1} (caloric equivalent) and then by 30 min of exercise, which will give you 310 kcal total for the exercise session.

37—A.   Resistance training composed exclusively of eccentric contractions conducted at very high intensities

The ACSM issued a position statement in 2009 regarding progression models in resistance training for healthy adults that discussed this very topic. Eccentric training at very high intensities (*i.e.*, >100% 1-RM) should absolutely be avoided. Rhabdomyolysis is muscle damage resulting in excretion of myoglobin into the urine that may harm kidney function.

38—C.   Stimulate appetite

Older people who exercise regularly report greater life satisfaction (older people who exercise regularly have a more positive attitude toward their work and generally are in better health than sedentary persons), greater happiness (strong correlations have been reported between the activity level of older adults and self-reported happiness), higher self-efficacy (older persons taking part in exercise programs commonly report that they can do everyday tasks more easily than before they began exercising), improved self-concept and self-esteem (older adults improve their score on self-concept questionnaires following participation in an exercise program), and reduced psychological stress (exercise is effective in reducing psychological stress without unwanted side effects).

39—B.   Children should perform 30 min of moderate-intensity and 30 min of vigorous-intensity physical activity on most days of the week.

This is according to the *2008 Physical Activity Guidelines for Americans*. Activity that is intermittent in nature is preferred for children over continuous exercise because this is the type of activity they naturally self-select. Active play versus exercise should be emphasized. Children should attempt to accumulate 60 or more minutes of physical activity daily, this may be continuous or discontinuous activity. Children should not focus on just one or two modes. Exposing them to a wide variety of physical activities is suggested to enhance adherence. Finally, children should not have prolonged periods during the day that are sedentary because this may promote negative health consequences.

40—C. Frequency, intensity, time, type, volume, and progression

Frequency (how often), intensity (how hard), time (duration or how long), type (mode or what kind), total volume (amount), and progression (advancement) or the FITT-VP principle of Ex R_x provides recommendations on exercise pattern to be consistent with the ACSM recommendations made in its companion evidence-based position stand (Garber CE, Blissmer B, Deschenes MR, et al. 2011).

41—A. Cardiorespiratory fitness, muscular strength, muscular endurance, flexibility, body composition, and neuromotor fitness

The optimal Ex R_x should address cardiorespiratory (aerobic) fitness, muscular strength and endurance, flexibility, body composition, and neuromotor fitness.

42—C. 5 d · wk^{-1}

Moderate-intensity aerobic exercise done at least 5 d · wk^{-1}, or vigorous-intensity aerobic exercise done at least 3 d · wk^{-1}, or a weekly combination of 3–5 d · wk^{-1} of moderate- and vigorous-intensity exercise is recommended for most adults to achieve and maintain health/fitness benefits.

43—D. 3 d · wk^{-1}

Moderate-intensity aerobic exercise done at least 5 d · wk^{-1}, or vigorous-intensity aerobic exercise done at least 3 d · wk^{-1} or a weekly combination of 3–5 d · wk^{-1} of moderate- and vigorous-intensity exercise is recommended for most adults to achieve and maintain health/fitness benefits.

44—B. 40%–59% HRR or $\dot{V}O_2R$

Moderate (*e.g.*, 40%–59% HRR or $\dot{V}O_2R$) to vigorous (*e.g.*, 60%–89% HRR or $\dot{V}O_2R$) intensity aerobic exercise is recommended for most adults, and light (*e.g.*, 30%–39% HRR or $\dot{V}O_2R$) to moderate intensity aerobic exercise can be beneficial in individuals who are deconditioned.

45—D. 60%–89% HRR or $\dot{V}O_2R$

Moderate (*e.g.*, 40%–59% HRR or $\dot{V}O_2R$) to vigorous (*e.g.*, 60%–89% HRR or $\dot{V}O_2R$) intensity aerobic exercise is recommended for most adults, and light (*e.g.*, 30%–39% HRR or $\dot{V}O_2R$) to moderate intensity aerobic exercise can be beneficial in individuals who are deconditioned.

46—A. 30–60 min · d^{-1}

Most adults are recommended to accumulate 30–60 min · d^{-1} ($\geq$150 min · wk^{-1}) of moderate-intensity exercise, 20–60 min · d^{-1} ($\geq$75 min · wk^{-1}) of vigorous-intensity exercise, or a combination of moderate- and vigorous-intensity exercise per day to attain the volumes of exercise recommended (Garber CE, Blissmer B, Deschenes MR, et al. 2011; U.S. Department of Health and Human Services. 2008 Physical Activity Guidelines for Americans [Internet] 2008).

47—C. 7,000 steps · d^{-1}

The goal of 10,000 steps · d^{-1} is often cited, but achieving a pedometer step count of at least 5,400–7,900 steps · d^{-1} can meet recommended exercise targets, with the higher end of the range showing more consistent benefit (Garber CE, Blissmer B, Deschenes MR, et al. 2011; Tudor-Locke C, Hatano Y, Pangrazi RP, Kang M. 2008). For this reason and the imprecision of step counting devices, a target of at least 7,000 steps is recommended for most people.

48—B. Muscular endurance, muscular power, and muscular strength

The ACSM uses the phrase "muscular fitness" to refer collectively to muscular strength, endurance, and power.

49—A. 2–4 sets with 8–12 repetitions

Ideally, adults should train each muscle group for a total of 2–4 sets with 8–12 repetitions per set.

50—C. Antihyperlipidemics

Nitrates and nitroglycerine are antianginals (used to reduce chest pain associated with angina pectoris). β-Blockers are antihypertensives (used to reduce BP by inhibiting the action of adrenergic neurotransmitters at the β-receptor, thereby promoting peripheral vasodilation). β-Blockers also are designed to reduce BP by inhibiting the action of adrenergic neurotransmitters at the β-receptors, thereby decreasing . Antihyperlipidemics control blood lipids, especially cholesterol and low-density lipoprotein (LDL). Aspirin is used to control for blood platelet stickiness.

51—C. Triglycerides

Dietary fats include triglycerides, sterols (*e.g.*, cholesterol), and phospholipids. Triglycerides represent more than 90% of the fat stored in the body. A *triglyceride* is a glycerol molecule connected to three fatty acid molecules. The fatty acids are identified by the amount of "saturation" or the number of single or double bonds that link the carbon atoms. Saturated fatty acids only have single bonds. Monounsaturated fatty acids have one double bond, and polyunsaturated fatty acids have two or more double bonds.

52—D. 118/84 mm Hg

The prehypertensive category is 120–139 mm Hg/80–89 mm Hg. To be classified as hypertensive, the SBP must equal or exceed 140 mm Hg or the diastolic pressure must equal or exceed 90 mm Hg as measured on two separate occasions, preferably days apart. An elevation of either the systolic or diastolic pressure is classified as hypertension.

53—A. Approximately 10 mm Hg

During dynamic exercise, SBP will increase in a direct proportion to exercise intensity. The increase in SBP is due to the increase in which helps to facilitate increase in blood flow to the exercising muscles. The increase in SBP is expected to rise 5–10 mm Hg per MET of effort. By definition, 1 MET being roughly equivalent to the energy expended during rest.

54—C. A slight decrease in diastolic pressure

During dynamic exercise, DBP may not change much or even decrease slightly because it represents the pressure in heart during diastole (rest).

55—C. 60% and 90%

Several methods are available to define exercise intensity objectively. The ACSM recommends that exercise intensity be prescribed within a range of 64%–70% and 94% of HR_{max} or between 40% and 50% and 85% of $\dot{V}O_2R$. Lower intensities will elicit a favorable response in individuals with very low fitness levels. Because of the variability in estimating HR_{max} from age, it is recommended that, whenever possible, an actual HR_{max} from a GXT be used. Factors to consider when determining appropriate exercise intensity include age, fitness level, medications, overall health status, and individual goals.

56—B. 15–25

Per *ACSM's Guidelines For Exercise Testing and Prescription* (GETP), 10th edition, "To improve muscular endurance rather than strength and mass, a higher number of repetitions, perhaps 15–25, should be performed per set along with shorter rest intervals and fewer sets (*i.e.*, 1 or 2 sets per muscle group) (American College of Sports Medicine. American College of Sports Medicine position stand. Progression models in resistance training for healthy adults. 2009; Garber CE, Blissmer B, Deschenes MR, et al. 2011). This regimen necessitates a lower intensity of resistance, typically of no more than 50% 1-RM."

57—B. The risk of orthopedic and cardiovascular complications is increased.

The risk of orthopedic and, perhaps, cardiovascular complications can be increased with high-intensity activity. Factors to consider when determining exercise intensity include the individual's level of fitness, presence of medications that may influence exercise performance, risk of cardiovascular or orthopedic injury, and individual preference for exercise and individual program objectives.

58—C. 8–12

Eight to 12 repetitions represent a relatively low intensity of 67%–80% of 1-RM. This low intensity allows the development of muscular endurance and reduces the risk of musculoskeletal related injuries.

59—B. Intrinsic reward

Reinforcement is the positive or negative consequence for performing or not performing a behavior. *Positive consequences* are rewards that motivate behavior. This can include both intrinsic and extrinsic rewards. *Intrinsic rewards* are the benefits gained because of the rewarding nature of the activity. *Extrinsic* or external rewards are the positive outcomes received from others, which may include encouragement and praise or material reinforcements such as T-shirts and money.

60—C. 150–2

The *2015–2020 Dietary Guidelines for Americans* recommends that adults need at least 150 minutes of moderate-intensity physical activity and should perform muscle-strengthening exercises on 2 or more days each week.

61—A. There is a perceived threat of disease.

The health belief model assumes that people will engage in a behavior (*e.g.*, exercise) when there exist a perceived threat of disease and a belief of susceptibility to disease, and the threat of disease is severe. This model also incorporates cues to action as critical to adopting and maintaining behavior. The concept of self-efficacy (confidence) is also added to this model. Motivation and environmental considerations are not a part of the health belief model.

62—A. An overuse injury

Overuse injuries become more common when people participate in more cardiovascular exercise by increasing time, duration, or intensity too quickly. A client exercises too much without time for rest and recovery or develops a minor injury and does not reduce or change that exercise allowing the injury to heal.

63—C. Negligence, improper test administration, inadequate personnel qualifications, and insufficient safety procedures are all items that are expressly covered by the informed consent.

Negligence, improper test administration, inadequate personnel qualifications, and insufficient safety procedures are all items that are expressly *not* covered by the informed consent. The informed consent is also not a legal document; it does not provide legal immunity to a facility or individual in the event of injury to a person, and it does not relieve the facility or individual of the responsibility to do everything possible to ensure the safety of an individual.

64—B. Application of cognitive-behavioral or motivational principles

Psychological theories are the foundations for effective use of strategies and techniques of effective counseling and motivational skill building for exercise adoption and maintenance. Theories provide a conceptual framework for development rather than management, of programs or interventions. Psychological theories facilitate evaluation of program effectiveness, not just measurement of outcomes. Within the field of behavioral change, a theory is a set of assumptions that accounts for the relationships between certain variables and the behavior of interest.

65—A. Flexibility of equipment to allow for different body sizes

Creating a safe environment in which to exercise is a primary responsibility of any fitness facility. In developing and operating facilities and equipment for use by exercisers, the managers and staff are obligated to meet a standard of care for exerciser safety. The equipment to be used includes not only testing, cardiovascular, strength, and flexibility pieces but also rehabilitation, pool, locker room, and emergency equipment. You must evaluate several criteria when selecting equipment. These criteria include correct anatomic positioning, ability to adjust to different body sizes, quality of design and materials, durability, repair records, and then price.

66—C. Facility operator or program director

The characteristics of a good facility operator or program director include designing programs and monitoring the implementation of programs. He or she also guides the staff or clients through the program. He or she is a good communicator who also purchases equipment and supplies. A good facility operator monitors the safety of the program or facility and surveys clients and staff to assess the success and value of the program.

67—A. To inform the client of participation risks as well as the rights of the client and the facility

Agreements, releases, and consents are documents that clearly describe what the client is participating in, the risks involved, and the rights of the client and the facility. If signed by the client, he or she is accepting some of the responsibility and risk by participating in this program. All fitness facilities are strongly encouraged to have program or service agreements and informed consents drafted by a lawyer for their protection.

68—D. All of the above

Possible medical emergencies during exercise include heat exhaustion or heat stroke, fainting, hypoglycemia, hyperglycemia, simple or compound fractures, bronchospasm, hypotension or shock, seizures, bleeding, and other cardiac symptoms.

69—D. Isometric

Isometric muscle action, also known as static muscle action, occurs when muscle tension increases with no overt muscular or limb movement; the length of the muscle does not change. These actions occur when with an attempt to push or pull against an immovable object. Measures of static strength are specific to both the muscle group and joint angle being tested; therefore, these tests' usefulness to generalize overall muscular strength is limited.

70—D. Walking

Large muscle group activity performed in rhythmic fashion over prolonged periods facilitates the greatest improvements in aerobic fitness. Walking, running, cycling, swimming, stair climbing, aerobic dance, rowing, and cross-country skiing are examples of these types of activities. Weight training should not be considered an appropriate activity for enhancing aerobic fitness but should be part of in a comprehensive exercise program to improve muscular strength and muscular endurance. The mode of activity should be selected based on the principle of specificity — that is, with attention to the desired outcomes — and to maintain the participation and enjoyment of the individual.

71—D. All of the above

Initial causes of coronary artery disease (CAD) are thought to be an irritation of, or an injury to, the tunica intima (the innermost of the three layers in the wall) of the blood vessel. Sources of this initial injury are thought to be caused by dyslipidemia (elevated total blood cholesterol), hypertension (chronic high BP, either an elevation of SBP or DBP measured on two different days), immune responses, smoking, tumultuous and nonlaminar blood flow in the lumen of the coronary artery (turbulence), vasoconstrictor substances (chemicals that cause the smooth muscle cells in the walls of the vessel to contract, resulting in a reduction in the diameter of the lumen), and viral infections.

72—D. <40 mg $\cdot$ dL^{-1}

Risk factors that contribute to the development of CAD include age (men, >45 yr; women, >55 yr), a family history of myocardial infarction or sudden death (male first-degree relatives <55 yr and female first-degree relatives <65 yr), cigarette smoking, hypertension (arterial BP $>140/90$ mm Hg measured on two separate occasions), hypercholesterolemia (total cholesterol >200 mg $\cdot$ dL^{-1} or 5.2 mmol $\cdot$ L^{-1}, or HDL <40 mg $\cdot$ dL^{-1} or 1.04 mmol $\cdot$ L^{-1}), and diabetes mellitus in individuals older than 30 yr or in individuals who have had Type 1 diabetes more than 15 yr or Type 2 diabetes in individuals older than 35 yr. Other risk factors contribute to the development of CAD but are not primary risk factors.

73—A.   Increase

SBP is an indicator of the amount of blood pumped out of the heart in 1 min in a healthy vascular system and normally increases as workload increases because the peripheral and central stimuli that control this specific process also normally increase with an increase in workload. Thus, SBP should increase with an increase in workload. Failure of the SBP to increase as workload increases indicates an abnormal response to increasing workload. Additionally, an abnormally elevated SBP response to aerobic exercise indicates an unhealthy vascular system.

74—A.   Developing the Ex R$_x$

The purpose of the fitness assessment is to develop a proper Ex R$_x$ (the data collected through appropriate fitness assessments assist the health fitness specialist in developing safe, effective programs of exercise based on the individual client's current fitness status), to evaluate the rate of progress (baseline and follow-up testing indicate progression toward fitness goals), and to motivate (fitness assessments provide information needed to develop reasonable, attainable goals). Progress toward or attainment of a goal is a strong motivator for continued participation in an exercise program.

75—D.   All of the above are examples of progressive overload.

By definition, *progressive overload* is a principle of training that states that the stress on the musculoskeletal system needs to progressively increase in order to keep producing greater force. This could be achieved by increasing the intensity (resistance), the number of rep or sets, and/or the number of exercise session per week.

76—E.   All of the above

Different factors affect exercise adherence. Some are situational in nature such as social support and time commitment, whereas others are personal (individualized). In order for a trainee to "stick" to an exercise routine, many of these factors must be met.

77—D.   All of the above

The effects of regular (chronic) exercise can be classified or grouped into those that occur at rest, during moderate (or submaximal) exercise, and during maximal effort work. For example, you can measure an untrained individual's HR$_{rest}$, train the person for several weeks or months, and then measure HR$_{rest}$ again to see what change has occurred. HR$_{rest}$ declines with regular exercise probably because of a combination of decreased sympathetic tone, increased parasympathetic tone, and decreased intrinsic firing rate of the sinoatrial node. Stroke volume increases at rest as a result of increased time for ventricular filling and an increased myocardial contractility. Little or no change occurs in cardiac output at rest because the decline in HR is compensated for by the increase in stroke volume.

78—C.   Self-reevaluation

Key components of the transtheoretical model are the processes of behavioral change. These processes include five cognitive processes (consciousness raising, dramatic relief, environmental reevaluation, self-reevaluation, and social liberation) and five behavioral processes (counterconditioning, helping relationships, reinforcement management, self-liberation, and stimulus control).

79—C.   Number of curl-ups in 1 min

Three common assessments for muscular endurance include the bench press, for upper body endurance (a weight is lifted in cadence with a metronome or other timing device; the total number of lifts performed correctly and in time with the cadence); the push-up, for upper body endurance (the client assumes a standardized beginning position with the body held rigid and supported by the hands and toes for men and the hands and knees for women; the body is lowered to the floor and then pushed back up to the starting position; the score is the total number of properly performed push-ups completed without a pause by the client, with no time limit); and the curl-up (crunch), for abdominal muscular endurance (the client begins in the bent-knee sit-up with knees at 90 degrees, the arms at the side, palms facing down with middle fingers touching masking tape. A second piece of tape is placed 10 cm apart. OR set a metronome to 50 bpm and the client performs slow, controlled curl-ups to lift the shoulder blades off the mat with the trunk making a 30-degree angle, in time with the metronome at a rate of 25 per minute done for 1 min. OR the client performs as many curl-ups as possible in 1 min).

80—C. Rest, ice, compression, elevation, and stabilization

Basic principles of care for musculoskeletal injuries include the objectives for care of exercise-related injuries, which are to decrease pain, reduce swelling, and prevent further injury. These objectives can be met in most cases by following "RICES" guidelines. RICES stands for rest, ice, compression, elevation, and stabilization. Rest will prevent further injury and ensure that the healing process will begin. Ice is used to reduce swelling, bleeding, inflammation, and pain. Compression also helps to reduce swelling and bleeding. Compression is achieved by the use of elastic wraps or tape. Elevation helps to decrease the blood flow and excessive pressure to the injured area. Stabilization allows musculature surrounding the injury to relax.

81—D. Management and staff

When an emergency or injury occurs, safe and effective management of the situation will assure the best care for the individual. Implementing emergency procedures is an important part of the training of the staff. In-services, safety plans, and emergency procedures should be a part of the staff training. In addition, all exercise staff should be CPR-certified and knowledgeable of first aid. Therefore, the fitness center management and staff all are included in the implementation of an emergency plan.

82—A. Lowering the center of gravity

Lowering the center of gravity will increase stability. Stability would also be increased by increasing the size of the base of support, by moving the center of gravity closer to the center of the base of support, or both.

83—D. Increased DBP

Because of the vasodilation associated with exercise-induced stimulation of the sympathetic nervous system, DBP remains unchanged, or even slightly decreased, during exercise. In those with known CVD, aerobic exercise may illicit increases in DBP at the beginning of exercise.

84—A. Frequency

Increased frequency of exercise is generally recommended for older adults to optimize cardiovascular as well as balance and flexibility adaptations. The recommended duration of exercise depends on the intensity of the activity because higher intensity activity should be conducted over a shorter period of time.

85—B. Arteriosclerosis

Arteriosclerosis, also called hardening of the arteries, is a loss of arterial elasticity and is associated with aging. Atherosclerosis is a form of arteriosclerosis characterized by an accumulation of obstructive lesions within the arterial wall. The *adventitia*, the outermost layer of the artery wall, provides the media and intima with oxygen and other nutrients.

86—B. Health belief model

The health belief model is a theoretical framework to help explain and predict interventions to increase physical activity. The model originated in the 1950s based on work by Rosenstock. Learning theories assume that an overall complex behavior arises from many small simple behaviors. By reinforcing partial behaviors and modifying cues in the environment, it is possible to shape the desired behavior.

87—C. Shorter duration, lower intensity, and higher frequency of exercise

The number of times per day or per week that a person exercises is interrelated with both the intensity and the duration of activity. Generally, sedentary persons or those with poor fitness may benefit from multiple short-duration, low-intensity exercise sessions per day. Individual goals, preferences, limitations, and time constraints also will determine frequency and the relationship between duration, frequency, and intensity.

88—D. All of the above

Different types of health screenings are used for various purposes. In commercial settings, clients should be screened more extensively for potential health risks. At minimum, a personal medical history should be taken. In addition, present medical status should be examined and questions asked regarding the use of medications (both prescription and over-the-counter).

89—B. Strategic plan

The strategic plan addresses strategic decisions of the organization in defining short- and long-term goals and serves as the overarching planning tool. Health and fitness programs, financial plans, risk management efforts, and marketing plans only address subsegments within the overall strategic plan.

90—B. Gradually increase in distance weekly with a slight lower distance Sunday every fourth week or so

The runner could become overtrained if he or she just built up to a longer distance each week without a down week built in periodically, even if done gradually. Doing the same distance weekly will not allow the runner to reach the race distance, therefore never allowing them to prepare for the actual race mileage. Periodization must be done gradually. If increased too rapidly, the runner may become injured or overtrained.

91—D. All modes of weight-bearing exercise

Regularly participating in weight-bearing exercises such as walking or running is important to keep bone mineral density high in order to decrease risk of developing osteoporosis. Water exercise is not considered weight-bearing because of the buoyancy effect of the water. Intensity, whether it is high or low, is not relevant in this case. What matters is if the exercise involves supporting the weight.

92—A. Estimated HR_{max}

The number that you subtract from originally is the estimated HR_{max}. With each year of life (age), we estimate that we lose one beat in terms of our HR_{max} (*i.e.*, 220 − age). It has nothing to do with SBP, weight, or gender.

93—D. Overload, specificity, progression

The three training principles are overload, specificity, and progression. Redundancy does not have anything to do with it. Although frequency, intensity, and duration are important items to consider with exercise programming, they are not considered training principles. *Overload* is pushing the body beyond what it is used to, *specificity* is being careful to choose exercises that closely relate to the outcome goal, and *progression* has to do with developing a systematic method of improving.

94—B. 108–137 bpm

You begin by subtracting her age of 24 yr from 220, which is her estimated HR_{max} at her current age. Then multiply both 0.55 and 0.70 to 196 bpm to get your answers. Answer letter A is incorrect because it subtracted her age from 200 instead of 220. Answer letter C is incorrect because it used 200 with no age adjustment, and answer letter D is incorrect because it used 220 with no age adjustment, which gave too high of a value.

95—C. PNF

PNF is a stretching technique that combines the use of isometric contractions with passive static stretching. This stretching technique involves the use of a partner and a few cycles and, therefore, is more time-consuming than the other stretching techniques (static and dynamic).

96—A. Physical Activity Readiness Questionnaire + (PAR-Q+)

The PAR-Q+ is a screening tool for self-directed exercise programming. The HSQ is a screening tool with similarities to the PAR-Q+, but it takes longer to complete versus the quick completion of the PAR-Q+. The RPE-Borg scale is used to measure or to RPE during exercise or during an exercise test. The E-ECG would involve continuous electrical heart monitoring during exercise stress test used in a clinical setting when deemed appropriate by a physician.

97—D. Body composition, cardiorespiratory fitness, muscular fitness, and flexibility

To get the most accurate and appropriate information, the following order of testing is recommended: resting measurements (*e.g.*, HR, BP, blood analysis), body composition, cardiorespiratory fitness, muscular fitness, and flexibility. Often, several methods of body composition assessment are sensitive to hydration status, and some tests of cardiorespiratory and muscular fitness may affect hydration. Therefore, it is inappropriate to administer those specific tests before the body composition assessment. Assessing cardiorespiratory fitness often uses measures of HR. Some tests of muscular fitness and flexibility affect HR. Hence, they are inappropriate to administer before cardiorespiratory fitness testing because the elevated HR from those assessments may have a negative impact on the cardiorespiratory fitness testing results.

98—C. Be higher

When engaging in physical activity or exercise at high altitude, HR will be higher than at sea level for the same perceived exertion because of the decreased supply of oxygen available. If one was to compete in endurance-oriented events at high altitude, it would be wise to properly acclimate to the "competition or event" altitude prior to the actual competitive event. Also note that dehydration is often an issue at high altitude, so it is important to adequately hydrate before, during, and after training or competing.

99—A. Walking (transferring)

Out of the list of possible choices, walking is the only choice that is considered an ADL. The six ADL are eating, bathing, dressing, toileting, transferring (walking), and continence. Although it is great to be able to lift a medium to moderately heavy weights, sing, read, and write, it is not necessary for ADL.

100—D. Supine position exercises

Exercises in the supine (lying on your back) position could cause mild obstruction of venous return, which decreases, and may cause BP to drop dangerously low. Exercise in the prone position may be uncomfortable if not contraindicated. Walking is a good exercise for most pregnant women with no other special conditions. Sitting exercises such as riding an upright stationary bicycle (*i.e.*, leg ergometer) may be fine to do at an adequate comfort level, but caution should occur with semirecumbent cycling to ensure that the knees are not hitting the torso of the pregnant woman.

EP-C EXAMINATION QUESTIONS BY DOMAIN

Use the following table as a guide to assist you in your studying process. It is important to note that some questions can be classified as testing multiple domains by the knowledge and skills (KSs).

Domain Number	I	II	III	IV	V
Domain Name	Health and Fitness Assessment	Exercise Prescription and Implementation	Exercise Prescription, Implementation, and Ongoing Support	Legal and Professional	Management
Percentage of Questions from Domain	30%	30%	15%	10%	15%
Question Numbers	1, 2, 3, 4, 5, 6, 7, 8, 9, 10, 12, 13, 14, 22, 24, 25, 26, 27, 28, 29, 30, 50, 51, 52, 53, 54, 71, 72, 73, 74, 96, 97	15, 16, 17, 18, 19, 20, 33, 34, 35, 36, 37, 40, 41, 42, 43, 44, 45, 46, 47, 48, 49, 55, 56, 57, 58, 68, 69, 70, 82, 83, 84, 85	21, 23, 38, 39, 59, 60, 61, 62, 75, 76, 77, 78, 86, 87, 90, 91, 92, 93, 94, 95, 98, 99, 100	11, 31, 32, 63	64, 65, 66, 67, 79, 80, 81, 88, 89

EP-C

3

ACSM Certified Clinical Exercise Physiologist (CEP)

PAUL SORACE, MS, FACSM, ACSM-RCEP
Associate Editor

Note: CEP certification candidates may also review the case studies found in Part 1, ACSM Certified Personal Trainer (CPT) and Part 2 ACSM Certified Exercise Physiologist (EP-C).

DOMAIN I: PATIENT/CLIENT ASSESSMENT

CASE STUDY CEP.I	Author: **Trent A. Hargens, PhD** Author's Certifications: **FACSM, ACSM-CEP**

You are a certified clinical exercise physiologist (CEP) at a wellness center with a physician-referred exercise program. Grant is a 42-yr-old male who works as a computer information technology specialist. His physician has referred Grant to the facility and has already cleared him for all exercise activity. He currently weighs 250 lb and is 6 ft 1 in tall, and his waist circumference (WC) is 40.5 in. Bioelectrical impedance estimated a body fat percentage of 35.5%. His resting heart rate (HR_{rest}) was 72 bpm, and his average resting blood pressure (BP) was 128/86 mm Hg. Results from his most recent (within 1 mo) blood measures were the following: total cholesterol = 209 mg $\cdot$ dL^{-1}, high-density lipoprotein cholesterol (HDL-C) = 36 mg $\cdot$ dL^{-1}, low-density lipoprotein cholesterol (LDL-C) = 115 mg $\cdot$ dL^{-1}, triglycerides = 292 mg $\cdot$ dL^{-1}, and glucose = 112 mg $\cdot$ dL^{-1}. Grant reports on his health history questionnaire that he is not on any medications and no symptoms suggestive of cardiovascular, metabolic, or pulmonary disease. His 67-yr-old father has been on BP medication for the previous 20 yr and was recently diagnosed with Type 2 diabetes mellitus (DM).

During your initial consultation with Grant, he reports that he spends most of his workdays sitting behind the computer and that he walks his dog around the neighborhood two to three times per week for approximately 10 min. He has been doing this since his dog was a puppy several years ago. He also reports that it was not his idea to join your wellness center. His doctor, who told him that he needs to improve his lifestyle, referred him to the program. He expresses to you that he is not very motivated about the program, but pressure from his doctor and his family are why he is here. He feels that his current health status is just "part of getting old."

MULTIPLE-CHOICE QUESTIONS FOR CASE STUDY CEP.I

1. Grant's body mass index (BMI) is
   A) 27.6 kg $\cdot$ m^{-2}
   B) 33.1 kg $\cdot$ m^{-2}
   C) 40.1 kg $\cdot$ m^{-2}
   D) 61.4 kg $\cdot$ m^{-2}

2. According to the most recent edition of the *American College of Sports Medicine's* (ACSM) *Guidelines For Exercise Testing and Prescription* (GETP), which of the

following would not be part of the decision-making process for referral to a health care provider prior to initiating a moderate-to-vigorous intensity exercise program for Grant?
   A) Current lipid values
   B) Dog walking
   C) Report of signs and symptoms
   D) Health history concerning diagnosed cardiovascular, metabolic, or renal disease

3. According to the most recent edition of the *ACSM's GETP*, what is recommended prior to his beginning exercise at a light-to-moderate intensity in your facility?
   A) Signed informed consent form only
   B) Signed informed consent form and additional medical clearance from physician
   C) Signed informed consent form and graded exercise test (GXT)
   D) Signed informed consent form, additional medical clearance from physician, and GXT with physician supervision

4. Based on what Grant has expressed during his initial consultation, he is in which stage of change?
   A) Precontemplation
   B) Contemplation
   C) Preparation
   D) Action

5. According to the most recent edition of *ACSM's GETP*, which of the following would classify Grant as having fasting blood glucose level?
   A) Grant would be classified as having normal fasting blood glucose.
   B) Grant would be classified as having impaired fasting glucose (IFG).
   C) Grant would be classified as having insulin-dependent DM.
   D) Grant would be classified as having noninsulin-dependent DM.

DISCUSSION QUESTIONS FOR CASE STUDY CEP.I

1. What do you believe should be the primary goal for Grant as he begins his exercise program?

2. As exercise capacity increases, Grant will need an adjustment in his exercise prescription. What would be an appropriate progression in his frequency, intensity, time, and type (FITT) of activity?

DOMAIN II: EXERCISE PRESCRIPTION

CASE STUDY CEP.II(1)

Author: **Donald M. Cummings, PhD**

You are a CEP in a cardiopulmonary rehabilitation department at a medical facility. A new patient, Nancy, a 58-yr-old female, has been referred by her physician. Her physician would like her to participate in a 12-wk exercise rehabilitation program due to her risk factor profile for cardiovascular disease (CVD) and a positive GXT result that was positive for ST depression. A brief synopsis of Nancy's medical history, fasting blood laboratory report, and recent GXT results is provided below.

MEDICAL HISTORY

Nancy is a 58-yr-old female who has a height of 5 ft 3 in, weighs 158 lb, (28.05 kg $\cdot$ m^{-2} BMI), and has a WC of 36 in. She reports a family history of CVD on her father's side. She reports him having a three-vessel bypass at the age of 58 yr and was deceased at the age of 75 yr. Her mother is still living at the age of 75 yr with a 20-year history of Type 2 diabetes. She reports that she has one older sibling, a sister, who underwent a percutaneous coronary intervention (PCI) with a stent in her right coronary artery (RCA) at the age of 60 yr. Nancy reports a smoking history of one pack per day for 20 yr. She claims that she has not smoked for 15 yr. She is currently being treated for hypertension. She has been prescribed a diuretic (spironolactone 50 mg twice a day), and a calcium channel blocker (amlodipine 100 mg once a day). She states that she saw her physician because she desires to lose weight by diet and participation in an exercise program. Nancy denies any other significant medical history. She was referred by her physician for blood analysis and a GXT.

Blood Laboratory Analysis (Fasting)

Glucose	110 mg · dL^{-1}
Urea nitrogen	12 mg · dL^{-1}
Creatinine	1.1 mg · dL^{-1}
Sodium	136 mmol · L^{-1}
Potassium	3.6 mmol · L^{-1}
Chloride	105 mmol · L^{-1}
Carbon dioxide	28 mmol · L^{-1}
Calcium	8.8 mg · dL^{-1}
Cholesterol	184 mg · dL^{-1}
Triglycerides	185 mg · dL^{-1}
HDL-C	46 mg · dL^{-1}
Glycolated hemoglobin (HbA1C)	45 mmol · mol^{-1}
Albumin	3.7 g · dL^{-1}
Aspartate aminotransferase (AST)	36 U · L^{-1}
Alanine aminotransferase (ALT)	42 U · L^{-1}
Alkaline phosphatase (ALKP)	98 U · L^{-1}
Total bilirubin	0 .6 mg · dL^{-1}
Unconjugated bilirubin	0.7 mg · dL^{-1}
Direct bilirubin	0 mg · dL^{-1}
LDL	101 mg · dL^{-1}
Very low-density lipoprotein (VLDL)	37 mg · dL^{-1}
Cholesterol/HDL	4.0 mg · dL^{-1}

GXT Results:	Name:	Nancy
	Age:	58 yr
	HR$_{rest}$	78 bpm
	Resting electrocardiogram (ECG)	Normal sinus rhythm (NSR)
	Resting BP	
	Supine	138/84 mm Hg
	Standing	140/84 mm Hg

Time (min)	Speed (mph)	Grade (%)	Heart Rate (HR) (bpm)	BP (mm Hg)	Rating of Perceived Exertion (RPE)	Metabolic Equivalent (MET)	Symptoms (scales all out of 4)	ECG
1	1.7	10	88				1+ shortness of breath (SOB)	Sinus rhythm
2	1.7	10	94				1+ SOB	0.5 mm horizontal ST depression

Time (min)	Speed (mph)	Grade (%)	Heart Rate (HR) (bpm)	BP (mm Hg)	Rating of Perceived Exertion (RPE)	Metabolic Equivalent (MET)	Symptoms (scales all out of 4)	ECG
3	1.7	10	107	154/84	14	4.7	2+ SOB	0.5 mm horizontal ST depression
4	2.5	12	125				2+ SOB	1.0 mm horizontal ST depression
5	2.5	12	136				2+ SOB	1.0 mm horizontal ST depression
6	2.5	12	150	176/84	19	7.0	3+ SOB	1.0 mm horizontal ST depression
7	Recovery	Supine	136	182/84			2+ SOB	1.0 mm horizontal ST depression
8	Recovery	Supine	115	166/84			2+ SOB	0.5 mm horizontal ST depression
9	Recovery	Supine	107	148/84			2+ SOB	0.5 mm horizontal ST depression
10	Recovery	Supine	94	136/82			1+ SOB	Normalized ST
11	Recovery	Supine	79	136/80			1+ SOB	NSR
12	Recovery	Supine	68	132/80			SOB Resolved	Sinus Rhythm

MULTIPLE-CHOICE QUESTIONS FOR CASE STUDY CEP.II(1)

1. According to the most recent edition of the *ACSM's GETP* and based on Nancy's medical history and GXT results, the approximate maximum "safe" goal-oriented exercise MET level she should exercise would be approximately
   A) 2.5 METs
   B) 3.5 METs
   C) 4.5 METs
   D) 5.5 METs
   E) 6.5 METs

2. According to the most recent edition of the *ACSM's GETP* and based on Nancy's GXT results, a good index of exercise intensity would be an exercise RPE on the Borg 6–20 scale of approximately
   A) 12
   B) 14
   C) 16
   D) 18
   E) 20

3. According to the most recent edition of the *ACSM's GETP*, which classes of medications prescribed to Nancy may have adverse side effects during exercise?
   A) Diuretics only may have adverse effects during exercise testing or programming.
   B) Dihydropyridine calcium channel blockers only may have adverse effects during exercise testing or programming.
   C) Both of Nancy's medications may have adverse effects during exercise testing or programming.
   D) Neither of Nancy's medications have possible reported adverse effects during exercise testing or programming.

4. According to the most recent edition of the *ACSM's GETP*, which classes of medications prescribed to Nancy may have an effect on her HR during exercise?
   A) Diuretic
   B) Dihydropyridine calcium channel blockers
   C) All of the medications that Nancy is prescribed may effect HR during exercise.
   D) None of Nancy's medication classes may have an effect on her HR during exercise.

5. Assuming that the GXT is a true positive test, the use of ACSM's metabolic calculations for the treadmill would suggest which of the following as a maximal safe workload for Nancy's exercise training?
   A) 2.0 mph and 7.0% grade
   B) 3.0 mph and 3.0% grade
   C) 4.0 mph and 1.0% grade
   D) 5.0 mph and 0.0% grade
   E) Either A or B would be an appropriate treadmill workload for Nancy.

6. Assuming that the GXT is a true positive test, the use of ACSM's metabolic calculations for the cycle ergometer would suggest which of the following as a maximal safe workload for Nancy's exercise training?
   A) 275 kgm $\cdot$ min^{-1}
   B) 350 kgm $\cdot$ min^{-1}
   C) 550 kgm $\cdot$ min^{-1}
   D) 700 kgm $\cdot$ min^{-1}
   E) Cannot be determined from the data given

7. Based on Nancy's medical history and according to the most recent edition of the *ACSM's GETP*, what frequency of exercise would you recommend?
   A) 2–3 d $\cdot$ wk^{-1}
   B) 3–5 d $\cdot$ wk^{-1}
   C) 3–7 d $\cdot$ wk^{-1}
   D) 5–7 d $\cdot$ wk^{-1}

8. According to the most recent edition of the *ACSM's GETP*, a resistance program may be initiated for Nancy incorporating which range of repetitions based on her % 1-RM?
   A) one repetition maximum (1-RM)
   B) 4–6 RM
   C) 6–10 RM
   D) 10–15 RM
   E) Any of the above levels of RM would be appropriate for Nancy.

9. Based the medical history, laboratory report, and GXT, which of the following pathologies would *not* be a consideration when developing and exercise program for Nancy?
   A) Prediabetes
   B) Coronary heart disease (CHD)
   C) Obesity
   D) Hypertension
   E) All of the above pathologies should be a consideration for Nancy's exercise program.

10. Assuming the GXT was a maximum test and based on the maximum exercise MET level as determined in question 1, at what approximate percentage of reserve volume of oxygen consumed per unit of time ($\dot{V}O_2R$) is Nancy working?
    A) 40%
    B) 50%
    C) 60%
    D) 70%
    E) 80%

DISCUSSION QUESTIONS FOR CASE STUDY CEP.II(1)

1. Based upon the information provided in the medical history and the results of the GXT are there any indications that this may be a false-positive test for obstructive coronary artery disease (CAD)? If you believed the test to be a false positive test, would you change the exercise prescription you have prescribed for Nancy?

2. The *ACSM's GETP* give guidelines for exercise intensity, duration, frequency, mode, and progression. Based on the information that you have been provided for this client, outline considerations in your development of Nancy's initial exercise program in order to achieve the most favorable outcomes and why?

DOMAIN II: EXERCISE PRESCRIPTION

CASE STUDY CEP.II(2)

Author: **David E. Verrill, MS, FAACVPR**

You are a CEP employed in the medical fitness program at a local health/fitness facility. You have a new client joining your program. He is a 57-yr-old male who currently weighs 193 lb and is 66 in tall (BMI = 31.2 kg $\cdot$ m^{-2}). His body composition by skinfolds was estimated at 32% body fat, and his waist (abdominal) circumference was 42 in. He is a current smoker (smokes one pack a day). His HR$_{rest}$ was 72 bpm, and his resting BP was 142/88 mm Hg. Fasting blood values were measured 2 wk ago as the following: total cholesterol = 227 mg $\cdot$ dL^{-1}; HDL-C = 33 mg $\cdot$ dL^{-1};

triglycerides = 156 mg $\cdot$ dL^{-1}; glucose = 132 mg $\cdot$ dL^{-1}; and HbA1C = 7.2%. He has been walking his "older" dog daily for the last 4 wk but reports no other physical activity. He reports no symptoms of exercise intolerance except SOB when walking up hills. His brother died of a fatal heart attack at age 60 yr. Currently, he is only taking a diuretic (hydrochlorothiazide [HCTZ], 25 mg once daily) to control his BP. He also takes rosuvastatin (Crestor) 10 mg once daily and metformin (Glucophage XR) 1,500 mg once daily. He has recently joined your medical fitness program to increase his fitness level and manage his body weight, dyslipidemia, diabetes, and hypertension safely.

Your client recently had a modified Bruce (5% grade) maximal exercise test ordered by his physician due to his SOB concerns. The physician interpreted the test as equivocal, as he did not reach 85% of predicted maximal heart rate (HR$_{max}$). The test interpretation also indicated ~0.5–1 mm of ST depression in the lateral leads at peak exercise only, but no symptoms of ischemia. His HR$_{max}$ and peak BP were 132 bpm and 224/94 mm Hg, respectively. His maximal oxygen consumption was estimated to be 23.1 mL $\cdot$ kg^{-1} $\cdot$ min^{-1} (6.6 METs). His physician ordered a pulmonary function test with the following results: forced expiratory volume in one second (FEV$_{1.0}$) = 2.1 L (54% predicted) and his forced vital capacity (FVC) = 3.2 L (64% predicted) immediately following bronchodilator administration. His FEV$_{1.0}$/FVC ratio = 0.66.

Based on these clinical findings, his physician has cleared him to exercise in a medically supervised health and fitness program.

MULTIPLE-CHOICE QUESTIONS FOR CASE STUDY CEP.II(2)

1. According to the most recent edition of the *ACSM's GETP*, when prescribing exercise, the optimal intensity of exercise for aerobic fitness benefits for this client would be set at
   A) Light; 30%–<40% of heart rate reserve (HRR)
   B) Light to moderate; 30%–<60% of HRR
   C) Moderate to vigorous; 40%–≥60% of HRR
   D) Vigorous; ≥60% of HRR

2. According to the most recent edition of the *ACSM's GETP*, the recommended frequency of exercise to achieve health benefits would optimally be
   A) 1–2 d $\cdot$ wk^{-1}
   B) 2–3 d $\cdot$ wk^{-1}
   C) 3–4 d $\cdot$ wk^{-1}
   D) ≥5 d $\cdot$ wk^{-1}

3. Metformin (Glucophage) is a
   A) Sulfonylureas drug for Type 1 DM
   B) Meglitinide drug for Type 2 DM
   C) Biguanide drug for Type 2 DM
   D) Glucagon-like peptide 1 receptor agonist drug for Type 2 DM

4. Based on your client's fasting blood levels,
   A) He currently has his medical conditions under adequate control.
   B) He may need to see his physician for follow-up of his current medication dosages.
   C) He may be noncompliant with taking his medications.
   D) Both B and C

5. Given the health information provided, your client very likely has
   A) Metabolic syndrome
   B) Pulmonary disease
   C) Peripheral vascular disease
   D) All of the above
   E) Only A and B of the above

6. An appropriate target heart rate (THR) for your client on his *first* day of exercise would be
   A) 90–96 bpm
   B) 99–115 bpm
   C) 115–124 bpm
   D) 124–130 bpm

7. The use of ACSM's metabolic calculations for the treadmill would suggest which of the following workloads as appropriate for an initial workload for exercise training?
   A) 5.0 mph and 4% grade
   B) 1.5 mph and 2% grade
   C) 3.0 mph and 2% grade
   D) 3.3 mph and 7% grade

8. Muscle strengthening and flexibility exercises for this client should include _____ d $\cdot$ wk^{-1} at a _____ intensity.
   A) 4–5; moderate
   B) 6–7; light
   C) 2–3; moderate
   D) 1–2; vigorous

9. Resistance exercise training has been shown to
   A) Enhance insulin sensitivity
   B) Diminish glucose tolerance
   C) Decrease total fat-free mass (FFM)
   D) Increase insulin resistance

10. According to the most recent edition of the *ACSM's GETP*, what would your recommended weekly MET-minute exercise prescription be for your client?
    A) $\geq$100–500 MET-min $\cdot$ wk^{-1}
    B) $\geq$2,000–4,000 MET-min $\cdot$ wk^{-1}
    C) $\geq$500–1,000 MET-min $\cdot$ wk^{-1}
    D) $\leq$200–400 MET-min $\cdot$ wk^{-1}

DISCUSSION QUESTIONS FOR CASE STUDY CEP.II(2)

1. What questions or recommendations will you have for your client prior to developing his exercise prescription?

2. What would you tell your client about the exercise benefits for those with his medical conditions?

DOMAIN II: EXERCISE PRESCRIPTION

CASE STUDY CEP.II(3)

Author: **Joselyn M. Rodriguez, MSH**
Author's Certifications: **ACSM EP-C**

You are a CEP in the cardiopulmonary department of a hospital. Joe is a new patient who has been referred by his physician to participate in your monitored phase II cardiac rehabilitation program. An initial review of his medical history states that he is a 52-yr-old male who currently weighs 253 lb and is 72 in in height (34.3 kg $\cdot$ m^{-2} BMI). He reports a family history of his father having died from a heart attack at the age of 50 yr. He quit smoking 4 mo ago after having smoked one pack per day for 34 yr. During his initial evaluation appointment, his resting vitals were measured as HR$_{rest}$ = 68 bpm, and his resting BP for both right and left arm were 148/84 mm Hg and 142/76 mm Hg, respectively. His WC was 50 in. His body fat (BF) percentage was measured as 34 percent using a bioelectrical impedance analysis scale. A recent report of his fasting blood values read as follows: glucose = 110 mg $\cdot$ dL^{-1}, total cholesterol = 203 mg $\cdot$ dL^{-1}, LDL = 137 mg $\cdot$ dL^{-1}, HDL-C = 44 mg $\cdot$ dL^{-1}, and triglycerides = 168 mg $\cdot$ dL^{-1}. He is currently taking metoprolol and atorvastatin to treat his hypertension and dyslipidemia. Joe claims that he attains most of his physical activity through his job as a mover, which is why he has not been exercising regularly. He states that he has been experiencing tightness in his chest on the job for the past several months. His physician referred him to have a GXT (Bruce protocol). A positive GXT indicated a need for a cardiac catheterization, which confirmed a 78% and 75% occlusion of the circumflex and RCAs, both requiring stenting. His ejection fraction (EF) was determined to be 52%. He refrained from taking medication prior to his GXT.

GXT Results:

Name:	Joe
Age:	52 yr
HR$_{rest}$:	64 bpm
Resting ECG:	NSR
Resting BP	
SUPINE:	146/82 mm Hg
STANDING:	140/72 mm Hg

Time (min)	Speed (mph)	Grade (%)	HR (bpm)	BP (mm Hg)	RPE	MET	Symptoms (scales are all out of 4)	ECG
1	1.7	10	82					NSR
2	1.7	10	94					NSR
3	1.7	10	114	170/74	11	4.7		NSR
4	2.5	12	126					NSR
5	2.5	12	136					NSR, 2 premature ventricular contraction (PVC)
6	2.5	12	144	182/84	15	7.0	2+ chest pain (CP) 1+ SOB	1.0 mm horizontal ST depression
7	3.4	14	150				2+ CP 1+ SOB	1.0 mm horizontal ST depression, 1 PVC
8	3.4	14	154				2+ CP 1+ SOB	1.5 mm horizontal ST depression
9	3.4	14	158	198/92	18	10.1	3+ CP 2+ SOB	1.5 mm horizontal ST depression, 2 PVC
10	Recovery	Supine	150	184/84			3+ CP 2+ SOB	1.5 mm horizontal ST depression
11	Recovery	Supine	138	178/82			2+ CP 1+ SOB	1.5 mm horizontal ST depression
12	Recovery	Supine	120	164/78			1+ SOB	1.0 mm horizontal ST depression
13	Recovery	Supine	100	156/76				NSR
14	Recovery	Supine	74	148/80				NSR

MULTIPLE-CHOICE QUESTIONS FOR CASE STUDY CEP.II(3)

1. According to Joe's body fat percentage, calculate his FFM.
   A) 21 kg
   B) 39 kg
   C) 76 kg
   D) None of the above

2. According to Joe's GXT results, which method for prescribing exercise intensity would be most appropriate?
   A) RPE of 11–16 on a scale of 6–20
   B) 40%–80% of HRR
   C) HR below the ischemic threshold (<10 beats)
   D) None of the above

3. Determine an appropriate index of exercise intensity with reference to question 2.
   A) 102–140 bpm
   B) No greater than 134 bpm
   C) 112 bpm
   D) Cannot be determined from the data given

4. According to the most recent edition of the *ACSM's GETP* and Joe's GXT results, what maximal workload would be most suitable for exercise training on a leg cycle ergometer?
   A) 124 W
   B) 157 W
   C) 146 W
   D) Cannot be determined from the data given

5. Joe wants to drop his body fat percentage to 22%. Calculate his target body weight.
   A) 167 lb
   B) 213 lb
   C) 236 lb
   D) Cannot be determined from the data given

6. During Joe's cardiac catheterization, his EF was measured to be 52%. Under which category does his EF fall under?
   A) Normal
   B) Below normal
   C) Congestive heart failure
   D) None of the above

7. According to the table depicting Joe's GXT results, under which circumstance was his test terminated?
   A) Hypertensive response
   B) Excessive ST depression
   C) Development of bundle branch block
   D) Moderately severe angina

8. What would Joe's estimated maximum exercise MET level be based on his GXT results?
   A) 6 METs
   B) 7 METs
   C) 8 METs
   D) 9 METs

9. According to Joe's GXT results, which of the following would be a safe maximal workload for exercising on a treadmill?
   A) 3.0 mph and 2.5% grade
   B) 3.2 mph and 3% grade
   C) 3.6 mph and 4.5% grade
   D) 4.0 mph and 5% grade

10. Estimate Joe's caloric expenditure if he is exercising at his maximal safe workload on a treadmill for a duration of 30 min.
    A) 261 kcal
    B) 288 kcal
    C) 362 kcal
    D) 461 kcal

DISCUSSION QUESTIONS FOR CASE STUDY CEP.II(3)

1. Explain why outpatient cardiopulmonary rehabilitation centers use a multidisciplinary team approach.

2. Sustained weight loss is one of Joe's goals after the completion of monitored phase II cardiac rehabilitation. What adjustments in Joe's exercise prescription are necessary?

3. BMI is a common method of assessing body composition. Discuss the reasons why this method is recommended for Joe's particular case.

4. Explain why the Bruce protocol was chosen as the primary method of GXT for this patient.

5. Joe's job is very physical and involves heavy lifting. Discuss how you would go about prescribing resistance exercise for Joe.

DOMAIN II: EXERCISE PRESCRIPTION

CASE STUDY CEP.II(4)

Author: **Joselyn M. Rodriguez, MSH**
Author's Certifications: **ACSM EP-C**

You are a CEP in an outpatient cardiopulmonary rehabilitation department at a hospital. Steve is a 66-yr-old male patient who currently weighs 145 lb and is 70 in in height. He was referred by his physician to participate in your monitored phase II cardiac rehabilitation program. Steve is a current smoker. He has smoked two packs a day for the past 50 yr. He stated that his father was a smoker and suffered a stroke at the age of 54 yr. During his initial evaluation, several measurements were attained and a recent report of fasting blood levels were discussed.

WC: 38 in

Resting vitals: HR_{rest} = 78 bpm, resting BP = 150/82 mm Hg (left arm) and 144/76 mm Hg (right arm)

Peripheral capillary oxygen saturation (SpO_2): 93% (on room air)

CEP

Fasting blood levels:

Glucose (mg $\cdot$ dL^{-1})	89
Total cholesterol (mg $\cdot$ dL^{-1})	195
LDL (mg $\cdot$ dL^{-1})	129
HDL-C (mg $\cdot$ dL^{-1})	43
Triglycerides (mg $\cdot$ dL^{-1})	147

He is currently taking an angiotensin-converting enzyme (ACE) inhibitor (ramipril), a platelet inhibitor (clopidogrel), and a statin (pravastatin) to treat his hypertension, prevent formation of clots, and treat his dyslipidemia, respectively. He states that he has not been exercising for several years due cramping and burning sensation in his calf muscles with exertion. He was recently hospitalized for an inferior wall myocardial infarction (MI), for which he was submitted to a cardiac catheterization and had his RCA stented. Steve was administered a physician-supervised modified treadmill GXT 1 wk after his event. The GXT consisted of walking at a constant speed of 2.0 mph, increasing the grade 2.0% every 2 min. Steve's test was terminated due to sharp bilateral burning pain in his calf muscles (4 on the intermittent claudication [IC] scale at the sixth minute). Note: IC scale is a 1–4 scale. His maximum HR and BP were measured at 110 bpm and 182/78 mm Hg, respectively. His ankle/brachial systolic pressure index (ABI) at the completion of the test was 0.66 versus his ABI of 0.76 at rest (pretest). Steve had no silent or clinical signs of myocardial ischemia during the duration of the GXT. His estimated maximal oxygen consumption was 3.6 METs using ACSM's walking treadmill metabolic calculations (having stopped the test at 2.0 mph and 4.0% after completing this stage).

MULTIPLE-CHOICE QUESTIONS FOR CASE STUDY CEP.II(4)

1. Steve was administered a 12-lead ECG during his recent hospitalization. Which leads would display ST elevation for an inferior wall MI?
   A) I, aVL, V_5, V_6
   B) V_1–V_4
   C) II, III, aVF
   D) None of the above

2. Steve's medical history, fasting blood levels, and GXT results indicate that he most likely has
   A) Congestive heart failure
   B) Chronic obstructive pulmonary disease (COPD)
   C) Peripheral arterial disease (PAD)
   D) Aortic stenosis

3. Prior to ending Steve's GXT as a result of a rating of 4 on the IC scale, he experienced bilateral calf pain/burning that he rated as a 3 on the IC scale at minute 4. As a CEP, how would you go about determining exercise intensity for Steve?
   A) <10 beats below is maximum HR
   B) 40%–60% HRR or $\dot{V}O_2R$, allowing him to walk until he reaches an IC pain rating of 3
   C) RPE of 16
   D) Cannot be determined from the data given

4. What type of modality would be most appropriate for this patient?
   A) Water aerobics
   B) Interval training exercise bike protocol
   C) Rowing machine interval training protocol
   D) IC treadmill protocol

5. As a CEP, what would your recommendation be regarding aerobic exercise frequency for this particular patient?
   A) 2–4 d $\cdot$ wk^{-1}
   B) 3–5 d $\cdot$ wk^{-1}
   C) 5–7 d $\cdot$ wk^{-1}
   D) None of the above

6. What would Steve's caloric expenditure be if he walked 15 min at his estimated maximal oxygen consumption?
   A) 44 kcal
   B) 63 kcal
   C) 71 kcal
   D) Cannot be determined from data given

7. What was Steve's measured systolic BP in his posterior tibial artery if his ABI was 0.66 at the end of his GXT?
   A) 110 mm Hg
   B) 112 mm Hg
   C) 120 mm Hg
   D) Cannot be determined from the data given

8. What is this patient's pack year history of smoking?
   A) 40
   B) 75
   C) 100
   D) 125

9. Steve is walking on a treadmill during one of his monitored cardiac rehabilitation sessions and develops bilateral cramping and burning sensation in his calves at minute 6 of his exercise time. He tells the CEP that he has reached a pain rating of 3 on the IC scale. The CEP should
   A) Cease exercise to allow ischemic pain to resolve before resuming exercise
   B) Continue to have Steve walk from the remainder of his exercise time
   C) Switch Steve from the treadmill to the leg cycle ergometer at the point of his reporting of ischemic pain
   D) None of the above

10. Which of the following is a *primary goal* to effectively treat and manage PAD?
    A) Controlling his hypertension through medications and behavior modification
    B) Quit smoking
    C) Lowering lipids
    D) Both A and B

11. Which of the following best describes the benefits of drug-eluting stents as compared to bare-metal stents?
    A) Release antibiotics preventing infection
    B) Release anticoagulants preventing clot reformation
    C) Inhibit cell proliferation and inflammation reducing restenosis
    D) Both B and C

DISCUSSION QUESTIONS FOR CASE STUDY CEP.II(4)

1. Discuss FITT recommendations for aerobic exercise for individuals with PAD.

2. Discuss the importance of using a modified treadmill GXT versus Bruce protocol for this patient.

3. Resistance exercise is recommended to enhance and maintain muscular strength and endurance. Use the FITT principle of exercise prescription to design a resistance exercise regimen for Steve.

4. Identify barriers that may impact exercise compliance for this patient.

5. Explain strategies to overcome these barriers and discuss goals for effective management and treatment of PAD.

DOMAIN II: EXERCISE PRESCRIPTION

CASE STUDY CEP.II(5)

Author: **David E. Verrill, MS, FAACVPR**

Mr. Kyle, a 63-yr-old bank executive, is entering your phase II cardiac rehabilitation program 3 wk following an anterior ST-segment elevation myocardial infarction (STEMI) and stent placements in his left anterior descending (LAD) and left circumflex (LCX) arteries. He also has intermittent periods of atrial fibrillation with slow to moderate ventricular rates. A predischarge hospital resting adenosine radionuclide study showed improved areas of myocardial perfusion in the anterior, lateral, and apical walls of his left ventricle. He began smoking at age 17 yr and continues to smoke one and a half packs a day. He was a recreational exerciser until 3 yr ago, at which time he hurt his back when he fell off a ladder at home. Since then, he has gained weight, continued smoking, been diagnosed with hypertension and dyslipidemia, and leads a sedentary lifestyle. He is somewhat noncompliant taking his medications. He has a "type A" personality and refuses to relax at any time (he has an upper level corporate position). The only symptom of exercise intolerance he reports is dyspnea when walking up hills. His brother died of an MI at age 60 yr. He also has developed low back pain from a bulging disc compressing a nerve at L5.

Mr. Kyle's weight is 218 lb and height is 70 in. His body fat measured by skinfolds was estimated at 35%, and his WC is 44 in. His coronary catheterization report revealed the following information prior to his percutaneous transluminal coronary angioplasty (PTCA) with stent placement procedure: LAD 85% lesion prior to the first diagonal branch, LCX 90% proximal lesion, minimal lesions to branches of LAD, nondominant RCA with minimal plaque, and EF = 45%. Upon examination, his HR_{rest} and BP were 76 bpm and 148/82 mm Hg, respectively. Fasting blood values were measured 2 wk ago and were as follows: total cholesterol: 244 mg · dL^{-1} (6.3 mmol · L^{-1}), LDL-C: 178 mg · dL^{-1} (4.6 mmol · L^{-1}), HDL-C: 34 mg · dL^{-1} (0.9 mmol · L^{-1}), triglycerides: 202 mg · dL^{-1} (2.3 mmol · L^{-1}), and glucose: 120 mg · dL^{-1} (6.8 mmol · L^{-1}). Currently, he is taking the following medications: diltiazem (Cardizem) 120 mg twice daily, furosemide (Lasix) 20 mg twice daily, atorvastatin (Lipitor) 20 mg twice daily, nicotinic acid (Niacin) 500 mg four times daily, aspirin (Ecotrin) 325 mg once daily, digoxin (Lanoxin) 750 mg once daily, warfarin (Coumadin) 2.5 mg once daily, and nitroglycerine spray as needed. Mr. Kyle reports not taking diltiazem or digoxin prior to his GXT per physician request. Below is his cardiac rehabilitation entry GXT data (summarized):

Modified Bruce 0% Protocol	Workload	Blood pressure (mm Hg)	Heart rate (bpm)	Percent Saturation of Arterial Oxygen (SaO₂) (%)	METs (estimated)	Angina (1–4 scale)	Treadmill Time	RPE (6–20 scale)
Rest	—	148/82	72	94%	1.0	None	—	6
Peak Exercise	1.7 mph, 10% grade	202/96	142	84%	4.6	1+	9:00	19
Active Recovery	1.5 mph, 2% grade	164/86	118	88%	2.6	None	—	12

Mr. Kyle has been given medical clearance from his physician to begin exercise and education in your cardiac rehabilitation program.

MULTIPLE-CHOICE QUESTIONS FOR CASE STUDY CEP.II(5)

1. Mr. Kyle takes diltiazem (Cardizem) for his CVD. This drug
   A) May reduce resting and exercise HR and BP
   B) Is likely to cause a false-positive ECG during a GXT
   C) Is a commonly used β-blocker
   D) Is a combined calcium channel blocker and $α_1$ antagonist
   E) Is rarely given for atrial fibrillation

2. Mr. Kyle had an 85% blockage in his LAD artery prior to his PTCA and stenting procedure. Which region of the heart does this artery supply?
   A) The anterior wall of the left ventricle
   B) The intraventricular septum
   C) The sinoatrial (SA) node in the right atrium
   D) The entire right ventricle
   E) Only A and B

3. Mr. Kyle has a resting EF of 45%. According to the most recent edition of the *ACSM's GETP*, what level of cardiovascular risk would he fall under with regard to exercise training?
   A) Lowest risk
   B) Moderate risk
   C) Highest risk
   D) None of the above

4. According to the most recent edition of the *ACSM's GETP*, when prescribing his exercise the optimal *initial* intensity of exercise for cardiopulmonary fitness benefits would be set at
   A) 10%–<20% HRR or $\dot{V}O_2R$, 1–<2 METs, RPE 7–9, an intensity that causes minimal increases in HR and breathing
   B) 30%–<40% HRR or $\dot{V}O_2R$, 2–<3 METs, RPE 9–11, an intensity that causes slight increases in HR and breathing
   C) 40%–<60% HRR or $\dot{V}O_2R$, 3–<6 METs, RPE 12–13, an intensity that causes noticeable increases in HR and breathing
   D) ≥60% HRR or $\dot{V}O_2R$, ≥6 METs, RPE ≥14, an intensity that causes substantial increases in HR and breathing

5. Mr. Kyle has a smoking history of _____ pack years.
   A) 30
   B) 40
   C) 50
   D) 69

6. During your initial assessment, you give Mr. Kyle various surveys to assess his quality of life (QOL), dietary habits, and depression. One commonly used survey that assesses QOL in cardiac rehabilitation participants is
   A) The Medical Outcomes Study Short Form-36 (SF-36)
   B) The Center for Epidemiologic Studies-Depression (CES-D) scale
   C) The Patient Health Questionnaire (PHQ-9)
   D) The Physical Activity Readiness Questionnaire (PAR-Q)

7. Mr. Kyle's BMI classifies him as _____ by expert panel normative data.
   A) Underweight
   B) Normal weight
   C) Overweight
   D) Obese (class I)

8. An initial exercise prescription for Mr. Kyle would include which of the following recommendations?
   A) Level treadmill walking at 2.5 mph at an HR of 128–136 bpm and an RPE of 14–17
   B) Rowing ergometer exercise at 15 W at an HR of 98–106 bpm and an RPE of 8–11
   C) Cycle ergometer exercise at 0.5 kg (180 kgm · min^{-1}) at an HR of 114–128 bpm and an RPE of 11–16
   D) Stepping on a 5-in bench, 20 steps per minute at an HR of 122–134 bpm and an RPE of 16–18

9. According to the most recent edition of the *ACSM's GETP*, the recommended frequency of exercise to achieve health benefits for Mr. Kyle would be
   A) 1–2 d · wk^{-1}
   B) 2–3 d · wk^{-1}
   C) At least 3 d · wk^{-1} but preferably most days of the week
   D) Twice daily, 7 d · wk^{-1}

10. Mr. Kyle currently weighs 218 lb (99 kg) and has a body fat level of ~35%. He would like to lose weight to achieve a realistic goal body fat percentage of ~28%. What is Mr. Kyle's goal body weight at this ideal body fat percentage?
    A) 204 lb (92.5 kg)
    B) 197 lb (89.3 kg)
    C) 182 lb (82.6 kg)
    D) 176 lb (79.8 kg)

DISCUSSION QUESTIONS FOR CASE STUDY CEP.II(5)

1. What two undiagnosed diseases (comorbidities) might Mr. Kyle have at the present time that were not discussed between Mr. Kyle and his physician? How would you address these undiagnosed conditions?

2. How would you address Mr. Kyle's noncompliance with his medicines, his continuation of smoking, and his level of stress?

3. List six purposes for performing GXT after acute MI.

4. Studies show that lack of muscular strength and endurance is of particular concern for the patient with post-MI. What type of resistive exercise training regimen and modalities would you recommend for Mr. Kyle during his stay in your cardiac rehabilitation program?

5. Mr. Kyle has intermittent periods of atrial fibrillation. However, this appears to be under control with his current medications. Which three medications is Mr. Kyle taking for his atrial fibrillation? What are some physiologic concerns for the cardiac patient with atrial fibrillation? What are some exercise concerns for the patient with atrial fibrillation?

DOMAIN III: PROGRAM IMPLEMENTATION AND ONGOING SUPPORT

CASE STUDY CEP.III Author: **David E. Verrill, MS, FAACVPR**

You are the CEP for a local hospital pulmonary rehabilitation program. A new patient, Cassidy, is a 64-yr-old retired female elementary school teacher just starting the program and you are performing her initial assessment. She arrives from a small town outside of the county (a 50-min drive). Her husband drove her and stated that the only times Cassidy can attend her rehab sessions is when he can drive her and when he is "not on a job" (he is a part-time plumber). She was short of breath when she entered the rehab facility, and her husband stated that she has not been feeling "up to par" over the past few weeks. Cassidy has stage 2 (moderate) COPD manifested by a combination of emphysema, chronic bronchitis, and bronchiectasis. She has been told that she has a "mild" asthmatic component to her lung disease. Cassidy also has a history of blood clots in her lungs, PAD, dyslipidemia, obesity, and knee osteoarthritis. She does not report any symptoms suggestive of myocardial ischemia. She was admitted to a local hospital for exacerbation of respiratory symptoms approximately 1 mo ago. She reports increasing fatigue and dyspnea with exertion in recent weeks as well as feeling more depressed. Her score on the CES-D indicated a score of 22, or "possibility of major depression." She is on $2 \text{ L} \cdot \text{min}^{-1}$ of oxygen by nasal cannula in resting (sedentary) conditions. She increases her oxygen liter flow to $4 \text{ L} \cdot \text{min}^{-1}$ with exertional activities per physician order. The patient currently weighs 155 lb and is 5 ft 3 in in height (BMI = $27.5 \text{ kg} \cdot \text{m}^{-2}$). You measured her body composition using skinfold calipers, and her estimated body fat value is 38%. Her waist (abdominal) circumference is 41 in. She quit smoking 2 mo ago and is on nicotine replacement therapy. Over her lifespan, she smoked approximately one and a half packs of cigarettes per day for 48 yr. During her initial assessment (while on $2 \text{ L} \cdot \text{min}^{-1}$ oxygen), the following resting physiologic data was assessed and recorded: HR = 98 bpm; BP = 146/94 mm Hg; SaO_2 = 93%; chest sounds = coarse (but mild) bilateral crackles during inspiration; heart sounds = regular pulse with no murmurs, gallops or bruits noted. The patient describes a sedentary lifestyle, rarely walking outside of the home and not participating in any recreational activities. She states that one reason for this is that she becomes unsteady when she walks due to balance issues. She uses either a rollator or a cane when she ambulates both inside and outside of the home. She reports a very low QOL based on her scores from the Ferrans and Powers QOL Index—Pulmonary Version. Her score on the dyspnea subscale of the Chronic Respiratory Disease Questionnaire was 5 (on a 1–7 scale) corresponding to "some shortness of breath" when performing her activities of daily living (ADL). She has a BODE Index score of 5. Her overall nutrition score on the Diet Habit Survey (DHS) was low and indicated poor nutritional habits.

Six months ago, Cassidy had a resting pulmonary function testing and performed a maximal cycle ergometer exercise test with metabolic analysis while on oxygen utilizing a ramp protocol. These studies yielded the following information: FVC = 2.2 L (60% predicted), $FEV_{1.0}$ = 1.8 L (52% predicted), $\dot{V}O_{2peak}$ = 4.8 METs, HR_{max} = 155 bpm, maximal BP (BP_{max}) = 158/84 mm Hg, and peak SaO_2 = 88%. No significant ECG abnormalities or signs of myocardial ischemia were noted, although she did have frequent premature atrial contractions (PACs) throughout the exercise test.

Cassidy currently takes the following medications: prednisone (Deltasone) 10 mg twice a day, theophylline (Theo-Dur) 75 mg four times a day, baby aspirin 80 mg once a day, simvastatin (Zocor) 40 mg once a day, formoterol (Foradil) nebulizer, 20 μg $\cdot 2 \text{ mL}^{-1}$ inhalation solution two times a day (10–12 h apart), ipratropium bromide and albuterol (Combivent MDI) two puffs four times a day, budesonide (Pulmicort Turbuhaler) 200 μg two inhalations two times a day, nicotine nasal spray (Nicotrol NS) 1 mg each nostril every 2 h, clopidogrel (Plavix) 75 mg once a day, citalopram (Celexa) 20 mg once a day, and bupropion HCL (Wellbutrin) 100 mg once a day.

You conducted a 6-min walk test (6MWT) test today on the patient immediately after her initial assessment. Her highest HR and BP achieved were 138 bpm and 164/96 mm Hg, respectively. Her peak exercise SaO_2 was 82% on $4 \text{ L} \cdot \text{min}^{-1}$ of oxygen, which returned back to 92% within 5 min of recovery. She walked 1,401 ft with one rest break using a rollator for balance and to push her oxygen tank. She rated her peak level of exertion as 17 on the Borg category scale. She had moderate-to-marked dyspnea (2–3 on a 0–4 point scale) at test termination and moderate calf pain in both legs (2 or "moderate pain" on a 0–4 point scale). Other fitness tests you conducted demonstrated "below average" scores for both upper body (handgrip dynamometer and 30-s bicep curl test) and lower body (30-s sit-to-stand test and 3-RM leg extension) muscular strength and endurance. To assess her balance, she performed the Timed Up and Go (TUG) Test and scored a time of 19 s, indicating an increased risk of future falls.

MULTIPLE-CHOICE QUESTIONS FOR CASE STUDY CEP.III

1. The *first* action for developing Cassidy's initial treatment plan (ITP) would be to
   A) Formulate her exercise prescription based on her metabolic GXT results
   B) Call her pulmonologist and discuss her 6MWT results with the medical staff
   C) Increase her supplemental oxygen flow to 6 L · min^{-1} during her rehabilitation exercise to compensate for her lower exercise SaO_2 values seen during her 6MWT
   D) Develop her individual short- and long-term goals that she wishes to strive for during program participation

2. The initial exercise prescription for Cassidy should
   A) Be deferred until her pulmonologist provides follow-up recommendations based on her initial assessment
   B) Include recumbent cycling of 15–20 W at 30–40 rpm for 8 min
   C) Include treadmill walking at 2.2 mph with a 1% incline for 10 min
   D) Include arm ergometry exercise of 10 W at 20–30 rpm for 8 min

3. Prednisone is a drug prescribed to
   A) Help provide immediate airway relief in the event of an asthma attack
   B) Help loosen mucus in the airways for easier removal
   C) Help shrink the swelling and inflammation of the airways
   D) Help provide long-term relief of dyspnea through dilation of the airways

4. Cassidy has a smoking history of _____ pack years.
   A) 72
   B) 154
   C) 32
   D) 90

5. Which of the following is an example of a short-acting anticholinergic pharmacologic agent?
   A) Theophylline (Theo-Dur)
   B) Albuterol (Proventil)
   C) Fluticasone/salmeterol (Advair)
   D) Ipratropium (Atrovent)

6. Cassidy complains of recent fatigue, worsening dyspnea, and frequent periods of depression. To address these problems, you would
   A) Orally explore her level of depression and self-refer her to a psychologist or psychiatrist, if indicated
   B) Have Cassidy perform a follow-up metabolic GXT to see if she has any further cardiac and/or pulmonary involvement that might be contributing to these issues

   C) Collect as much information as possible in your initial assessment about these issues and contact her physician with this information
   D) Ask Cassidy's pulmonologist to refer her to the hospital pulmonary function testing laboratory to reassess her FVC and $FEV_{1.0}$ values

7. During your initial assessment, you give Cassidy various surveys to assess her QOL, level of dyspnea with ADL, dietary habits, and depression. One commonly used survey that specifically assesses dyspnea with ADL in pulmonary rehabilitation participants is
   A) The University of California, San Diego Shortness of Breath Questionnaire
   B) The Beck Depression Inventory-II survey
   C) The Ferrans and Powers QOL Index (Pulmonary Version)
   D) The Physical Activity Readiness Questionnaire (PAR-Q+)

8. Cassidy's BMI classifies her as _____ by expert panel normative data.
   A) Underweight
   B) Normal weight
   C) Overweight
   D) Obese (class I)

9. Which of the following statements is true regarding factors to consider for Cassidy's ITP?
   A) Since she quit smoking 2 mo ago, there is no longer a need to focus on smoking cessation interventions.
   B) Once cleared for program participation, Cassidy should exercise at a level of 100 W for 10 min on the cycle ergometer as one component of her exercise prescription.
   C) Cassidy should avoid walking as part of her exercise regimen to avoid exacerbating her leg claudication pain.
   D) Once cleared for program participation, Cassidy should exercise at a level of 25 W for 8 min on the arm ergometer as one component of her exercise prescription.

10. Cassidy's ITP would consist of all of the following components *except*
    A) A plan to address her worsening depression
    B) Additional vitamins B and D supplementation to help improve her $FEV_{1.0}$ and FVC values
    C) A diet and exercise plan to help decrease her body weight and increase her lean body mass
    D) Pursed-lip breathing training to help her lessen her daily dyspnea

DISCUSSION QUESTIONS FOR CASE STUDY CEP.III

1. List and discuss some short- and long-term goals that Cassidy should be trying to achieve throughout her pulmonary rehabilitation program.

2. What problems do you foresee Cassidy having with program participation, compliance, and completion?

3. What undiagnosed medical conditions that your initial consult screening brought to light might Cassidy have? How would you treat these new (or preexisting) underlying medical conditions?

4. How would you compare the results of Cassidy's 6MWT to her previous metabolic GXT? Were the results similar with regard to her physiologic responses? How did her physical work capacity compare on both tests?

5. How would you develop Cassidy's exercise prescription from the results of her initial evaluation and her 6MWT? How would you estimate her functional capacity from her 6MWT?

6. Assuming Cassidy completes 12–16 wk of phase II pulmonary rehabilitation, what types of assessments would you administer for her follow-up outcomes documentation to provide feedback to her physician and other rehab staff? What other types of information would you track during this initial phase of rehabilitation?

DOMAIN IV: LEADERSHIP AND COUNSELING

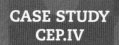 **CASE STUDY CEP.IV**   Author: **Shala E. Davis, PhD, FACSM**

Kimberly is a 43-yr-old woman (65 in tall and 159 lb) who is an office manager at a large shipping company. She is divorced and has two school-aged children (8 and 11 yr old). Kimberly has no known cardiovascular, pulmonary, or metabolic disease but considers herself to be highly deconditioned. Kimberly has been diagnosed with fibromyalgia syndrome (FMS). She works 45 h $\cdot$ wk^{-1} and commutes 30 min each way daily. Her medications are limited to over-the-counter sleep aids and nonsteroidal anti-inflammatory drugs (NSAIDs). Kimberly has initiated multiple exercise programs with little success over the past 2 yr and complains of low motivation and depression-like symptoms.

MULTIPLE-CHOICE QUESTIONS FOR CASE STUDY CEP.IV

1. Which of the following are common symptoms of clients diagnosed with FMS?
   A) Sleep disturbances
   B) Undue fatigue
   C) Diffuse soft tissue pain
   D) Depression
   E) All of the above

2. FMS symptoms may be increased by which of the following?
   A) Emotional stress
   B) Low-intensity exercise
   C) Poor sleep
   D) Both A and B
   E) Both A and C
   F) Both B and C

3. Which of the following theories related to exercise behavior is based on the principle that the person, behavior, and environment all influence future behavior?
   A) Transtheoretical model
   B) Social cognitive theory
   C) Health behavior model
   D) Self-determination model

4. Which of the following is not a strategy or strategies used to increase self-efficacy?
   A) Experiencing successful completion of tasks
   B) Modeling experiences
   C) Social persuasion
   D) Challenging self with difficult goals

5. Which of the following is not part of the SMART principles of goal setting?
   A) Goals should be realistic.
   B) Goals should have a reasonable time frame.
   C) Goals should be challenging.
   D) Goals should be specific.

DISCUSSION QUESTIONS FOR CASE STUDY CEP.IV

1. Identify three barriers and elaborate on how each barrier impacts exercise compliance for this client.

2. Provide strategies to address the barriers identified.

3. How would you approach goal setting for this client?

DOMAIN V: LEGAL AND PROFESSIONAL CONSIDERATIONS

CASE STUDY CEP.V(1)	Author: **Mandy J. Van Hofwegen, BS** Author's Certifications: **ACSM-RCEP, ACSM-CEP**

When it comes to health care, protecting patients' privacy is a high priority. Health care providers have access to detailed, personal information about their patients. Keeping this information confidential is important, which is why in 1996, the federal government passed the Health Insurance Portability and Accountability Act (HIPAA). This led to the development of the Privacy Rule in 2000. The Privacy Rule established a set of national standards for the protection, use, and disclosure of certain health information by organizations as well as standards for the privacy rights of individuals.

A central aspect of the Privacy Rule is "minimum necessary" use. Organizations may share health information with others directly involved in the care or treatment of a patient but must only disclose the minimum amount of protected information to accomplish the intended purpose.

Health care organizations must develop policies and procedures to establish privacy practices within their facilities. They must then educate all health care providers in their organization and help them comply with HIPAA regulations. Organizations that violate HIPAA Privacy Rules are subject to monetary fines and civil or criminal charges.

TRUE OR FALSE AND MULTIPLE-CHOICE QUESTIONS FOR CASE STUDY CEP.V(1)

1. A nurse from a patient's primary care office calls your facility requesting a record of recent BP readings to see if a medication change is necessary for the patient. She also asks for an update on the patient's progress because she knows the patient personally and would like to give an update to her book club tonight. What should you do?
    A) Fax the requested BP readings and give her an updated report on his progress
    B) Tell the nurse that you cannot give out any of that information
    C) Fax the BP readings and let the nurse know that you may not give out other personal information on the patient's progress
    D) Ask the nurse to contact the patient directly for all of the information requested

2. True or False: The HIPAA Privacy Rule grants individuals the right to access other family member's health information without further consent.

3. A coworker calls you from home and states that he forgot to check for an e-mail from a physician regarding a patient before he left work. He asks you to log on to the computer using his passwords and check for the e-mail. He says it is okay because you know the patient situation and the information that needs to be communicated from the physician. What should you do?
    A) Put him on hold and ask another coworker to take the call
    B) Tell your coworker that you cannot share passwords, but you will call the physician office and obtain the information needed
    C) Log on to the computer using your coworkers passwords, get the information, and then ask your coworker to change his passwords the next time he works
    D) Contact the patient and see if the physician's office possibly contacted them

4. True or False: A physician asks you to pull up a report on a mutual patient. He scans the room and sees that no one else is around. He then asks you to turn the computer toward him, now in public view, so he can see it. When he is finished discussing the report with you, he turns the computer back around. This is a violation of the patient's privacy.

5. Which of the following information is considered to be protected under the Privacy Rule?
A) Names and addresses
B) Birthdates and social security numbers
C) Past, present, and future medical diagnoses
D) All of the above

6. True or False: A patient is graduating from your rehabilitation program today and asks for a photo of himself with your staff to share with his family and friends. Later that night, you check your social media account and see that he has posted this picture with the caption, "Thanks to the rehab facility for the helping me recover after my heart attack." The patient has violated the Privacy Rule.

7. A coworker knows that she will be running late tomorrow morning and would like to get the patient charts out tonight that will be needed first thing in the morning. She wants to leave them on the desk overnight. This will save 10 extra minutes in the morning, and therefore, it will not matter if she is running late. What should you do?
A) Tell her that you cannot do that and offer to come in earlier to help out
B) Help her get the charts out and organized for the morning
C) Leave the charts on the desk with a note on each one stating "Confidential"
D) Tell her you don't think it's a good idea, but she can do what she thinks is best

DOMAIN V: LEGAL AND PROFESSIONAL CONSIDERATIONS

CASE STUDY CEP.V(2)

Author: **Shenelle E. Higbee, MS**
Author's Certifications: **ACSM-RCEP, ACSM-CEP, ACSM EP-C**

The benefits of regular exercise outweigh the risks. Exercise professionals in clinical and fitness facilities have an obligation to provide the safest possible training and testing environments while minimizing the legal and personal liability associated with adverse outcomes. The best approach to preventing emergencies is through proper screening, selection of appropriate exercise protocols, and supervision and monitoring. Structured participant education, proper placement of exercise equipment, and development of evidence-based exercise prescriptions are additional measures that will enhance the efficacy of patient safety.

Health/fitness facilities should also have policies and procedures to manage medical emergencies. Policy and procedure manuals are an integral part of the day to day operations of clinical and wellness facilities. Written emergency plans should list the specific responsibilities of each staff member, emergency equipment, and predetermined contact for emergency response.

TRUE OR FALSE AND MULTIPLE-CHOICE QUESTIONS FOR CASE STUDY CEP.V(2)

1. Which one of the following is not a common piece of emergency equipment or supply for a health/fitness facility?
A) Cardiopulmonary resuscitation (CPR) barrier masks
B) Glucometer
C) First aid kit
D) Automated external defibrillator (AED) with adult and pediatric attenuator pads (as appropriate)

2. True or False: All health/fitness facilities (levels 1–5) should have an emergency plan in place.

3. A middle-aged man at your fitness facility is currently walking on the treadmill and waves you over to him. He reports that he has suddenly started getting pressure and discomfort in his jaw and upper back. What should you do first?
A) Check his pulse
B) Check his BP
C) Have him stop exercising
D) Give the patient aspirin

4. John is attending his third cardiac rehab session today and is exercising on the treadmill without complaint. You are monitoring his ECG, and he starts having ventricular ectopy. You quickly review his chart and note that he has never had ventricular ectopy before. You ask him how he is feeling and he states he feels great. What should you do?
   A) Call a code
   B) Stop exercise and notify his physician, check and document his vitals, and continue to observe him
   C) Let him continue at the current workload and finish his exercise session
   D) Decrease his workload and continue to monitor him for the rest of his exercise session

5. An individual at your fitness facility waves you over to him while he is resting in a chair. He reports that he just tripped and has severe pain in wrist from catching himself when he fell. You notice his wrist is extremely bruised and swollen. He states he is unable to move his wrist or put any weight on it. Select the most appropriate acute response to manage this musculoskeletal emergency.
   A) Have the patient rest while you call his physician.
   B) Immediately immobilize his wrist, implement RICE (rest, ice, compress, and elevate), and promptly notify his physician.

C) Apply ice and ask if the patient if he feels comfortable going home and instruct him to contact his physician if he has any increased in symptoms.
D) Perform a range of motion test on the patient to see if his pain increases or decreases with different positions. Note any information regarding his pain and relay it to his physician.

6. Jane arrives today at phase III cardiac rehabilitation and states, "I just don't feel right." During your discussion with her, you recognize the signs of a possible transient ischemic attack (TIA) or stroke. What should you do next?
   A) Activate EMS; note the time the symptoms started
   B) Hook her up to your telemetry system and monitor her ECG
   C) Call her husband to take her to the emergency room
   D) Place in a supine position and give administer oxygen

ECG CASE STUDIES

CEP.ECG(1)　Authors: **Dennis Kerrigan (DK), PhD, and Clinton A. Brawner (CAB), PhD, MS, FACSM**
Authors' Certifications: **DK: ACSM-CEP; CAB: ACSM-RCEP, ACSM-CEP**

A 25-yr-old male was referred for a clinical exercise stress test following two witnessed episodes of syncope. Both episodes were preceded by vigorous physical activity. The following ECG was recorded at 5 min 11 sec postexercise.

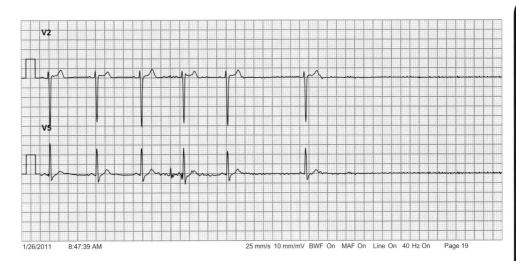

1/26/2011　8:47:39 AM　25 mm/s 10 mm/mV BWF On MAF On Line On 40 Hz On　Page 19

SHORT-ANSWER QUESTION FOR CEP.ECG(1)

1. What is the disorder? _____

MULTIPLE-CHOICE QUESTIONS FOR CEP.ECG(1)

1. What should be the first response to this ECG?
   A) Activate emergency procedures
   B) Defibrillate
   C) Check the BP
   D) Check the patient

2. Which of the following is *not* true?
   A) A patient can be stable with a sustain presentation of this disorder.
   B) This ECG could be the result of a disconnected lead.

C) Unless transient, this disorder will cause the patient to become unstable.
D) If this disorder is sustained and a normal rhythm does not return, cardiopulmonary resuscitation will be necessary.

3. This ECG could also be which of the following?
   A) Fine atrial fibrillation
   B) Course atrial fibrillation
   C) Fine ventricular fibrillation
   D) Course ventricular fibrillation

CEP.ECG(2)	Authors: **Dennis Kerrigan (DK), PhD, and Clinton A. Brawner (CAB), PhD, MS, FACSM** Authors' Certifications: **DK: ACSM-CEP; CAB: ACSM-RCEP, ACSM-CEP**

A 41-yr-old male police officer presented to cardiology for a clinical exercise stress test with the following rhythm.

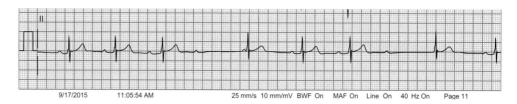

9/17/2015   11:05:54 AM   25 mm/s   10 mm/mV   BWF On   MAF On   Line On   40 Hz On   Page 11

SHORT-ANSWER QUESTIONS FOR CEP.ECG(2)

1. What is the rhythm? _____

2. What is the disorder? _____

3. What is the ventricular rate? _____

MULTIPLE-CHOICE QUESTIONS FOR CEP.ECG(2)

1. What is an important determinant of whether to conduct this test in the presence of this rhythm?
   A) According to the American Heart Association, this is a contraindication to exercise testing.
   B) According to the American Heart Association, a physician should be consulted before conducting the test.
   C) It is okay to perform the test if this is *not* a new finding.
   D) The patient's medical and symptom history as well as the presence of signs or symptoms of poor perfusion should guide whether the test can be performed.

2. Where is the origin of the impulse that conducts the ventricles?
   A) SA node
   B) Atrioventricular (AV) node
   C) Bundle of His
   D) Ventricles

3. What are the implications if this rhythm was not observed at rest but presented during the exercise test?
   A) According to the American Heart Association, the test should be terminated.
   B) According to the American Heart Association, the test should be terminated if the ventricular rate decreases by 10 beats.
   C) According to the American Heart Association, the test should be terminated if it interferes with maintenance of cardiac output (CO).
   D) According to the American Heart Association, it is not an indication to terminate a test.

CEP.ECG(3)	Authors: **Dennis Kerrigan (DK), PhD, and Clinton A. Brawner (CAB), PhD, MS, FACSM** Authors' Certifications: **DK: ACSM-CEP; CAB: ACSM-RCEP, ACSM-CEP**

A 74-yr-old woman presented to phase III (maintenance) cardiac rehabilitation without complaints and resting vitals within normal limits. During exercise, she complained of mid-upper back pain and fatigue. It was also noted that her HR did not increase with exercise. Because of these symptoms, an ECG was obtained (shown below).

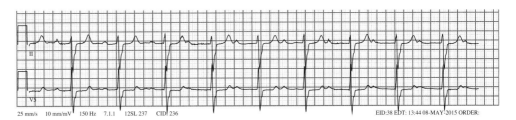

25 mm/s   10 mm/mV   150 Hz   7.1.1   12SL 237   CID 236   EID:38 EDT: 13:44 08-MAY-2015 ORDER:

SHORT-ANSWER QUESTIONS FOR CEP.ECG(3)

1. What is the disorder? _____

2. What the atrial rate? _____

3. What is the ventricular rate? _____

MULTIPLE-CHOICE QUESTIONS FOR CEP.ECG(3)

1. According to the American Heart Association,
   A) Presence of this disorder at rest is an absolute contraindication to exercise testing/training
   B) Presence of this disorder at rest is a relative contraindication to exercise testing/training
   C) If this develops during exercise, it is an absolute indication to end an exercise testing/training
   D) If this develops during exercise, it is a relative indication to end an exercise testing/training
   E) Both A and C are correct.
   F) Both B and D are correct.
   G) Both A and D are correct.
   H) Both B and C are correct.

2. Where is the origin of the impulse that conducts the ventricles?
   A) SA node
   B) AV node
   C) Bundle of His
   D) Ventricles

3. Which of the following is *not* correct?
   A) Patients are usually asymptomatic with this disorder.
   B) This disorder can compromise CO.
   C) This disorder can present due to transient ischemia.
   D) This disorder can be an indication for a permanent pacemaker.

CEP.ECG(4)   Authors: **Dennis Kerrigan (DK), PhD, and Clinton A. Brawner (CAB), PhD, MS, FACSM**
Authors' Certifications: **DK: ACSM-CEP; CAB: ACSM-RCEP, ACSM-CEP**

A 75-yr-old male patient with a recent history (2 mo ago) of coronary bypass surgery presents to cardiac rehabilitation for his initial visit with the following rhythm. His vitals are as follows: weight = 230 lb, BP = 102/84 mm Hg.

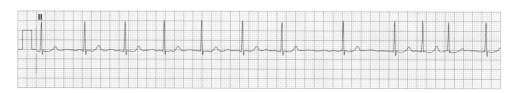

SHORT-ANSWER QUESTIONS FOR CEP.ECG(4)

1. What is the rate? _____

2. Regular or irregular? _____

3. Interpret the rhythm. _____

MULTIPLE-CHOICE QUESTIONS FOR CEP.ECG(4)

1. Name the medication usually prescribed that prevents a common complication due to this arrhythmia.
    A) Lisinopril
    B) Warfarin
    C) Metoprolol
    D) Simvastatin

2. What effect does this arrhythmia typically have on CO?
    A) CO is elevated due to the increased contractions in the atria.
    B) The "atrial kick" has negligible effect on CO.
    C) CO is reduced.
    D) None of the above

3. How should exercise be prescribed in this patient, assuming he performed a sign- and symptom-limited exercise stress test prior to cardiac rehabilitation?
    A) RPE
    B) An HR 20–30 beats above rest
    C) 50%–85% of HRR
    D) The patient should not exercise with this arrhythmia.

CEP.ECG(5)   Authors: **Dennis Kerrigan (DK), PhD, and Clinton A. Brawner (CAB), PhD, MS, FACSM**
Authors' Certifications: **DK: ACSM-CEP; CAB: ACSM-RCEP, ACSM-CEP**

A patient with a history of cardiac arrest and MI is walking on the treadmill in cardiac rehabilitation when you observe this rhythm.

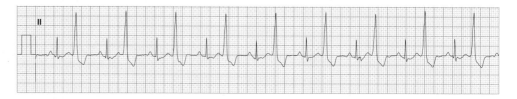

SHORT-ANSWER QUESTIONS FOR CEP.ECG(5)

1. What is the underlying rhythm? _____

2. What is the dysrhythmia? _____

MULTIPLE-CHOICE QUESTIONS FOR CEP.ECG(5)

1. Assuming this patient has a history of this dysrhythmia, what actions should be taken?
   A) Continue to monitor
   B) Stop the exercise immediately
   C) Call an emergency code and grab the automatic defibrillator
   D) Slow treadmill speed and call physician

2. What might be some potential causes of this dysrhythmia?
   A) Caffeine
   B) Anxiety/stress
   C) Forgetting to take medications
   D) All of the above

CEP.ECG(6)

Authors: **Dennis Kerrigan (DK), PhD, and Clinton A. Brawner (CAB), PhD, MS, FACSM**
Authors' Certifications: **DK: ACSM-CEP; CAB: ACSM-RCEP, ACSM-CEP**

A 52-yr-old male without a history of heart disease is scheduled in your laboratory for a standard sign- and symptom-limited exercise stress test with ECG to evaluate a recent episode of angina while performing yard work.

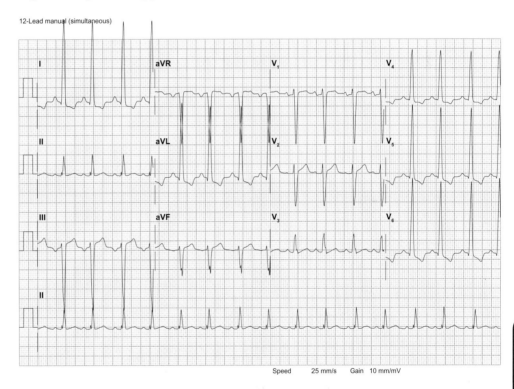

SHORT-ANSWER QUESTIONS FOR CEP.ECG(6)

1. What is the rate? _____

2. Regular or irregular? _____

3. Interpret the ECG. _____

TRUE OR FALSE AND MULTIPLE-CHOICE QUESTIONS FOR CEP.ECG(6)

1. Assuming the patient is asymptomatic at rest, what course of action would you follow?
   A) Proceed with the stress test using a low-level treadmill protocol
   B) Send patient directly to emergency department
   C) Attempt Valsalva maneuver
   D) Contact referring physician to verify the test ordered

2. True or False: If the aforementioned patient presented with the observed ECG abnormality *and* severe CP, this could indicate an acute MI.

CEP.ECG(7)

Authors: **Dennis Kerrigan (DK), PhD, and Clinton A. Brawner (CAB), PhD, MS, FACSM**
Authors' Certifications: **DK: ACSM-CEP; CAB: ACSM-RCEP, ACSM-CEP**

A 42-yr-old male with hypertension is undergoing a symptom-limited exercise stress test on a treadmill in response to a recent episode of syncope he experienced while running. The following ECG was taken during stage IV of the Bruce protocol.

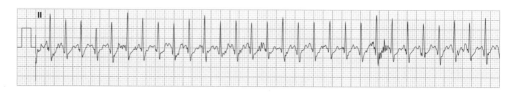

SHORT-ANSWER QUESTIONS FOR CEP.ECG(7)

1. What is the rate? _____

2. Regular or irregular? _____

3. Interpret the rhythm. _____

MULTIPLE-CHOICE QUESTIONS FOR CEP.ECG(7)

1. If the aforementioned ECG was taken during rest, what might you suspect?
   A) Second-degree AV block, type I
   B) Supraventricular tachycardia (SVT)
   C) Ventricular tachycardia
   D) Both A and B

2. Which of the following medications for hypertension is he likely *not* taking
   A) ACE inhibitor
   B) Diuretic
   C) Angiotensin II receptor antagonists
   D) β-Blocker

3. Based on the ECG alone and information given earlier, should the stress test be stopped?
   A) Yes
   B) No

CEP.ECG(8)

Authors: **Dennis Kerrigan (DK), PhD, and Clinton A. Brawner (CAB), PhD, MS, FACSM**
Authors' Certifications: **DK: ACSM-CEP; CAB: ACSM-RCEP, ACSM-CEP**

A 53-yr-old female with ischemic cardiomyopathy is performing a symptom-limited exercise stress test in your laboratory. During stage III of the Naughton protocol, you observe for the first time the following on the ECG.

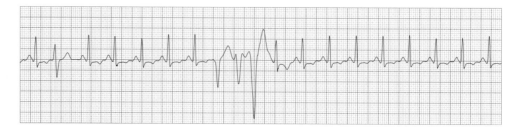

SHORT-ANSWER QUESTIONS FOR CEP.ECG(8)

1. What is the rate? _____

2. Regular or irregular? _____

3. Interpret the rhythm. _____

MULTIPLE-CHOICE QUESTIONS FOR CEP.ECG(8)

1. What course of action should you take?
   A) Stop the test immediately
   B) Continue with the test
   C) Take an immediate BP
   D) Administer a sublingual nitroglycerin

2. What can be said about the ectopic beats?
   A) They are multifocal.
   B) They are unifocal.
   C) They are junctional beats.
   D) They are both ventricular and supraventricular in nature.

CEP.ECG(9)

Authors: **Dennis Kerrigan (DK), PhD, and Clinton A. Brawner (CAB), PhD, MS, FACSM**
Authors' Certifications: **DK: ACSM-CEP; CAB: ACSM-RCEP, ACSM-CEP**

A 16-yr-old hockey player has an ECG as part of his preparticipation screening. The following is his resting ECG.

12-Lead manual (simultaneous)

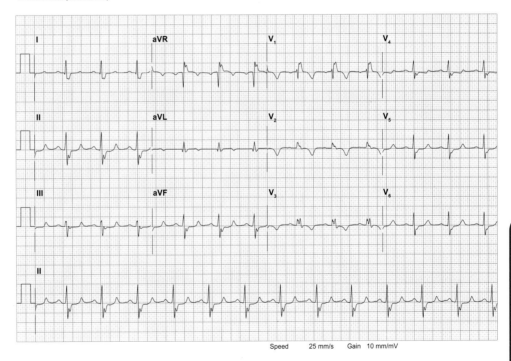

SHORT-ANSWER QUESTIONS FOR CEP.ECG(9)

1. What is the rate? _____

2. Regular or irregular? _____

3. Interpret the ECG. _____

MULTIPLE-CHOICE QUESTION FOR CEP.ECG(9)

1. Based on the ECG, what will likely happen with this athlete?
    A) The athlete will be cleared to participate without any further workup.
    B) The athlete will likely play hockey next year after receiving treatment.
    C) The athlete will no longer be able to participate in sports.
    D) The athlete will likely undergo additional evaluation before returning to play.

CEP.ECG(10)

Authors: **Dennis Kerrigan (DK), PhD, and Clinton A. Brawner (CAB), PhD, MS, FACSM**
Authors' Certifications: **DK: ACSM-CEP; CAB: ACSM-RCEP, ACSM-CEP**

A 32-yr-old apparently healthy male cyclist is self-referred for a maximal exercise test to assess his and anaerobic threshold in preparation for an upcoming race. The following is his resting ECG.

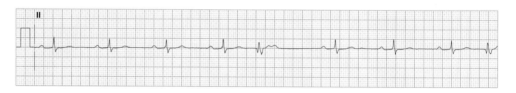

SHORT-ANSWER QUESTIONS FOR CEP.ECG(10)

1. What is the rate? _____

2. Regular or irregular? _____

3. Interpret the rhythm. _____

TRUE OR FALSE AND MULTIPLE-CHOICE QUESTIONS FOR CEP.ECG(10)

1. True or False: The length of the PR interval is directly responsible for the rate.

2. What are the testing implications of this ECG?
    A) Physician should be notified due to the likelihood of a complete heart block.
    B) Due to the decreased CO, $\dot{V}O_{2peak}$ will be blunted.
    C) This is a benign finding, which will have no effect on the test.
    D) There is a slight risk for atrial reentry tachycardia.

CEP.ECG(11)

Authors: **Dennis Kerrigan (DK), PhD, and Clinton A. Brawner (CAB), PhD, MS, FACSM**
Authors' Certifications: **DK: ACSM-CEP; CAB: ACSM-RCEP, ACSM-CEP**

An 84-yr-old female is exercising in cardiac rehabilitation for the first time. While on the recumbent cycle, you see the following on the monitor.

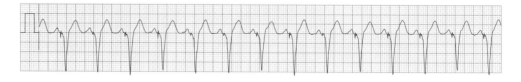

SHORT-ANSWER QUESTIONS FOR CEP.ECG(11)

1. What is the rate? _____

2. Regular or irregular? _____

3. Interpret the rhythm. _____

MULTIPLE-CHOICE QUESTIONS FOR CEP.ECG(11)

1. Which of the following conditions might be the reason she received a pacemaker?
   A) Sick sinus syndrome
   B) Ventricular tachycardia
   C) Third-degree AV block
   D) Both A and C

2. During her first three visits, she experiences CP. As a result, her physician sends her for a symptom-limited exercise stress test with nuclear imaging. Why was the nuclear imaging specified?
   A) She is unable to walk very long on a treadmill.
   B) Her pacemaker would interfere with an echocardiogram.
   C) If present, ischemia would not be undetectable by ECG alone due to the pacemaker depolarization.
   D) All of the above

CEP.ECG(12)

Authors: **Dennis Kerrigan (DK), PhD, and Clinton A. Brawner (CAB), PhD, MS, FACSM**
Authors' Certifications: **DK: ACSM-CEP; CAB: ACSM-RCEP, ACSM-CEP**

A 64-yr-old male with a history of an MI and stent 15 yr ago is exercising in your phase III cardiac rehabilitation program. While on the treadmill, he complains of jaw pain and nausea. You place him in a semisupine position with the upper body slightly elevated and attach an ECG.

12-Lead manual (simultaneous)

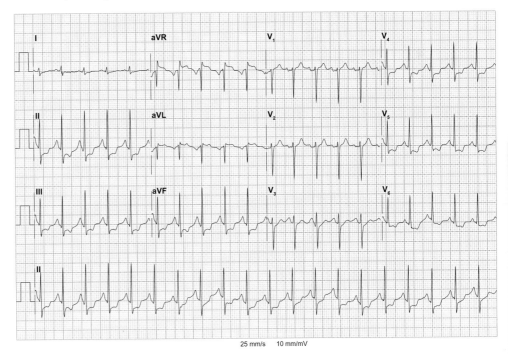

25 mm/s   10 mm/mV

CEP

SHORT-ANSWER QUESTIONS FOR CEP.ECG(12)

1. What is the rate? _____

2. Regular or irregular? _____

3. Interpret the rhythm. _____

MULTIPLE-CHOICE QUESTIONS FOR CEP.ECG(12)

1. Which of the following medications may improve his jaw pain?
   A) Nitroglycerin
   B) Plavix
   C) Epinephrine
   D) Both A and C

2. Based on the ECG, what regions of the heart are ischemic?
   A) Inferior
   B) Septal
   C) Lateral
   D) Both A and C

CEP.ECG(13)   Authors: **Dennis Kerrigan (DK), PhD, and Clinton A. Brawner (CAB), PhD, MS, FACSM**
Authors' Certifications: **DK: ACSM-CEP; CAB: ACSM-RCEP, ACSM-CEP**

A 58-yr-old female has just completed a low-level exercise test as a predischarge requirement following an STEMI a few days ago. While seated in recovery, you notice a change in the ECG.

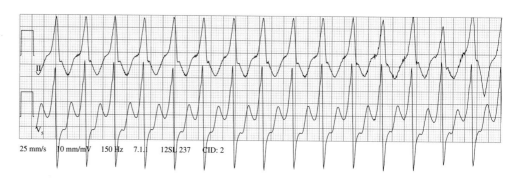

25 mm/s   10 mm/mV   150 Hz   7.1.1   12SL 237   CID: 2

SHORT-ANSWER QUESTIONS FOR CEP.ECG(13)

1. What is the rate? _____

2. Regular or irregular? _____

3. Interpret the rhythm. _____

MULTIPLE-CHOICE QUESTIONS FOR CEP.ECG(13)

1. What actions should you take?
   A) Check the patient
   B) Notify the physician
   C) Prepare the crash cart
   D) All of the above

2. Your patient suddenly loses consciousness, what was likely the cause of this?
   A) Low blood glucose
   B) Vasovagal response
   C) Seizure
   D) Low CO

CEP CASE STUDIES ANSWERS AND EXPLANATIONS

CASE STUDY CEP.I

Multiple-Choice Answers for Case Study CEP.I

1—B. $33.1 \text{ kg} \cdot \text{m}^{-2}$

250 lb / 2.2 = 113.64 kg. 6 ft 1 in = 73 in.
73 × 2.54 = 185.42 cm. 185.42 / 100 = 1.8524 m.
113.64 kg / $(1.8524)^2$ = 33.05 or $33.1 \text{ kg} \cdot \text{m}^{-2}$

2—A.   Current lipid values

The current preparticipation screening guidelines no longer include CVD risk factors as part of the decision-making process for referral to a health care provider prior to initiating a moderate- to vigorous-intensity exercise program. Grant's current lipid values are a CVD risk factor assessment. One that should still be part of an overall cardiovascular and metabolic disease prevention and management program.

Resource: Riebe D, senior editor. *ACSM's Guidelines for Exercise Testing and Prescription*. 10th ed. Philadelphia (PA): Wolters Kluwer; 2018.

3—A.   Signed informed consent form only

The preparticipation screening algorithm now takes into account three factors: (1) current level of physical activity, (2) presence of signs or symptoms and/or known cardiovascular, metabolic, or renal disease, and (3) desired exercise intensity, as these three factors have been identified as important risk modulators of exercise-related cardiovascular events. Grant does not regularly exercise; has no diagnosed cardiovascular, metabolic, or renal disease; and has no sign or symptoms suggestive of such. Medical clearance is not needed for light-to moderate-intensity exercise.

Resources: James PA, Oparil S, Carter BL, et al. 2014 evidence-based guideline for the management of high blood pressure in adults: report from the panel members appointed to the Eighth Joint National Committee (JNC 8). *JAMA*. 2014;311(5):507–20.

Riebe D, senior editor. *ACSM's Guidelines for Exercise Testing and Prescription*. 10th ed. Philadelphia (PA): Wolters Kluwer; 2018.

JNC7

Resource: Chobanian AV, Bakris GL, Black HR, et al. The Seventh Report of the Joint National Committee on Prevention, Detection, Evaluation, and Treatment of High Blood Pressure: the JNC 7 report. *JAMA*. 2003;289(19):2560–72.

4—A.   Precontemplation

Resource: Riebe D, senior editor. *ACSM's Guidelines for Exercise Testing and Prescription*. 10th ed. Philadelphia (PA): Wolters Kluwer; 2018.

5—B.   Grant would be classified as having impaired fasting glucose (IFG).

Resources: Riebe D, senior editor. *ACSM's Guidelines for Exercise Testing and Prescription*. 10th ed. Philadelphia (PA): Wolters Kluwer; 2018.

National Cholesterol Education Program (NCEP) Expert Panel on Detection, Evaluation, and Treatment of High Blood Cholesterol in Adults (Adult Treatment Panel III). Third Report of the National Cholesterol Education Program (NCEP) Expert Panel on Detection, Evaluation, and Treatment of High Blood Cholesterol in Adults (Adult Treatment Panel III) final report. *Circulation*. 2002;106(25):3143–421.

Discussion Question Answers for Case Study CEP.I

1. His main goal should be to adopt a more physically active lifestyle, increase his leisure-time physical activity, and exercise to maximize his caloric expenditure. This will benefit Grant in improving all aspects of his risk factor profile. His cardiometabolic risk profile is highly related to his obesity (overall and abdominal) and physical inactivity. By maximizing caloric expenditure and becoming more active, he can improve his body composition, which can aid in improving his blood lipids, glucose levels, and BP.

2. Individuals with metabolic syndrome should continually work toward maximizing energy expenditure; this favorably impacts cardiometabolic profile. Grant should progress to a frequency of $>5 \text{ d} \cdot \text{wk}^{-1}$, gradually increasing his intensity to vigorous ($>60\%$ of $\dot{V}O_2R$). Time spent exercising should be between >300 min of moderate or >150 min of vigorous intensity exercise per week, or a combination of both. Given his relatively low current motivation to exercise, modalities chosen should be those Grant enjoys, effectively increasing the likelihood that he will maintain his exercise program.

CEP

CASE STUDY CEP.II(1)

Multiple-Choice Answers for Case Study CEP.II(1)

1—C. 4.5 METs

If exercise test data is available, exercise can be prescribed at a workload below the ischemic threshold (~ 1 MET). Some considerations for this client are:

Is this a true positive or false positive test for CAD?

Her blood laboratory values indicate that she may have blood glucose control problems (prediabetes).

The GXT documentation provides real data at workloads that are equivalent to 4.7 and 7.0 METs.

Based on HR response, the 7 MET workload represents a near maximum test.

Given all of the aforementioned concerns, a workload equivalent at or near 4.7 METs would seem most appropriate for this client.

Resource: Riebe D, senior editor. *ACSM's Guidelines for Exercise Testing and Prescription*. 10th ed. Philadelphia (PA): Wolters Kluwer; 2018.

2—B. 14

If exercise test data is available, exercise can be prescribed at an RPE represented during the stage of testing for that MET level and can act as a calibration of the individual's subjective RPE rating.

Resource: Riebe D, senior editor. *ACSM's Guidelines for Exercise Testing and Prescription*. 10th ed. Philadelphia (PA): Wolters Kluwer; 2018.

3—C. Both of Nancy's medications may have adverse effects during exercise testing or programming.

Diuretics may produce hypotension through hypovolemia and therefore result in a higher HR. Caution in interpreting ECG ST-segment depression as representative of an ischemic response must be used due to the possibility of diuretics causing hypokalemia which can result in a depressed ST segment on the ECG. Dihydropyridine calcium channel blockers commonly used in treating hypertension are an effective vasodilator and may result in a higher HR response due to increased sympathetic compensation.

Resource: Riebe D, senior editor. *ACSM's Guidelines for Exercise Testing and Prescription*. 10th ed. Philadelphia (PA): Wolters Kluwer; 2018.

4—C. All of the medications that Nancy is prescribed may effect HR during exercise.

As previously noted in question 3, the medications that Nancy is taking may result in HR increases during exercise secondarily to potential hypovolemia (diuretics) and/or vasodilation (dihydropyridine calcium channel blockers).

Resource: Riebe D, senior editor. *ACSM's Guidelines for Exercise Testing and Prescription*. 10th ed. Philadelphia (PA): Wolters Kluwer; 2018.

5—E. Either A or B would be an appropriate treadmill workload for Nancy.

Calculations:

Treadmill = 2.0 mph and a 7% grade

Workload Equivalent = 4.5 METs

Resting Component = 3.5 mL $\cdot$ kg^{-1} $\cdot$ min

Walking Horizontal
Component = 0.1 $\times$ speed

$$= 0.1 \times (2.0 \text{ mph} \times 26.8)$$

$$= 0.1 \times 53.6 \text{ m min}$$

$$= 5.3 \text{ mL} \cdot \text{kg}^{-1} \cdot \text{min}$$

Walking Vertical
Component = 1.8 $\times$ speed $\times$ grade

$$= 1.8 \times 53.6 \text{ m} \cdot \text{min} \times .07$$

$$= 6.7 \text{ mL} \cdot \text{kg}^{-1} \cdot \text{min}$$

$\dot{V}O_2$ mL $\cdot$ kg^{-1} $\cdot$ min = Resting + Walking Horizontal + Vertical Components

$\dot{V}O_2$ mL $\cdot$ kg^{-1} $\cdot$ min = 3.5 + 5.3 + 6.7

$$= 15.5 \text{ mL} \cdot \text{kg}^{-1} \cdot \text{min}$$

METs = $\dot{V}O_2$ mL $\cdot$ kg^{-1} $\cdot$ min / 3.5 mL $\cdot$ kg^{-1} $\cdot$ min

METs = 15.5 mL $\cdot$ kg^{-1} $\cdot$ min / 3.5 mL $\cdot$ kg^{-1} $\cdot$ min

$$= 4.43 \text{ METs}$$

Treadmill = 3.0 mph and a 3% grade

Workload Equivalent = 4.5 METs

Resting Component = 3.5 mL $\cdot$ kg^{-1} $\cdot$ min

Walking Horizontal
Component = 0.1 $\times$ speed

$$= 0.1 \times (3.0 \text{ mph} \times 26.8)$$

$$= 0.1 \times 80.4 \text{ m} \cdot \text{min}$$

$$= 8.0 \text{ mL} \cdot \text{kg}^{-1} \cdot \text{min}$$

Walking Vertical
Component = 1.8 × speed × grade

$$= 1.8 \times 80.4 \text{ m} \cdot \text{min} \times .03$$

$$= 4.3 \text{ mL} \cdot \text{kg}^{-1} \cdot \text{min}$$

$\dot{V}O_2$ mL · kg^{-1} · min = Resting + Walking
Horizontal + Vertical Components

$\dot{V}O_2$ mL · kg^{-1} · min = 3.5 + 8.0 + 4.3

$$= 15.8 \text{ mL} \cdot \text{kg}^{-1} \cdot \text{min}$$

METs = $\dot{V}O_2$ mL · kg^{-1} · min / 3.5 mL · kg^{-1} · min

METs = 15.8 mL · kg^{-1} · min / 3.5 mL · kg^{-1} · min

$$= 4.51 \text{ METs}$$

The ACSM's metabolic equation for walking is most accurate for speeds of 1.9–3.7 mph. All speed units for equations should be in units of meter per minute, which is converted when you multiply miles per hour by the constant 26.8. All grades should be in decimal form, for example, 7% = 0.07.

The vertical component is only valid for estimating the metabolic cost of walking and running on a grade on a treadmill. The vertical component equation is *not* valid for the metabolic cost of ground walking or running on grades.

Resource: Riebe D, senior editor. *ACSM's Guidelines for Exercise Testing and Prescription.* 10th ed. Philadelphia (PA): Wolters Kluwer; 2018.

6—A.   275 kgm · min^{-1}

Calculations:

Workload Equivalent
(Treadmill) = 4.5 METs

$$= 4.5 \text{ METs} \times 3.5$$

$$= 15.75 \text{ mL} \cdot \text{kg}^{-1} \cdot \text{min}$$

Workload Equivalent
(Cycle Ergometer) = 15.75 mL · kg^{-1} · min × 0.90 (10% reduction)

$$= 14.18 \text{ mL} \cdot \text{kg}^{-1} \cdot \text{min}$$

Nancy's Body Weight = 158 lb × 0.454

$$= 71.7 \text{ kg}$$

Resting Component = 3.5 mL · kg^{-1} · min

Cycle Ergometer Horizontal Component = 3.5 mL · kg^{-1} · min

Cycle Ergometer Resistance Component = (1.8 × work rate kg · min^{-1}) / body mass kg

Cycle Ergometer Total Equation mL · kg^{-1} · min = Resistance + Horizontal + Resting

14.18 mL · kg^{-1} · min = (1.8 × work rate kg · min^{-1}) / 71.7 kg + 3.5 + 3.5

7.18 mL · kg^{-1} · min = (1.8 × work rate kg · min^{-1}) / 71.7 kg

514.8 mL · min^{-1} = 1.8 × work rate kg · min^{-1}

286.0 = work rate kg · min^{-1}

If the initial GXT was completed on a treadmill, then the conversion to similar physiological aerobic stress will be approximately 10%–15% less on a cycle ergometer. Therefore, either the functional capacity or the workload in MET needs to be reduced by 10%–15%. The metabolic equation is most accurate for work rates of 300–1,200 kg · min^{-1}.

Resource: Riebe D, senior editor. *ACSM's Guidelines for Exercise Testing and Prescription.* 10th ed. Philadelphia (PA): Wolters Kluwer; 2018.

7—D.   5–7 d · wk^{-1}

Nancy's medical history indicates that she has low fitness, is overweight, and meets the criteria for both prediabetes and metabolic syndrome. Her stated goal is to exercise to lose weight. Based on all of these criteria, it is recommended that Nancy exercise ≥5 d · wk^{-1}, and preferably she should exercise most days of the week.

Resource: Riebe D, senior editor. *ACSM's Guidelines for Exercise Testing and Prescription.* 10th ed. Philadelphia (PA): Wolters Kluwer; 2018.

8—D.   10–15 RM

Initial loads in beginning a resistance program should allow 10–15 repetitions that can be lifted comfortably (40%–50% of 1-RM, progressing to 60%–70% of 1-RM).

Resource: Riebe D, senior editor. *ACSM's Guidelines for Exercise Testing and Prescription.* 10th ed. Philadelphia (PA): Wolters Kluwer; 2018.

9—C.   Obesity

Nancy's BMI was calculated as 28.0 kg · m^{-2}. Although this places her in the "Overweight" category for BMI, her BMI does not achieve the criterion level for "Obesity" (≥30.0 kg · m^{-2}).

Resource: Riebe D, senior editor. *ACSM's Guidelines for Exercise Testing and Prescription.* 10th ed. Philadelphia (PA): Wolters Kluwer; 2018.

CEP

10—C. 60%

Calculations:

Maximum Functional Capacity = 7.0 METs

$\dot{V}O_2R$ = 7.0 METs − 1 MET

$\qquad$ = 6.0 METs

Maximum Workload Question 1 = 4.5 METs

$\dot{V}O_2R$ % = [(4.5 METs − 1.0 METs) / 6.0 METs]

$\qquad$ = 0.583

$\qquad$ = 0.583 × 100

$\qquad$ = 58.3 %

Resource: Riebe D, senior editor. *ACSM's Guidelines for Exercise Testing and Prescription*. 10th ed. Philadelphia (PA): Wolters Kluwer; 2018.

Discussion Question Answers for Case Study CEP.II(1)

1. Considerations of medical history, GXT, and patient goals in developing an exercise program:

   Medical History
   - Risk Factor Profile
     1. Family history
     2. Hypertension
     3. Abnormal fasting blood glucose and HbA1C
     4. Dyslipidemia (triglycerides)
     5. Fitness level
     6. BMI
     7. Predicted maximal volume of oxygen consumed per unit time ($\dot{V}O_{2max}$) from GXT
   - Medication Effects on Exercise Testing and Programming
     1. Diuretics
     2. ST-segment depression (possible)
     3. Hypovolemia
     4. Hypohydration
     5. Calcium channel blockers
     6. Dihydropyridine versus nondihydropyridine class effects on exercise
     7. Vasodilation compensatory sympathetic response (increased HR)
   - Laboratory Blood Analysis

   Graded Exercise Test as a Basis for Exercise Prescription
   - ECG Changes (ST-Segment Depression) during GXT
     1. Causes of abnormal ST changes in the absence of obstructive CAD
        A. Female gender
        B. Hypokalemia (diuretic induced)
   - Hemodynamic Responses to Exercise
   - Subjective RPE
   - Predicted $\dot{V}O_{2max}$ from GXT

   Patient Goals
   - Nancy expressed a desire to lose weight through exercise and diet.

2. **Outline of Discussion (II)**
   - Intensity of exercise that minimizes blood lactate accumulation
   - Intensity of exercise that minimizes frustration
   - Intensity/duration of exercise that maximizes caloric expenditure
   - Exercise bout and/or daily interval training
   - Frequency that establishes positive exercise patterns
   - Frequency that aids in blood glucose control
   - Mode in aerobic exercise that involves large muscle mass
   - Mode that minimizes orthopedic joint stress but utilizes bone stress (osteoporosis)
   - Mode in resistance exercise that minimizes delayed onset muscle soreness (DOMS)
   - Progression for a new, low-fit, overweight, middle-aged client with prediabetes

CASE STUDY CEP.II(2)

Multiple-Choice Answers for Case Study CEP.II(2)

1—B.   Light to moderate; 30%–<60% of HRR

Resource: Riebe D, senior editor. *ACSM's Guidelines for Exercise Testing and Prescription*. 10th ed. Philadelphia (PA): Wolters Kluwer; 2018.

2—D. $\geq$5 d · wk^{-1}

Resource: Riebe D, senior editor. *ACSM's Guidelines for Exercise Testing and Prescription*. 10th ed. Philadelphia (PA): Wolters Kluwer; 2018.

3—C.   Biguanide drug for Type 2 DM

Resource: Riebe D, senior editor. *ACSM's Guidelines for Exercise Testing and Prescription*. 10th ed. Philadelphia (PA): Wolters Kluwer; 2018.

4—D.   Both B and C

Resource: Riebe D, senior editor. *ACSM's Guidelines for Exercise Testing and Prescription*. 10th ed. Philadelphia (PA): Wolters Kluwer; 2018.

5—E.   Only A and B of the above

Resource: Riebe D, senior editor. *ACSM's Guidelines for Exercise Testing and Prescription*. 10th ed. Philadelphia (PA): Wolters Kluwer; 2018.

6—A. 90–96 bpm

Initial THR = 40%–<60% of exercise capacity using HRR. Initially, you would start the client at 40%–50% HRR for his metabolic syndrome and obesity.

$$THR = [(HR_{max} - HR_{rest}) \times \% \text{ intensity}] + HR_{rest}$$

$$THR = (132 - 72) \times 0.40 + 72 = \underline{96 \text{ bpm}}$$
$$(132 - 72) \times 0.50 + 72 = \underline{102 \text{ bpm}}$$

THR = 96–102 bpm

Resource: Riebe D, senior editor. *ACSM's Guidelines for Exercise Testing and Prescription.* 10th ed. Philadelphia (PA): Wolters Kluwer; 2018.

7—D. 3.3 mph and 7% grade

$$\dot{V}O_2 = (0.1 \times 3.3 \text{ mph} \times 26.8) + (1.8 \times 3.2 \times 26.8 \times .07) + 3.5$$

(Horizontal)   (Vertical)   (Rest)

$$\dot{V}O_2 = (8.84) + (10.8) + 3.5$$

$$\dot{V}O_2 = 23.14 \text{ mL} \cdot \text{kg}^{-1} \cdot \text{min}^{-1}$$

METs = 23.14 / 3.5 = 6.61 METs

Resource: Riebe D, senior editor. *ACSM's Guidelines for Exercise Testing and Prescription.* 10th ed. Philadelphia (PA): Wolters Kluwer; 2018.

8—C. 2–3; moderate

Resource: Riebe D, senior editor. *ACSM's Guidelines for Exercise Testing and Prescription.* 10th ed. Philadelphia (PA): Wolters Kluwer; 2018.

9—A. Enhance insulin sensitivity

Resource: Tresierras MA, Balady GJ. Resistance training in the treatment of diabetes and obesity: mechanisms and outcomes. *J Cardiopulm Rehabil Prev.* 2009;29:67–75.

10—C. ≥500–1,000 MET-min · wk^{-1}

Resource: Riebe D, senior editor. ACSM's Guidelines for Exercise Testing and Prescription. 10th ed. Philadelphia (PA): Wolters Kluwer; 2018.

Discussion Question Answers for Case Study CEP.II(2)

1. Questions or recommendations include the following:

   a. Ask him about his medication compliance.
   b. Refer him to a smoking cessation program.
   c. Have him schedule a follow-up visit with his physician concerning his abnormal fasting blood values and pulmonary function test values.
   d. Have him talk with the program dietician regarding weight loss strategies.
   e. Ask him about his compliance taking his daily blood glucose measurements.
   f. Ask him if his glucometer works properly.
   g. Ask him if he has a home automatic BP measuring device.
   h. Ask him about the amount of home exercise he is currently performing.
   i. Inquire about any potential orthopedic or musculoskeletal limitations that he may have.

2. Exercise benefits include the following:

   a. Enhanced muscle glucose uptake through improved insulin sensitivity and decreased insulin resistance
   b. Better weight control
   c. Lowered BP
   d. Improved blood lipid and lipoprotein values
   e. Better sleep
   f. Improved mood and outlook on life
   g. Decreased stress level
   h. Decreased fat mass and increased FFM
   i. Stronger bones
   j. Less SOB if he quits smoking
   k. Decreased overall body weight

CASE STUDY CEP.II(3)

Multiple-Choice Answers for Case Study CEP.II(3)

1—B. 39 kg

Resource: Riebe D, senior editor. *ACSM's Guidelines for Exercise Testing and Prescription.* 10th ed. Philadelphia (PA): Wolters Kluwer; 2018.

2—C. HR below the ischemic threshold (<10 beats)

Resource: Riebe D, senior editor. *ACSM's Guidelines for Exercise Testing and Prescription.* 10th ed. Philadelphia (PA): Wolters Kluwer; 2018.

3—B. No greater than 134 bpm

If exercise data is provided, exercise should be prescribed at an HR below the ischemic threshold (<10 bpm).

Resource: Riebe D, senior editor. *ACSM's Guidelines for Exercise Testing and Prescription.* 10th ed. Philadelphia (PA): Wolters Kluwer; 2018.

4—A.   124 W

If GXT is administered on a leg cycle ergometer, there is ~10%–15% less physiological stress than on a treadmill. Functional capacity needs to be reduced by 10%.

$\dot{V}O_2$ Relative = 6 METs × 3.5 mL · kg^{-1} · min^{-1} = 21.0 mL · kg^{-1} · min^{-1} × 0.90 = 18.9 mL · kg^{-1} · min^{-1}

Joe's body weight = 253 lb × 2.2 = 115 kg

1 W = 6.12 kgm

Resting component = 3.5 mL · kg^{-1} · min^{-1}

Leg cycle ergometer horizontal component = 3.5 mL · kg^{-1} · min^{-1}

$\dot{V}O_2$ Relative = $\dfrac{1.8 \times W}{M}$ + 7

18.9 mL · kg^{-1} · min^{-1} = $\dfrac{1.8 \times W}{115\ kg}$ + 7 → 760 kgm / 6.12 → 124 W

Resource: Riebe D, senior editor. *ACSM's Guidelines for Exercise Testing and Prescription.* 10th ed. Philadelphia (PA): Wolters Kluwer; 2018.

5—B.   213 lb

Joe's BF percentage = 34 percent

Joe's target BF percentage = 22 percent

Fat mass = 115 kg × 0.34 = 39 kg

Fat-free mass = 76 kg

Target body weight = Fat-free mass ÷ (1 − BF%)

76 kg ÷ (1 − 0.22) = 97 kg

97 kg × 2.2 = 213 lbs

Resource: Riebe D, senior editor. *ACSM's Guidelines for Exercise Testing and Prescription.* 10th ed. Philadelphia (PA): Wolters Kluwer; 2018.

6—A.   Normal

Resting EF of <55% is considered normal.

Resources: Ehrman JK, Gordon PM, Visich PS, Keteyian SJ. *Clinical Exercise Physiology.* 3rd ed. Champaign (IL): Human Kinetics; 2013.

Riebe D, senior editor. *ACSM's Guidelines for Exercise Testing and Prescription.* 10th ed. Philadelphia (PA): Wolters Kluwer; 2018.

7—D.   Moderately severe angina

3+ on a 1–4 scale

Resource: Riebe D, senior editor. *ACSM's Guidelines for Exercise Testing and Prescription.* 10th ed. Philadelphia (PA): Wolters Kluwer; 2018.

8—A.   6 METs

If exercise data is provided, exercise intensity should be prescribed at a workload 1 MET below the ischemic threshold.

Resource: Riebe D, senior editor. *ACSM's Guidelines for Exercise Testing and Prescription.* 10th ed. Philadelphia (PA): Wolters Kluwer; 2018.

9—C.   3.6 mph and 4.5% grade

mph to m · s^{-1} = 3.6 mph × 26.8 m · s^{-1} = 98.48 m · s^{-1}

grade % to decimal form = 4.5 % = 0.045

Resting component = 3.5 mL · kg^{-1} · min^{-1}

Horizontal component = (0.1 × speed) = (0.1 × 98.48 m · s^{-1}) = 9.848 mL · kg^{-1} · min^{-1}

Vertical component = (1.8 × speed × grade) = (1.8 × 98.48 × 0.045) = 7.976 mL · kg^{-1} · min^{-1}

MET = 21.324 mL · kg^{-1} · min^{-1} / 3.5 mL · kg^{-1} · min^{-1} = 6.093 = 6 METs

Resource: Riebe D, senior editor. *ACSM's Guidelines for Exercise Testing and Prescription.* 10th ed. Philadelphia (PA): Wolters Kluwer; 2018.

10—C.   362 kcal

Maximal MET level on treadmill is 6 MET.

VO_2Relative = 6 METs × 3.5 mL · kg^{-1} · min^{-1} = 21 mL · kg^{-1} · min^{-1}

Joe's weight in kg = 115 (253 lb / 2.2)

1 L · min^{-1} = 5 cal

Time = 30 min

$\dot{V}O_2$Absolute = 21 mL · kg^{-1} · min^{-1} × 115 kg = $\dfrac{2.415\ L \cdot min^{-1}}{1,000\ mL}$

2.415 L· min^{-1} × 5 cal × 30 min = 362 cal

Resource: Riebe D, senior editor. *ACSM's Guidelines for Exercise Testing and Prescription.* 10th ed. Philadelphia (PA): Wolters Kluwer; 2018.

Discussion Question Answers for Case Study CEP.II(3)

1.   Individuals diagnosed with CVD benefit from participation in regular exercise and lifestyle changes. Outpatient cardiopulmonary rehabilitation is commonly encouraged to promote exercise and lifestyle interventions. It generally consists of a coordinated, multifaceted program designed to reduce risk, promote healthy behaviors and compliance, reduce disability, and encourage an active lifestyle for patients

with CVD. Taking into account lifestyle modification, a cardiopulmonary rehabilitation program is composed of a medically supervised exercise and education program. The cardiopulmonary team is typically composed of a medical director (physician), program coordinator (registered nurse or CEP), registered nurses, CEPs, registered dieticians, and psychologists among other health care professionals. Individuals who participate in outpatient cardiopulmonary rehabilitation benefit from a multidisciplinary team due to comorbidities or conditions that accompany CVD such as that of obesity, diabetes, dyslipidemia, arthritis, and depression. A multidisciplinary approach assists patients with engaging in a physically active lifestyle, dietary changes, weight loss, smoking cessation, stress management, and overall education about their specific diagnoses.

2. Literature suggests that it may take more than the public health recommendation of 150 min $\cdot$ wk^{-1} or 30 min of physical activity on most days of the week to promote sustained weight loss. Adults such as Joe who bear overweight or obesity are likely to benefit from progression in their exercise routine to approximately >250 min $\cdot$ wk^{-1}, preferably 5–7 d $\cdot$ wk^{-1} of aerobic activity to maximize caloric expenditure. Eventual progression to more vigorous exercise intensity ($\geq$60% $\dot{V}O_2R$ or HRR) is advised and may result in further health benefits. From Joe's medical history and the information provided from his initial evaluation, it is likely that he is one of the individuals who will be encouraged to exercise at a higher than moderate intensity level. It is important to address Joe's capability and willingness to exercise at higher levels of physical exertion. They key is to enhance the likelihood of the adoption and maintenance of physical activity. This can be achieved by the accumulation of the suggested amount of physical activity in multiple daily bouts of at least 10 min in duration for those previously sedentary individuals. Resistance exercise should also be incorporated into Joe's routine to promote muscular strength and physical function. There may be additional benefits of participating in a resistance exercise routine such as that of improvements in CVD and DM.

3. Excess body mass (measured in kg $\cdot$ m^{-2} [$\geq$30 kg $\cdot$ m^{-2}]), specifically, abdominal adiposity is linked to stroke, hypertension, DM, metabolic syndrome, dyslipidemia, and overall CVD risk. BMI is used to assess weight relative to height. Joe forms part of the general population. That is, Joe is not an athlete such as a body builder, swimmer, or runner. Nevertheless, the rehabilitation center where he is undergoing his cardiac rehabilitation is unlikely have state-of-the-art equipment. This cardiopulmonary rehabilitation center is likely to only treat patients with various CVD and pulmonary issues between the ages of 38 and 90 yr; the simplistic approach

of assessing BMI is very convenient at the initial and post-program evaluation in terms of obtaining body composition statistics. Athletic population would benefit from having their body composition assessed by hydrodensitometry or air displacement plethysmography as the result of these methods being able to distinguish between fat mass and lean muscle mass unlike BMI.

4. The Bruce protocol is geared toward populations who are younger and physically capable of performing physical activity that involves walking. It is important to recall Joe's age and his line of work. Joe is fairly young and has a high activity occupational job as a mover. The Bruce protocol employs relatively large incremental workload adjustments (*i.e.*, 2–3 METs per stage) every 3 min. Joe's job as a mover likely elicits MET levels of $\geq$6 when pushing, pulling, and carrying heavy furniture on a daily basis. The Bruce protocol was the appropriate method of assessing his functional capacity as well as ischemic threshold because he had reported chest tightness/pressure while on the job. A submaximal GXT via leg cycle ergometry would have likely provided an underestimation of results in terms of overall functional capacity and ischemic threshold for this particular patient.

5. Patients who are undergoing cardiac rehabilitation should be considered for a resistance exercise routine geared toward improving ADL and recreational activities. The individual should have no evidence of congestive heart failure, uncontrolled arrhythmias, uncontrolled hypertension, and overall unstable symptoms.

- Equipment type should consist of elastic bands, hand weights, and weight machines.
- Proper techniques such as that of raising and lowering weights with controlled movements to full extension should be implemented.
- Joe is advised to maintain a regular breathing pattern and avoid holding his breath. Nonetheless, it is imperative that he avoids straining and sustained gripping, which may evoke an excessive BP response.
- An RPE of 11–14 (fairly light to somewhat hard) on a scale of 6–20 may be used as a subjective guide.
- Resistance exercise should be terminated if abnormal signs or symptoms occur including dizziness, arrhythmias, unusual SOB, or angina.
- The initial workload should allow for 10–15 repetitions that can be lifted without straining (40%–50% of 1-RM, progressing to 60%–70% of 1-RM).
- The determination of a 1-RM may be deemed inappropriate for individuals with CVD. Therefore, multiple trials using progressively higher loads can be performed until the patient can perform no more than 10 repetitions without straining.

- Resistance exercise intensity can be progressed by increasing the resistance, increasing the number of repetitions, or decreasing the rest period between sets or exercises.
- Joe should exercise each major muscle group, with at least 8–10 exercises (chest, shoulders, arms, abdomen, back, hips, and legs).
- Joe's regimen should exercise large muscle groups before small muscle groups and should include multijoint exercises that affect more than one muscle group.
- Joe should participate in resistance exercise 2–3 d $\cdot$ wk^{-1} with at least 48 h separating training sessions for the same muscle group.
- All muscle groups that are trained may be done in the same session or in a split routine.
- Two to four sets are recommended to improve muscular strength and power.
- Rest intervals of 2–3 min between each set provides sufficient recovery.

- Resistance exercise should be performed after the aerobic component of the exercise session allowing for adequate warm-up of the muscles.
- Joe's resistance exercise program progression should be based in slowly increasing ($\sim$2–5 lb $\cdot$ wk^{-1}) for upper body and ($\sim$5–10 lb $\cdot$ wk^{-1}) for lower body as tolerated.

> *Resources*: American Association of Cardiovascular and Pulmonary Rehabilitation. *Guidelines for Cardiac Rehabilitation and Secondary Prevention Programs*. 4th ed. Champaign (IL): Human Kinetics; 2004.
>
> Riebe D, senior editor. *ACSM's Guidelines for Exercise Testing and Prescription*. 10th ed. Philadelphia (PA): Wolters Kluwer; 2018.
>
> U.S. Department of Health and Human Services. *2008 Physical Activity Guidelines for Americans*. Rockville, MD: U.S. Department of Health and Human Services; 2008. Available from: http://www.health.gov/paguidelines/

CASE STUDY CEP.II(4)

Multiple-Choice Answers for Case Study CEP.II(4)

1—C.   II, III, aVF

> *Resource*: Dubin D. *Rapid Interpretation of EKG's*. 6th ed. Tampa (FL): Cover Publishing; 2000.

2—C.   Peripheral arterial disease (PAD)

> Steve displays frequent episodes of IC rated up to a 4 with exertion.
>
> *Resource*: Riebe D, senior editor. *ACSM's Guidelines for Exercise Testing and Prescription*. 10th ed. Philadelphia (PA): Wolters Kluwer; 2018.

3—B.   40%–60% HRR or $\dot{V}O_2R$, allowing him to walk until he reaches an IC pain rating of 3

> *Resource*: Riebe D, senior editor. *ACSM's Guidelines for Exercise Testing and Prescription*. 10th ed. Philadelphia (PA): Wolters Kluwer; 2018.

4—D.   IC treadmill protocol

> Leg cycle ergometer may be used as a warm-up but should not be the primary form of aerobic exercise. Weight-bearing exercise such as walking to improve/increase the length of time to ischemic threshold/claudication (patient providing a rating of 3 on IC scale) is recommended.
>
> *Resource*: Riebe D, senior editor. *ACSM's Guidelines for Exercise Testing and Prescription*. 10th ed. Philadelphia (PA): Wolters Kluwer; 2018.

5—B.   3–5 d $\cdot$ wk^{-1}

> *Resource*: Riebe D, senior editor. *ACSM's Guidelines for Exercise Testing and Prescription*. 10th ed. Philadelphia (PA): Wolters Kluwer; 2018.

6—B.   63 kcal

> Estimated maximal oxygen consumption = 3.6 METs (2.0 mph and 4.0% grade)
>
> 1 MET = 3.5 mL $\cdot$ kg^{-1} $\cdot$ min^{-1}
>
> $\dot{V}O_2$Relative = (3.6 METs $\times$ 3.5 mL $\cdot$ kg^{-1} $\cdot$ min^{-1}) = 12.6 mL $\cdot$ kg^{-1} $\cdot$ min^{-1}
>
> Steve's weight kg = 145 lb / 2.2 = 66 kg
>
> 1 L $\cdot$ min^{-1} = 5 kcal
>
> Time = 15 min
>
> $\dot{V}O_2$Absolute = 12.6 mL $\cdot$ kg^{-1} $\cdot$ min^{-1} $\times$ 66 kg = 0.8316 L $\cdot$ min^{-1}
>
> $$\frac{}{1{,}000 \text{ mL}}$$
>
> 0.8316 L $\cdot$ min^{-1} $\times$ 5 kcal $\times$ 15 min = 6 kcal
>
> *Resource*: Riebe D, senior editor. *ACSM's Guidelines for Exercise Testing and Prescription*. 10th ed. Philadelphia (PA): Wolters Kluwer; 2018.

CEP

7—C. 120 mm Hg

$$\text{ABI} = \frac{\text{Highest ankle systolic pressure}}{\text{Highest brachial systolic pressure}} \rightarrow 0.66 = X$$

Highest brachial systolic pressure	Highest brachial systolic pressure = (182)
$0.66 = \dfrac{X}{182}$ $\rightarrow$	$(0.66) \times (182 \text{ mm Hg})$ $= 120 \text{ mm Hg}$

Resources: Riebe D, senior editor. *ACSM's Guidelines for Exercise Testing and Prescription*. 10th ed. Philadelphia (PA): Wolters Kluwer; 2018.

Wennberg PW, Rooke TW. Diagnosis and management of diseases of the peripheral arteries and veins. In: Fuster V, Walsh RA, Harrington RA, editors. *Hurst's The Heart*. 13th ed. New York (NY): McGraw-Hill; 2011. p. 2331–46.

8—C. 100

2 packs a day $\times$ 50 yr = 100.

Resource: Riebe D, senior editor. *ACSM's Guidelines for Exercise Testing and Prescription*. 10th ed. Philadelphia (PA): Wolters Kluwer; 2018.

9—A. Cease exercise to allow ischemic pain to resolve before resuming exercise

An IC protocol would need to be established for this patient.

Resource: Riebe D, senior editor. *ACSM's Guidelines for Exercise Testing and Prescription*. 10th ed. Philadelphia (PA): Wolters Kluwer; 2018.

10—D. Both A and B

Resources: Riebe D, senior editor. *ACSM's Guidelines for Exercise Testing and Prescription*. 10th ed. Philadelphia (PA): Wolters Kluwer; 2018.

Wennberg PW, Rooke TW. Diagnosis and management of diseases of the peripheral arteries and veins. In: Fuster V, Walsh RA, Harrington RA, editors. *Hurst's The Heart*. 13th ed. New York (NY): McGraw-Hill; 2011. p. 2331–46.

11—C. Inhibit cell proliferation and inflammation reducing restenosis

Drug-eluting stents do not elute antibiotics or anticoagulants.

Resource: Puranik AS, Dawson ER, Peppas NA. Recent advances in drug eluting stents. *Int J Pharm*. 2013;441(1):665–79.

Discussion Question Answers for Case Study CEP.II(4)

1. Individuals with PAD should perform weight-bearing aerobic exercise 3–5 d $\cdot$ wk^{-1}. Patients should exercise at 40%–<60% $\dot{V}O_2R$ that allows the patient to walk until he or she reaches a pain rating of 3 (*i.e.*, intense pain) on the 4-point IC scale. Between bouts of activity, the CEP should allow for the subsiding of ischemic pain by resting prior to resuming exercise. Time for aerobic exercise should be aimed for 30–60 min $\cdot$ d^{-1}. However, someone like Steve may need to start with 10-min bouts and exercise intermittently to accumulate a total of 30–60 min $\cdot$ d^{-1}. Severely deconditioned patients may need to begin the program by accumulating only 15 min $\cdot$ d^{-1}, gradually increasing the time by 5 min $\cdot$ d^{-1} on a biweekly basis. Patients with this clinical history should focus on weight-bearing aerobic exercise in order to increase the length time to ischemic threshold versus a non–weight-bearing exercise such as a leg cycle ergometer (can be used as a warm-up).

2. Steve is a patient who is severely deconditioned. The Bruce protocol is geared toward populations who are younger and physically capable of performing physical activity that involves walking. The Bruce protocol employs relatively large incremental workload adjustments (*i.e.*, 2–3 METs stages) every 3 min. These large incremental workload adjustments would call for an early termination of the GXT had the Bruce protocol been administered to Steve due to possible early onset of IC during the first stage. A ramped treadmill protocol increases the work rate in a constant and continuous manner. Some of the primary advantages of a ramp protocol include

   - Avoidance of large and unequal increments in workload
   - Uniform increase in physiologic and hemodynamic responses
   - Individualized test protocol (ramp rate)
   - More accurate estimates of exercise capacity

   Ramp protocols should be individualized so that the treadmill speed and increments in grade are based on perceived functional capacity of the subject. Increments in work rate should be chosen relative to total test time between 8 and 12 min (assuming the termination point is volitional fatigue). Yet, with severely deconditioned individuals, this is not always the case.

3. There are various types of resistance exercise equipment that can effectively be used to improve muscular strength and endurance. Steve is an older individual who has a chronic condition such as PAD and is deconditioned. He would most likely benefit from using equipment that includes elastic bands, hand

CEP

weights, and weight machines. Proper techniques such as raising and lowering weights with controlled movements should be demonstrated. He should maintain a regular breathing pattern and avoid holding his breath, straining, and sustained gripping because these factors may induce an excessive BP response.

- Each major muscle group, at least 8–10 exercises (*i.e.*, chest, shoulders, legs, arms, back, etc.) should be trained between with 48 h separating each resistance exercise session, 2–3 d · wk^{-1}.
- Steve is an older individual and is very deconditioned. The CEP can also apply resistance exercise guidelines that are geared toward older individuals as well.
- His initial load should begin with 40%–50% of 1-RM, progressing to 60%–70% of 1-RM.
- The determination of a 1-RM may be deemed inappropriate for individuals with CVD. Therefore, multiple trials using progressively higher loads can be performed until the patient can perform no more than 10 repetitions without straining.
- If 1-RM is not measured, intensity can be prescribed according to his overall fitness level. Progression can be determined in terms of moderate (5–6) and vigorous (7–8) on an RPE scale of 0–10.
- One or more sets of 10–15 repetitions exercising each major muscle group should be performed.
- He should adhere to lower weight and higher repetitions, especially when initiating a resistance exercise regimen.
- Overall rest periods between sets can range from 2 to 3 min.

4. Those who have PAD may lack motivation in terms of establishing and adhering to an exercise program. Potential barriers regarding the development of a structured exercise regimen include not having the energy, fear of getting hurt, safety issues, and overall concerns with comorbidities. Many patients with PAD tend to have clustering of comorbidities such as diabetes, hypertension, obesity, musculoskeletal conditions, neuropathy, and foot ulcers that may affect exercise tolerance.

5. The CEP should focus on discussing modifications to FITT principles regarding an exercise program. Counseling and motivational interviewing should be emphasized ("smaller goals, to bigger goals"). Steve's attitude to exercise and lifestyle modifications should be addressed throughout the duration of his monitored phase II cardiac rehabilitation program. Maintenance of lifestyle modification and relapse prevention is highly recommended in this population.

The overall goals of treating PAD include the reduction of symptoms (IC), improvement of QOL, and the prevention of complications. Treatment for Steve is primarily based on his signs and symptoms, risk factors, results from various tests, as well as the outcomes of any interventions or procedures. The lack of aggressive treatment for PAD may lead to complications such as ulcers, sores, and gangrene, which may result in lower extremity amputation.

Ultimate lifestyle modifications include the cessation of smoking (smoking raises risk for other comorbidities such as stroke, lung cancer, COPD, etc.). Steve should adhere to his regimen of taking his medications as prescribed to control his hypertension and dyslipidemia. His maintenance of an exercise program will further improve the latter comorbidities and general symptoms (IC). A healthy diet plan should be followed as well (monitor sodium intake, trans fat, cholesterol intake, etc.)

Resources: Askew CD, Parmenter B, Leicht AS, Walker PJ, Golledge J. Exercise & Sports Science Australia (ESSA) position statement on exercise prescription for patients with peripheral arterial disease and intermittent claudication. *J Sci Med Sport*. 2014;17(6):623–9.

Riebe D, senior editor. *ACSM's Guidelines for Exercise Testing and Prescription*. 10th ed. Philadelphia (PA): Wolters Kluwer; 2018.

Wennberg PW, Rooke TW. Diagnosis and management of diseases of the peripheral arteries and veins. In: Fuster V, Walsh RA, Harrington RA, editors. *Hurst's The Heart*. 13th ed. New York (NY): McGraw-Hill; 2011. p. 2331–46.

CASE STUDY CEP.II(5)

Multiple-Choice Answers for Case Study CEP.II(5)

1—A.   May reduce resting and exercise HR and BP

Resource: Riebe D, senior editor. *ACSM's Guidelines for Exercise Testing and Prescription*. 10th ed. Philadelphia (PA): Wolters Kluwer; 2018.

2— E.   Only A and B

Resource: Riebe D, senior editor. *ACSM's Guidelines for Exercise Testing and Prescription*. 10th ed. Philadelphia (PA): Wolters Kluwer; 2018.

CEP

3— B. Moderate risk

Resource: Riebe D, senior editor. *ACSM's Guidelines for Exercise Testing and Prescription.* 10th ed. Philadelphia (PA): Wolters Kluwer; 2018.

4— B. 30%–<40% HRR or $\dot{V}O_2R$, 2–<3 METs, RPE 9–11, an intensity that causes slight increases in HR and breathing

Resource: Riebe D, senior editor. *ACSM's Guidelines for Exercise Testing and Prescription.* 10th ed. Philadelphia (PA): Wolters Kluwer; 2018.

5— D. 69

Pack Years = Number of Packs Smoked per Day × Number of Years Smoked.

Resource: Verrill D, Graham H, Vitcenda M, Peno-Green L, Kramer V, Corbisiero T. Measuring behavioral outcomes in cardiopulmonary rehabilitation—an AACVPR statement. *J Cardiopulm Rehabil Prev.* 2009;29:193–203.

6—A. The Medical Outcomes Study Short Form-36 (SF-36)

Resource: American Association of Cardiovascular and Pulmonary Rehabilitation. *Guidelines for Cardiac Rehabilitation and Secondary Prevention Programs.* 5th ed. Champaign (IL): Human Kinetics; 2014.

7— D. Obese (class I)

BMI = Body Weight (kg) / Height (m)^2

BMI = 218 lb × .4536 = 98.9 kg

70 ft × .0254 = 1.778 m

$(1.778)^2 = 3.16$

BMI = 98.9 / 3.16 = 31.3 (Obesity class I)

Resource: Riebe D, senior editor. *ACSM's Guidelines for Exercise Testing and Prescription.* 10th ed. Philadelphia (PA): Wolters Kluwer; 2018.

8—C. Cycle ergometer exercise at 0.5 kg (180 kgm · min^{-1}) at an HR of 114–128 bpm and an RPE of 11–16

RPE = <u>11–16</u>

THR = 40%–80% of exercise capacity using HRR method

THR = [(HR_{max} − HR_{rest}) × % intensity] + HR_{rest}

THR = (142 − 72) × .40 + 72 = <u>100 bpm</u>

THR = (142 − 72) × .80 + 72 = <u>128 bpm</u>

THR = <u>100–128 bpm</u>

Peak Treadmill Workload Estimated $\dot{V}O_2$ by Mr. Kyle at 1.7 mph, 10% grade

$\dot{V}O_2$ = (0.1 × 1.7 × 26.8) + (1.8 × 1.7 × 26.8 × 0.10) + 3.5

(Horizontal) (Vertical) (Rest)

$\dot{V}O_2$ = (0.1 × 45.56) + (1.8 × 45.56 × .10) + 3.5

$\dot{V}O_2$ = 4.556 + 8.2 + 3.5

$\dot{V}O_2$ = 16.26 mL · kg^{-1} · min^{-1}

METs = 16.26 / 3.5 = 4.64

Training Cycle Workload Estimated $\dot{V}O_2$ at 0.5 kp:

$\dot{V}O_2$ (mL · kg^{-1} · min^{-1}) = 1.8 (work rate / body mass) + 3.5 mL · kg^{-1} · min^{-1} + 3.5 mL · kg^{-1} · min^{-1}

(resting $\dot{V}O_2$) (unloaded cycling $\dot{V}O_2$)

Work rate (WR) = 0.5 kg × 6 m × 60 rpm

WR = 180 kg · m · min^{-1}

$\dot{V}O_2$ (mL · kg^{-1} · min^{-1}) = 1.8 (180/98.9 kg) + 3.5 + 3.5

$\dot{V}O_2$ = 10.3 mL · kg^{-1} · min^{-1}

METs = 10.3 mL · kg^{-1} · min^{-1} / 3.5 = 2.94 METs

2.94 METs / 4.64 METs = 63% $\dot{V}O_{2peak}$ (in the range of 40%–80% of $\dot{V}O_{2peak}$)

Resource: Riebe D, senior editor. *ACSM's Guidelines for Exercise Testing and Prescription.* 10th ed. Philadelphia (PA): Wolters Kluwer; 2018.

9—C. At least 3 d · wk^{-1} but preferably most days of the week

Resource: Riebe D, senior editor. *ACSM's Guidelines for Exercise Testing and Prescription.* 10th ed. Philadelphia (PA): Wolters Kluwer; 2018.

10—B. 197 lb (89.3 kg)

218 lb (99 kg) male

35% estimated body fat

28% goal body fat

Fat-free weight = Body weight × ([100 − % Body fat] / 100)

= 218 lb × ([100 − 35] / 100) = 141.7 lb

Goal body weight (ideal body weight [IBW]) = 141.7 lb / (1 − [28 / 100]) = X lb

X = 141.7 / 0.72 = 196.8 lb (89.3 kg) ~ 197 lb

CEP

Discussion Question Answers for Case Study CEP.II(5)

1. Mr. Kyle may have some form of chronic lung disease (*e.g.*, COPD or restrictive lung disease) as demonstrated by his oxygen desaturation levels during his rehab entry GXT. He may also have IFG (pre-DM) as demonstrated by a fasting blood glucose level of 120 mg · dL^{-1}.

   Send the results of the GXT that shows the oxygen desaturation levels during exercise to the patient's medical office and discuss these results with the physician or the physician's nurse. Also, inform his medical office of his elevated fasting glucose values, which may represent prediabetes and require further medical testing and analysis. COPD and diabetes are often comorbid conditions with CVD due to the common risk factors of smoking, obesity, and poor diet. The presence of COPD in current or former smokers is also an independent predictor of overall cardiovascular events.

   > **Resources**: Riebe D, senior editor. *ACSM's Guidelines for Exercise Testing and Prescription*. 10th ed. Philadelphia (PA): Wolters Kluwer; 2018.
   >
   > de Barros e Silva PG, Califf RM, Sun JL et al. Chronic obstructive pulmonary disease and cardiovascular risk: insights from the NAVIGATOR trial. *Int J Cardiol*. 2014;176(3):1126–8.

2. Because Mr. Kyle may not be compliant with his medications at the present time, you should inform his medical office (*e.g.*, physician) of potential noncompliance issues with regard to his medication usage. You should talk to Mr. Kyle about the purpose and importance of taking each medication as prescribed in a one-on-one consultation. Discuss barriers that he encounters when taking his medications (*e.g.*, undesirable side effects, inconvenience, difficulty swallowing pills). You should also discuss potential side effects for each of his medications, and whether or not he is experiencing any associated side effects should be discussed with him. Finally, you should record Mr. Kyle's daily medication compliance at rehab entry and at each follow-up evaluation with established medication compliance surveys.

   You should inform Mr. Kyle's medical office (*e.g.*, physician) of his current smoking status. His physician may want to consider some form of nicotine replacement therapy or medications such as bupropion to help Mr. Kyle with his tobacco cravings. You should also suggest that Mr. Kyle see the staff rehab psychologist (with permission from his personal physician) to address the barriers to smoking cessation that currently exist. You should monitor and record his number of cigarettes smoked daily at rehab entry and at each follow-up evaluation to demonstrate progress or regression in his smoking cessation efforts. Finally, you should recommend the hospital's smoking cessation program to Mr. Kyle and check on his smoking status during each cardiac rehabilitation visit.

   You should inform Mr. Kyle's medical office (*e.g.*, physician) of his current level of high stress status. His physician may want to consider some form of antianxiety or antidepressant medication as well as professional counseling. He should take an established depression or anxiety survey (*e.g.*, Beck Depression Inventory-II) at rehab entry and at each follow-up evaluation to help determine if he is suffering from clinical depression and/or anxiety. You should also suggest that he see the staff rehab psychologist (with permission from his personal physician) to discuss stress management techniques. He should also attend the cardiac rehab educational classes on stress management and participate in the relaxation sessions offered weekly during the exercise sessions. Mr. Kyle may also want to pursue tai chi, yoga, or other form of relaxation-inducing exercise program that you present to him.

   > **Resource**: Verrill D, Graham H, Vitcenda M, Peno-Green L, Kramer V, Corbisiero T. Measuring behavioral outcomes in cardiopulmonary rehabilitation—an AACVPR statement. *J Cardiopulm Rehabil Prev*. 2009;29:193–203.

3. The six purposes for performing GXT after acute MI include the following:

   1. To evaluate signs, symptoms and potential myocardial ischemia
   2. To determine the need for coronary angiography in patients treated initially with a noninvasive strategy
   3. To determine the effectiveness of medical therapy
   4. To assess future level of cardiovascular risk and prognosis
   5. To develop the initial exercise prescription for cardiac rehabilitation participation with regard to training HR and MET level
   6. To objectively determine the patient's functional capacity for return to work and vocational and avocational activities

   > **Resource**: Ehrman JK, Gordon PM, Visich PS, Keteyian SJ. *Clinical Exercise Physiology*. 3rd ed. Champaign (IL): Human Kinetics; 2013.

4. Recommendations include the following:

   - Modalities: free weights, dumbbells, elastic bands, wall or weight machine pulleys, stability balls, weighted wands, machines (*i.e.*, resistive machines specific to avoid further injury to Mr. Kyle's lower back); light dumbbell weights (2–5 lb) or moderate resistance elastic bands performed during each rehab session during his early rehabilitation sessions.
   - Frequency: 2–3 d · wk^{-1} with at least 48 h separating training sessions for the same muscle group.

- Intensity:
  - Initial workloads of 10–15 repetitions at an RPE of 11–14 (6–20 scale)
  - Initial workloads of 40%–50% of 1-RM (if 1-RM testing performed)
  - If 1-RM technique is not used, multiple trials using progressively higher workloads performed until the patient can perform >10 repetitions without straining
  - One to three sets of resistive exercises, increasing up to four sets over time if indicated
- Progression: Increase weight slowly as the patient adapts to the program (*e.g.*, ~2–5 lb · wk^{-1} for the upper body and 510 lb · wk^{-1} for the lower body).
- Resistance exercises for each major muscle group of the upper and lower body
- Exercise large muscle groups before small muscle groups.
- Circuit weight training may be incorporated with low-level resistance stations to better prepare Mr. Kyle to perform his occupational and leisure time activities.

> *Resource*: Riebe D, senior editor. *ACSM's Guidelines for Exercise Testing and Prescription.* 10th ed. Philadelphia (PA): Wolters Kluwer; 2018.

5. Medications: diltiazem (Cardizem), digoxin (Lanoxin), warfarin (Coumadin)

Physiologic Concerns:
- Increased risk of thromboembolic events
- Rapid ventricular rates when the AV node is inadequately suppressed
- Incomplete ventricular filling causing reduced CO
- Decreased functional capacity
- Fatigue
- Arrhythmic symptoms (*e.g.*, palpitations, rapid HR, slow HR)

Exercise Concerns:
- Decreased exercise tolerance
- Difficult to determine systolic BP due to variability in diastolic filling
- Difficult to determine pulse due to rapid, irregular ventricular response
- Marked variability in maximal HR response—age-predicted maximal HR targets not valid
- Longer sampling of pulse may be needed for reliable target HR determination
  - May need to be on continuous electrocardiographic monitoring

> *Resource*: Moore GE, Durstine JL, Painter PL. *ACSM's Exercise Management for Patients with Chronic Disease and Disabilities.* 4th ed. Champaign (IL): Human Kinetics; 2016.

CASE STUDY CEP.III

Multiple-Choice Answers for Case Study CEP.III

1—B. Call her pulmonologist and discuss her 6MWT results with the medical staff

> *Resource*: American Association of Cardiovascular and Pulmonary Rehabilitation. *Guidelines for Cardiac Rehabilitation and Secondary Prevention Programs.* 4th ed. Champaign (IL): Human Kinetics; 2004.

2—A. Be deferred until her pulmonologist provides follow-up recommendations based on her initial assessment

> *Resource*: Riebe D, senior editor. *ACSM's Guidelines for Exercise Testing and Prescription.* 10th ed. Philadelphia (PA): Wolters Kluwer; 2018.

3—C. Help shrink the swelling and inflammation of the airways

> *Resource*: Riebe D, senior editor. *ACSM's Guidelines for Exercise Testing and Prescription.* 10th ed. Philadelphia (PA): Wolters Kluwer; 2018.

4—A. 72

> *Resource*: Verrill D, Graham H, Vitcenda M, Peno-Green L, Kramer V, Corbisiero T. Measuring behavioral outcomes in cardiopulmonary rehabilitation—an AACVPR statement. *J Cardiopulm Rehabil Prev.* 2009;29:193–203.

5—D. Ipratropium (Atrovent)

> *Resource*: Riebe D, senior editor. *ACSM's Guidelines for Exercise Testing and Prescription.* 10th ed. Philadelphia (PA): Wolters Kluwer; 2018.

6—C. Collect as much information as possible in your initial assessment about these issues and contact her physician with this information

> *Resource*: American Association of Cardiovascular and Pulmonary Rehabilitation. *Guidelines for Cardiac Rehabilitation and Secondary Prevention Programs.* 4th ed. Champaign (IL): Human Kinetics; 2004.

7—A. The University of California, San Diego Shortness of Breath Questionnaire

> *Resource*: American Association of Cardiovascular and Pulmonary Rehabilitation. *Guidelines for Cardiac Rehabilitation and Secondary Prevention Programs.* 4th ed. Champaign (IL): Human Kinetics; 2004.

CEP

8—C.   Overweight

   Resource: Riebe D, senior editor. *ACSM's Guidelines for Exercise Testing and Prescription*. 10th ed. Philadelphia (PA): Wolters Kluwer; 2018.

9—D.   Once cleared for program participation, Cassidy should exercise at a level of 25 W for 8 min on the arm ergometer as one component of her exercise prescription.

   Resource: Riebe D, senior editor. *ACSM's Guidelines for Exercise Testing and Prescription*. 10th ed. Philadelphia (PA): Wolters Kluwer; 2018.

10—B.   Additional vitamins B and D supplementation to help improve her $FEV_{1.0}$ and FVC values

   Resource: Riebe D, senior editor. *ACSM's Guidelines for Exercise Testing and Prescription*. 10th ed. Philadelphia (PA): Wolters Kluwer; 2018.

Discussion Question Answers to Case Study CEP.III

1.   The following are some of the short- and long-term goals that Cassidy should be trying to achieve throughout her pulmonary rehabilitation program:

Short-Term Goals Of Pulmonary Rehabilitation Program:

- Have physician evaluate her depression issues and refer her for a psychosocial consult (if indicated)
- Have physician evaluate her exercise SaO_2 desaturation issues and adjust oxygen liter flow (if indicated)
- Maintain smoking cessation with group support if available and desired
- Incorporate stretching program for osteoarthritis
- Incorporate nutrition education, including consult with the program dietician
- Incorporate stress intervention techniques
- Decrease levels of resting and exercise dyspnea (*i.e.*, reduce the work of breathing)
- Improve SaO_2 levels during exercise
- Improve perception of physical exertion level during exercise (*i.e.*, decrease RPE)

Long-Term Goals Of Pulmonary Rehabilitation Program:

- Increase upper and lower body strength
- Decrease overall body weight/BMI
- Increase maximal exercise capacity
- Reduce heart rate, $\dot{V}O_2$, and pulmonary ventilation during submaximal exercise
- Improve QOL
- Lower resting and exercise BP
- Improve nutritional habits
- Improve emotional state and restore a positive outlook

- Increase 6MWT distance
- Decrease leg pain with exercise prescription for PAD
- Reduce pulmonary exacerbations to help to decrease recurrent unscheduled physician and hospital visits
- Be able to drive herself to her rehab sessions

2.   Cassidy could potentially have problems with program participation, compliance, and completion related to the following factors:

   a.   Travel distance, reliance on someone to drive to her rehab sessions, and her husband's work schedule
   b.   Lack of spousal support
   c.   Potential for future pulmonary exacerbations due to disease progression and smoking history
   d.   Socioeconomic variables that may be related to additional program costs (*e.g.*, her being retired, husband working part-time)
   e.   Low exercise compliance if she resumes smoking
   f.   Obesity, resulting in poor mobility and increased risk of lower body injury
   g.   Her depression
   h.   Her level of dyspnea with activity
   i.   Her leg pain from PAD and osteoarthritis
   j.   Daily fatigue

3.   Cassidy could have the following undiagnosed medical conditions: (1) hypertension and (2) worsening (severe) depression. One would address these underlying medical conditions as follows:

   a.   Hypertension
   - Contact her physician with her BP responses at rest and during her 6MWT.
   - Incorporate exercise and nutrition education for weight loss.
   - Have her cut back on sodium and high-salt products.
   - Advocate a healthy diet with high-fiber and low–saturated fat and sugar consumption.
   - Provide education in daily mechanical efficiency of movement for less acute energy expenditure.

   b.   Depression
   - Contact her physician with her depression survey scores and your initial assessment personal observations.
   - Stress the importance exercise compliance.
   - Have her perform stress management and relaxation techniques.
   - Offer her the services of the staff psychologist.

4.   Her peak SaO_2 was significantly lower on her 6MWT compared to her metabolic cycle ergometer test on the same oxygen liter flow. Her diastolic BP was higher during the 6MWT compared to her cycle exercise test. It is important to monitor her BP during exercise due to her potential hypertensive response to activity. Her exercise HR was significantly lower

on the 6MWT than her cycle exercise test. This is understandable because the 6MWT was a submaximal exercise test. Her measured functional capacity (METs) from the metabolic GXT was quite close to her estimated METs from the 6MWT. An effective exercise prescription considering medications should be able to be developed due to measured and estimated functional capacity being close.

5. Use the FITT principle for patients with COPD:

    - **Frequency:** At least 3–5 d · wk^{-1}
    - **Intensity:** Exercise at 30%–40% of peak work rate has been recommended by ACSM for improvements in QOL and ADL. However, exercise at 60%–80% of peak work rate has been recommended to provide physiologic improvements (*e.g.*, reduced minute ventilation and HR at a given workload). As Cassidy's peak work rate has not been determined, one may estimate Cassidy's current work capacity from the results of her 6MWT and calculate her estimated MET value using the following equation (*ACSM's GETP* 2014, p. 78):

    Predicted $\dot{V}O_{2max}$ (mL · kg^{-1} · min^{-1}) = (0.02 × distance [m]) − (0.191 × age [yr]) − (0.07 × weight [kg]) + (0.09 × height [cm]) + (0.26 × [RPP × 10^{-3}]) + 2.45

    Where:

    - m = distance in meters
    - yr = year
    - kg = kilogram
    - cm = centimeter
    - RPP = rate pressure product (HR × systolic BP [SBP] in mm Hg)

    For this patient:

    - Predicted $\dot{V}O_{2max}$ (mL · kg^{-1} · min^{-1}) = [0.02 × distance (m)] − [0.191 × age (yr)] − [0.07 × weight (kg)] + [0.09 × height (cm)] + [0.26 × (RPP × 0.001)] + 2.45
    - Predicted $\dot{V}O_{2max}$ (mL · kg^{-1} · min^{-1}) = [0.02 × distance (427.0248 m)] − [0.191 × age (64)] − [0.07 × weight (70.31 kg)] + [0.09 × height (160.02 cm)] + [0.26 × RPP (138 × 164 × 0.001)] + 2.45
    - 8.54 − 12.224 − 4.9216 + 14.4018 + 5.884 + 2.45 = 14.2 mL · kg^{-1} · min^{-1} or 4 METs

Exercise would be prescribed anywhere from 30% to 80% of the MET level above. This would depend on the CEP's philosophy and the patient's individual health status because there are currently no solid evidence-based recommendations to support an actual entry starting MET level for patients with COPD. From this peak 6MWT MET level, one could determine training MET workload levels for each modality used from the ACSM metabolic equations. Exercise should also be prescribed at a target RPE level of 12–14 on the Borg category scale, and at a target dyspnea level of 4–6 on the Borg 10-point dyspnea scale. Once a follow-up metabolic GXT is performed, the exercise prescription can be more accurately refined.

Determining a target exercise HR could prove difficult because those with COPD often have higher resting and exercise HRs due to the nature of the disease and pulmonary medications taken. Although one could take a percentage of the peak HR observed during the 6MWT, it may be more prudent to rely on RPE and dyspnea ratings as well as exercise SaO$_2$ levels (*e.g.*, ≥88%).

- **Time:** Cassidy's initial exercise prescription duration will depend on her individual tolerance level. Typically, patients entering a pulmonary rehab program may exercise for 4–7 min on various modalities. They may also perform track and/or treadmill walking, as tolerated. She will have to use her rollator (at least initially) due to her balance issues and to help move her oxygen tank.
- **Type:** Typical exercise modalities for pulmonary rehabilitation phase II patients include the arm ergometer, NuStep machine, stairs or stair stepper, upright cycle ergometer, recumbent cycle ergometer, and elliptical trainer. Because the stair stepper and elliptical trainer both elicit a higher metabolic cost, these modalities are often reserved for "maintenance" pulmonary exercise when the patient is better conditioned. Water exercise may be incorporated (if available) including swimming, "water walking," and water aerobics. Walking on either the track or treadmill should be strongly reinforced. Inspiratory muscle training may also prove useful when performed a minimum of 4–5 d · wk^{-1} for 30 min · d^{-1} (*e.g.*, two 15-min sessions). Breathing retraining exercises including pursed-lip breathing should be incorporated during warm-up or cool-down exercise or at a specified time during the exercise session.
- Because patients with COPD may experience greater dyspnea while performing ADL with the upper extremities, it is very beneficial to incorporate resistive exercise using light dumbbells/hand weights and/or elastic bands of varying intensities. Over time, the patient can progress to machine weight exercise for both the upper and lower body. Flexibility exercise training should be also prescribed, following the same ACSM FITT principle as that for healthy and/or older adults to help improve her range of motion and balance and alleviate her joint pain from osteoarthritis.

CEP

6. Types of assessments include the following:

Fitness Assessments

a. 6MWT (walking distance in feet or meters and physiologic parameters such as HR, BP, SaO$_2$, and RPE)

b. 30-s sit-to-stand test (number of reps)

c. Handgrip dynamometer test (pounds or kilogram)

d. 3-RM leg extension weight lifted (pounds or kilogram)

e. 30-s biceps curl test (number of reps, both arms)

f. TUG Test (seconds)

Health Surveys

g. Chronic Disease Respiratory Questionnaire score (dyspnea)

h. CES-D scale score (depression)

i. Ferrans and Powers QOL Index—Pulmonary Version survey score (overall QOL)

j. DHS score (nutritional habits)

k. BODE Index (COPD status)

Body Composition

l. Height (inches or centimeters)

m. Weight (pounds or kilogram)

n. BMI (kg · m^{-2})

o. Abdominal circumference (inches or centimeters)

p. Skinfold assessment (total number of millimeters and estimated fat percentage)

Other

q. Number of unscheduled hospital, physician, and emergency room visits due to pulmonary exacerbations (if any)

r. Number of cigarettes smoked per day (if patient resumes smoking)

s. Oxygen liter flow (rest and exercise)

t. Number of exercise sessions attended

u. Number of educational sessions attended

v. Number of exercise untoward events (if any)

w. Patient satisfaction survey with area for comments

> **Resources**: American Association of Cardiovascular and Pulmonary Rehabilitation. *Guidelines for Cardiac Rehabilitation and Secondary Prevention Programs*. 4th ed. Champaign (IL): Human Kinetics; 2004.
>
> Ehrman JK, Gordon PM, Visich PS, Keteyian SJ. *Clinical Exercise Physiology*. 3rd ed. Champaign (IL): Human Kinetics; 2013.
>
> Riebe D, senior editor. *ACSM's Guidelines for Exercise Testing and Prescription*. 10th ed. Philadelphia (PA): Wolters Kluwer; 2018.
>
> Verrill D, Barton C, Beasley W, Lippard W. The effects of short-term and long-term pulmonary rehabilitation on functional capacity, perceived dyspnea, and quality of life. *Chest*. 2005;128:673–83.

CASE STUDY CEP.IV

Multiple-Choice Answers for Case Study CEP.IV

1—E.   All of the above

2—E.   Both A and C

3—B.   Social cognitive theory

4—D.   Challenging self with difficult goals

5—C.   Goals should be challenging.

> **Resource**: Swain D, senior editor. *ACSM's Resource Manual for Guidelines for Exercise Testing and Prescription*. 7th ed. Baltimore (MD): Lippincott Williams & Wilkins; 2014. 896 p.

Discussion Question Answers for Case Study CEP.IV

1. The following are the three barriers and its impact on exercise compliance:

a. Time: A full-time job and primary child care responsibilities place a time crunch on the client. Discontinuous bouts of activity with a focus on walking may alleviate the burden of time as a significant barrier. In addition, this mode of activity can be completed in various convenient settings, thereby matching the work and commuter schedule.

b. Fatigue/pain: Patients with FMS often complain of multiple tender points, undue fatigue, and morning stiffness. In addition, the client's sleep disturbances

CEP

coupled with chronic soft tissue discomfort may make some exercise intensities and types of exercise difficulty. Consideration of using low-intensity exercise with shorter bouts may reduce the fatigue and pain response. Remind the client that discomfort during exercise may occur, but that pain may require exercise termination or selection of various modalities of exercise.

c. Depression/motivation: Due to the primary symptoms associated with FMS and life demands currently placed on Kimberly, it is not uncommon to see a significant reduction in motivation toward physical activity. In addition, the incidence of depression is higher in patients with FMS as compared to their apparently healthy counterparts.

2. Selecting types of exercise that Kimberly enjoys and has easy access to may alleviate some of the barriers that she presents. Little skill and equipment (good

walking shoes, pedometer, polar heart monitor) are necessary to implement an effective exercise program.

In addition, shorter, discontinuous bouts of exercise may be warranted considering the numerous demands on Kimberly's time. Suggestions to include her children in the exercise plan (biking alongside) would increase her social support, which has been demonstrated to increase adherence.

3. The client should be part of the goal-setting process with the health care team to develop realistic goals, timeline for implementation, periodic measures, and revisions to goals as warranted. Developing a goal-setting contract with signature for client and CEP provides a public proclamation, which often may enhance the effectiveness of the goal-setting plan. In addition, both short- and long-term goals should be included with regular assessment to allow for new strategies if necessary.

CASE STUDY CEP.V(1)

True or False and Multiple-Choice Answers for Case Study CEP.V(1)

1—C. Fax the BP readings and let the nurse know that you may not give out other personal information on the patient's progress

You may fax the requested BP readings to the patient's primary care office because this is a continuation of care and necessary for treatment of the patient. You may not give out a status update to the nurse who is planning to share this information with others and which is not directly related to the care of this patient. Follow the "minimum necessary" use guidelines when sharing information with others involved in the care of the patient.

2—False.

Unless the individual has legal authority to make decisions for the patient, he or she does not have access to other family member's health information without written consent from the patient. In some states, even minors have certain rights to privacy from their parents. Be familiar with your state laws regarding release of health information to others.

3—B. Tell your coworker that you cannot share passwords, but you will call the physician office and obtain the information needed

Sharing computer passwords or posting them in a public place is a HIPAA violation. When individuals share passwords, they pose a direct threat to

patient privacy. The recipient, even if a coworker, can use your passwords to access confidential information in an unauthorized way, for which you will be held responsible.

4—False.

The physician scanned the room first to make sure that no unauthorized individuals would hear or see confidential patient information. Turning the screen to view it in a public location is acceptable when only authorized individuals are in the room. If others were present who should not hear or see this information, the physician would need to go behind the desk to view the information.

5—D. All of the above

All information that identifies an individual is protected under the Privacy Rule. This includes, but is not limited to, name, address, e-mail address, date of birth, social security numbers, phone and fax numbers, medical record number, and photographs. It also includes past, present, and future medical records as well as billing information.

6—False.

A patient has the right to disclose his or her own personal health information and diagnosis to anyone he or she wants. A patient sharing information about himself or herself is not a violation of the Privacy Rule.

7—A. Tell her that you cannot do that and offer to come in earlier to help out

Under the Privacy Rule, organizations are required to have reasonable safeguards in place for the protection of confidential patient information. This includes storing patient records in a locked file cabinet or record room. Leaving the charts out on the desk at night, even if they are labeled confidential, is allowing for the potential of unauthorized access to private patient information. There may be other individuals that enter your facility when you are not there, including housekeeping staff, maintenance workers, and security staff. These individuals may be authorized to access your work area but not the confidential information on patients that is stored there. The safest place for medical records is safely locked in a storage file or records room.

Resource: Health Insurance Portability and Accountability Act of 1996 Web site [Internet]. Washington, DC: U.S. Department of Health and Human Services; [cited 2016 Jan 28]. Available from: http://www.hhs.gov/hipaa/for-professionals/index.html

CASE STUDY CEP.V(2)

True or False and Multiple-Choice Answers for Case Study CEP.V(2)

1—B. Glucometer

A glucometer is not a common piece of emergency equipment or supply found in a health/fitness facility.

2—True.

All health/fitness facilities should have emergency plans in place regardless of their level.

3—C. Have him stop exercising

The first action when an individual reports possible angina for the first time is to stop activity.

4—B. Stop exercise and notify his physician, check and document his vitals, and continue to observe him

The patient is asymptomatic, but the ventricular ectopy is new and needs to be treated.

5—B. Immediately immobilize his wrist, implement RICE (rest, ice, compress, and elevate), and promptly notify his physician.

The correct response is to immediately immobilize this type of injury, implement RICE, and notify the individual's physician. Promptly dealing musculoskeletal injury is extremely important to decrease pain and stabilize the individual.

6—A. Activate EMS; note time the symptoms started

The acute action that should be taken is to notify EMS and note the time the symptoms started.

Resources: Tharrett SJ, Peterson JA, senior editors. *ACSM's Health/Fitness Facility Standards and Guidelines*. 4th ed. Champaign (IL): Human Kinetics; 2012.

ECG CASE STUDIES ANSWERS AND EXPLANATIONS

CEP.ECG(1)

Short Answers for CEP.ECG(1)

1. Asystole

Multiple-Choice Answers for CEP.ECG(1)

1—D. Check the patient

2—A. A patient can be stable with a sustain presentation of this disorder.

3—C. Fine ventricular fibrillation

Teaching points: Syncope is a common diagnosis, occurring at least once in a lifetime in approximately 40% of individuals. The majority of syncopal episodes are vasovagal-related which can lead to sudden drops in both BP and HR. Often, if the individual is monitored during the syncopal event, the presenting rhythm can be pronounced bradycardia, an advanced AV block (type 2 or 3), or transient asystole, as defined as a ventricular pause of >3 s (*i.e.*, 75 mm at 25 mm $\cdot$ s^{-1}). Typically, such syncopal episodes carry a low mortality rate and are considered benign. However, such events can reoccur, which can impact QOL and possibly lead to trauma. In some individuals, the placement of a permanent pacemaker has helped to reduce recurrence. Other treatments include adequate fluids and sodium as well as medications such as β-blockers, selective serotonin reuptake inhibitors, and fludrocortisone. Although the case presented here was benign, prolonged asystole is the most grave rhythm indicating end of life. Often, the latter is precipitated by ventricular tachycardia and/or fibrillation and could be mistaken for fine ventricular fibrillation.

Resource: Ganzeboom KS, Mairuhu G, Reitsma JB, Linzer M, Wieling W, van Dijk N. Lifetime cumulative incidence of syncope in the general population: a study of 549 Dutch subjects aged 35-60 years. *J Cardiovasc Electrophysiol.* 2006;17:1172–6.

CEP.ECG(2)

Short Answers for CEP.ECG(2)

1. Sinus

2. Second-degree AV block (Mobitz type I)

3. 45–50 bpm

Multiple-Choice Answers for CEP.ECG(2)

1—D. The patient's medical and symptom history as well as the presence of signs or symptoms of poor perfusion should guide whether the test can be performed.

2—A. SA node

3—C. According to the American Heart Association, the test should be terminated if it interferes with maintenance of cardiac output (CO).

Teaching points: Unlike a second-degree type II AV block, a second-degree type I AV block generally does not progress to a complete heart block (*i.e.*, third-degree AV block). Therefore, unless an individual with a second-degree type I AV block (also known as Wenckebach) becomes symptomatic due to bradycardia, a pacemaker is not usually indicated. When the ventricular rhythm is irregular, as in second-degree AV block or atrial fibrillation, the ventricular rate can be estimated by counting the number of ventricular complexes that appear over a given time. As displayed on this ECG, the standard ECG paper speed is 25 mm $\cdot$ s^{-1}. That results in 50 large (5 mm) boxes (starting after the calibration mark) across a standard ECG for 10 s of time (50 $\times$ 5 mm $=$ 150 mm / 25 mm $\cdot$ s^{-1} $=$ 10 s). In this example, there are eight ventricular complexes during this 10-s period for an estimated ventricular rate of 48 bpm. The clinician could also use a millimeter ruler to measure 150 mm (30 large boxes) across an ECG which would represent 6 s (count the complexes and multiple by 10 for the rate). A standard Bic pen with the cap on can be a useful estimate of 150 mm.

CEP.ECG(3)

Short Answers for CEP.ECG(3)

1. Third-degree AV block

2. 60 bpm

3. 60–65 bpm

Multiple-Choice Answers for CEP.ECG(3)

1—H. Options B and C are correct.

2—B. AV node

3—A. Patients are usually asymptomatic with this disorder.

Teaching points: Often, patients with a third-degree AV block (*e.g.*, complete heart block) are symptomatic with pronounced hypotension and bradycardia. However, on occasion, patients may be hemodynamically stable at rest and present as asymptomatic or with mild complaints of fatigue or light-headedness. The defining characteristics of third-degree AV block are a regular atrial rhythm and a regular (but dissociated) ventricular rhythm which is very slow (*e.g.*, 30–60 bpm). P waves can be hidden within the QRS complex and/or T waves but still should "march out" to show an underlying regular sinus rhythm. Additionally, the QRS complex can be wide; however, the width of the QRS complex depends on where the escape rhythm originates (*e.g.*, AV node vs. ventricles). The treatment for a third-degree AV block is a permanent pacemaker.

CEP.ECG(4)

Short Answers for CEP.ECG(4)

1. Rate is approximately 70 bpm.

2. Irregular rhythm

3. Atrial fibrillation

Multiple-Choice Answers for CEP.ECG(4)

1—B.   Warfarin

2—D.   None of the above

3—A.   RPE

Teaching points: Warfarin is often prescribed in patients with atrial fibrillation to prevent the formation of and to treat existing thrombi that result due to the unorganized and weak contractions of the atria. It is important to confirm that the patient is on some type of anticoagulation therapy. Patients presenting with new onset atrial fibrillation should see a physician before resuming cardiac rehabilitation. Regarding exercise training, while compromised with this condition because of the reduced "atrial kick," patients can still improve fitness. Although HR does increase with exercise, the HR method is not reliable because of the irregular nature of this arrhythmia. Because of the irregular rhythm, when measuring the HR with atrial fibrillation, the number of cardiac cycles should be counted from a 6- or 10-s strip.

CEP.ECG(5)

Short Answers for CEP.ECG(5)

1. Sinus

2. Ventricular bigeminy

Multiple-Choice Answers for CEP.ECG(5)

1—A.   Continue to monitor

2—D.   All of the above

Teaching points: Ventricular bigeminy is a stable and non–life-threatening dysrhythmia. Patients with this may or may not report feeling "skipped beats." Regardless, as with any new-onset arrhythmias, the referring physician should be notified, but this does not warrant withholding exercise. Although emotional distress and stimulants, such as caffeine, can lead to increased rates and ectopic beats, some patients may regularly have frequent ventricular activity without precipitating factors. Regardless, the clinician should first "rule out" medication noncompliance before considering secondary causes in a new onset.

CEP.ECG(6)

Short Answers for CEP.ECG(6)

1. 98 bpm

2. Regular

3. Sinus rhythm with left ventricular hypertrophy (LVH) and a left bundle-branch block (LBBB)

True or False and Multiple-Choice Answers for CEP.ECG(6)

1—D.   Contact referring physician to verify the test ordered

2—True.

Teaching points: Both LVH as well as LBBB can mask changes due to myocardial ischemia that are typically seen on a standard 12-lead ECG. Therefore, a symptom-limited exercise stress test with ECG only is typically not administered due to the inability to diagnose ischemia. However, new-onset LBBB in the presence of angina may indicate an acute coronary event. Regardless of the presence (or lack) of angina, a new occurrence of LBBB should be reported to a physician to determine the underlying cause.

CEP.ECG(7)

Short Answers for CEP.ECG(7)

1. 176 bpm

2. Regular

3. Sinus tachycardia

Multiple-Choice Answers for CEP.ECG(7)

1—B. Supraventricular tachycardia (SVT)

2—D. β-Blocker

3—B. No

Teaching points: The HR response in the earlier ECG is normal for someone during stage IV of the Bruce protocol. Although his HR is close to his age-predicted maximum, percentage of age-predicted maximum HR is not a criterion for stopping at test. If this ECG were obtained at rest, it would be abnormal and likely an SVT, not emanating from the SA node. Finally, because of the normal HR response during exercise, if this individual was on antihypertensive medications, it would likely not be a type of β-blocker because they attenuate the chronotropic response to exercise.

CEP.ECG(8)

Short Answers for CEP.ECG(8)

1. 115 bpm

2. Irregular

3. Sinus tachycardia with a PVC and a ventricular triplet

Multiple-Choice Answers for CEP.ECG(8)

1—B. Continue with the test

2—A. They are multifocal.

Teaching points: An isolated ventricular triplet, although associated with a greater likelihood of ventricular tachycardia, is not by itself dangerous. Therefore, although an isolated triplet should be noted, it is not an indication for stopping a test, according to *ACSM's GETP*. The fact that these are multifocal PVC, thus originating at different ventricular areas does not change these guidelines. More than one observed ventricular triplet, however, is listed as a relative contraindication for stopping a stress test.

CEP.ECG(9)

Short Answers for CEP.ECG(9)

1. 78 bpm

2. Regular

3. Sinus rhythm with a right bundle-branch block (RBBB)

Multiple-Choice Answer for CEP.ECG(9)

1—D. The athlete will likely undergo additional evaluation before returning to play.

Teaching points: RBBB is not an uncommon finding in athletes. As long as there is no underlying structural heart disease, most athletes are cleared to return to play.

CEP.ECG(10)

Short Answers for CEP.ECG(10)

1. 50 bpm

2. Regular

3. Sinus bradycardia with a first-degree AV block and PVC

True or False and Multiple-Choice Answers for CEP.ECG(10)

1—False.

2—D. There is a slight risk for atrial reentry tachycardia.

Teaching points: First-degree AV block is a benign finding in healthy individuals. There is no known risk for individuals who have a first-degree AV block to develop more severe AV nodal disruptions that necessitate a pacemaker. The bradycardia is caused by enhanced vagal tone (*i.e.*, parasympathetic influence), which is common in endurance athletes. Isolated PVC are also benign.

CEP

CEP.ECG(11)

Short Answers for CEP.ECG(11)

1. 83 bpm

2. Regular

3. Sinus with ventricular-paced rhythm (notice pacemaker spike before QRS complex)

Multiple-Choice Answers for CEP.ECG(11)

1—C. Third-degree AV block

2—C. If present, ischemia would not be undetectable by ECG alone due to the pacemaker depolarization.

Teaching points: Pacemakers are indicated when the heart's natural pacemaker (*i.e.*, SA node) does not depolarize properly, as in sick sinus syndrome, or complete AV nodal block (*i.e.*, third-degree block). Due to the fact that this ECG is only ventricular paced, the cause was likely not sick sinus syndrome; otherwise, there would also be a pacer spike before the P wave. Similar to LVH and LBBB, ventricular pacemakers can hide ECG changes due to myocardial ischemia.

CEP.ECG(12)

Short Answer Answers for CEP.ECG(12)

1. 120 bpm

2. Regular

3. Sinus tachycardia with 2 mm of ST-segment depression in the inferior and lateral leads

Multiple-Choice Answers for CEP.ECG(12)

1—A. Nitroglycerin

2—D. Both A and C

Teaching points: This is an example of classic ST-segment depression due to myocardial ischemia. The ECG reveals 2 mm of ST-segment depression in both the inferior leads (II, III, and aVF) and the lateral leads (VL, V_5, and V_6). Although left-sided chest pressure along with concomitant left arm pain is considered classic angina by many, pain in the jaw, between the shoulder blades, indigestion-type sensation, or just excessive SOB can be anginal equivalents. If discontinuing exercise and rest do not relieve the angina, then the drug of choice would be nitroglycerin. Typically, given sublingually for rapid absorption, the main mechanism of nitroglycerin in reducing the ischemic burden is the reduction of preload on the heart from dilation of the veins.

CEP.ECG(13)

Short Answers for CEP.ECG(13)

1. 125 bpm

2. Regular

3. Ventricular tachycardia

Multiple-Choice Answers for CEP.ECG(13)

1—D. All of the above

2—D. Low CO

Teaching points: Ventricular tachycardia can be a lethal arrhythmia and is an indication for stopping a stress test. When a patient loses consciousness and a pulse cannot be obtained, immediate defibrillation is indicated. Although transient changes leading to wide QRS complexes are also seen with rate-dependent bundle-branch blocks and aberrancies, the clinician should always rule out ventricular tachycardia first because of its serious implications.

CEP Job Task Analysis

Note: CEP certification candidates may also review the knowledge and skills (KSs) found in Part 1, ACSM Certified Personal Trainer (CPT) and Part 2, ACSM Certified Exercise Physiologist (EP-C).

DOMAIN I: PATIENT/CLIENT ASSESSMENT

A. Determine and obtain the necessary physician referral and medical records to assess the potential participant.

Knowledge or Skill Statement	Explanation/Examples	Resources
Knowledge of the procedure to obtain informed consent from participant to meet legal requirements	• Participant and/or guardian should have verbal explanation and questions answered. • If the participant is a minor, a legal guardian must sign the consent. • Various components of informed consent (*e.g.*, purpose, risks, participant responsibilities, freedom to withdraw) • Purpose, legal concerns, content, administration	*ACSM's Guidelines for Exercise Testing and Prescription* (GETP), 10th edition (6) • Chapter 3
Knowledge of information and documentation required for program participation **Knowledge** of the procedure to obtain physician referral and medical records required for program participation **Knowledge** of the procedure to obtain participant's medical history through available documentation **Knowledge** of the components of a best practice-based physician referral form **Knowledge** of methods used to obtain a referral for clinical exercise physiology services **Knowledge** of the necessary medical records needed to properly assess a participant, given their diagnosis and/or reason for referral	• American Heart Association (AHA)/American College of Sports Medicine (ACSM) Health/Fitness Facility Preparticipation Screening Questionnaire, Physical Activity Readiness Questionnaire (PAR-Q+), medical history, informed consent • Must be treated as confidential and privileged information • Understand policy and procedures for obtaining medical records and Health Insurance Portability and Accountability Act (HIPAA) regulations.	*ACSM's Guidelines for Exercise Testing and Prescription* (GETP), 10th edition (6) • Chapter 2 and 3
Skill in assessing participant physician referral and medical records to determine program participation status	• Assess appropriateness of referral based on medical records/physician referral.	*ACSM's Guidelines for Exercise Testing and Prescription* (GETP), 10th edition (6) • Chapter 2

CEP

B. Perform a preparticipation health screening including review the participant's medical history and knowledge, their needs and goals, the program's potential benefits, and additional required testing and data.

Knowledge or Skill Statement	Explanation/Examples	Resources
Knowledge of normal cardiovascular, pulmonary, and metabolic anatomy and physiology **Knowledge** of best practice-based intake assessment tools and techniques **Knowledge** of the epidemiology, pathophysiology, progression, risk factors, key clinical findings, and treatments of chronic disease. **Knowledge** of instructional techniques to assess participant's expectations and goals **Knowledge** of commonly used medication for cardiovascular, pulmonary, and metabolic diseases **Knowledge** of the effects of physical inactivity, including bed rest, and methods to counteract these changes **Knowledge** of normal physiologic responses to exercise **Knowledge** of abnormal responses/signs and symptoms to exercise associated with different pathologies (*e.g.*, cardiovascular, pulmonary, metabolic) **Knowledge** of anthropometric measurements and their interpretation **Knowledge** of normal 12-lead and telemetry electrocardiogram (ECG) interpretation **Knowledge** of interpretation of ECGs for abnormalities (*e.g.*, arrhythmias, blocks, ischemia, infarction) **Knowledge** of normal and abnormal heart and lung sounds **Knowledge** of pertinent areas of a participant's medical history (*e.g.*, any symptoms since their procedure, description of discomfort/pain, orthopedic issues) **Knowledge** of validated tools for measurement of psychosocial health status **Knowledge** of various behavioral assessment tools (*e.g.*, SF-36, health-related quality of life, Chronic Respiratory Disease Questionnaire) and strategies for their use **Knowledge** of psychological issues associated with acute and chronic illness (*e.g.*, anxiety, depression, social isolation, suicidal ideation)	• Understand resting and exercise cardiovascular, pulmonary, and metabolic anatomy and physiology. • Understanding of how diagnostic testing and medical regimens/procedures can assess clinical progression of disease and/or exercise effects • Coaching techniques to set achievable goals and overcome potential obstacles • Understanding medication effects on resting and exercise related to cardiovascular, pulmonary, and metabolic diseases • Understanding of deconditioning effects of bed rest and inactivity on the various body systems (*e.g.*, cardiovascular, pulmonary, muscular) • Metabolic equivalent (MET) requirements for various physical activities; arm vs. leg exercise differences in hemodynamics; volume of oxygen consumed per unit of time ($\dot{V}O_2$); myocardial oxygen consumption; neuromuscular, vascular, and metabolic adaptations; muscle hypertrophy • Knowledge of absolute and relative contraindications to exercise and abnormal responses/signs and symptoms for cardiovascular, pulmonary, and metabolic disease states • Height, weight, circumferences, and body composition testing (*e.g.*, skinfolds, body mass index [BMI]); understand the difference between BMI and body fat percentage. • Know the anatomical landmarks for ECG lead placement, identify/minimize artifact, identify normal resting ECG and exercise ECG changes, and know/identify dangerous arrhythmias. • Understanding clinical descriptions and auscultation sounds for normal and abnormal heart and lung sounds • Issues that may alter exercise testing selection and/or the exercise prescription (*e.g.*, knee osteoarthritis may limit weight-bearing activity, previous injury, or surgery)	*ACSM's Guidelines for Exercise Testing and Prescription* (GETP), 10th edition (6) • Appendix A *ACSM's Exercise Management for Persons with Chronic Diseases and Disabilities*, 4th edition (2) *ACSM's Guidelines for Exercise Testing and Prescription* (GETP), 10th edition (6) • Chapter 5 *ACSM's Guidelines for Exercise Testing and Prescription* (GETP), 10th edition (6) • Chapters 3 and 5 "Exercise Standards for Testing and Training: A Statement for Healthcare Professionals from the American Heart Association" (10) *ACSM's Guidelines for Exercise Testing and Prescription* (GETP), 10th edition (6) • Chapter 4 *ACSM's Guidelines for Exercise Testing and Prescription* (GETP), 10th edition (6) • Chapter 4

B. Perform a preparticipation health screening including review the participant's medical history and knowledge, their needs and goals, the program's potential benefits, and additional required testing and data. (cont.)		
Knowledge or Skill Statement	**Explanation/Examples**	**Resources**
Knowledge of participant-centered goal setting **Knowledge** of functional and diagnostic exercise testing methods, including symptom-limited maximal and submaximal aerobic testing **Knowledge** of indications and contraindications to exercise testing **Knowledge** of normal and abnormal (*i.e.*, signs/symptoms) endpoints for termination of exercise testing **Knowledge** of testing and interpretation of muscle strength/endurance and flexibility **Knowledge** of current published guidelines for treatment of cardiovascular, pulmonary, and metabolic pathologies (*e.g.*, American College of Cardiology [ACC]/American Heart Association [AHA] Joint Guidelines, Global Initiative for Chronic Obstructive Lung Disease [GOLD], American Diabetes Association [ADA] guidelines)	• Five-factor model of personality, transtheoretical model, *Diagnostic and Statistical Manual of Mental Disorders* (*DSM*), classes of mood disorders, subtypes of anxiety disorders • Knowledge of health-related quality-of-life tools, their target populations, strategies for their use, and how results may effect program participation • Know how these conditions may affect exercise adherence and motivation; social support groups; referral to other health care professionals. • Set goals that are specific, measurable, and challenging but realistic (*e.g.*, specific, measurable, attainable, realistic, and time-bound [SMART] goals). • Knowledge of exercise test modalities, test protocols, disease diagnosis, severity and prognosis, functional testing, and return-to-work testing • Clinical understanding of absolute and relative indications for terminating exercise testing • Clinical understanding of what exercise testing termination does to normal (*i.e.*, target heart rate achieved) or abnormal (*i.e.*, signs/symptoms) physiological markers • One repetition maximum bench press and leg press, push-up test, curl up (crunch test), Young Men's Christian Association (YMCA) bench press test, sit and reach (trunk flexion), range of motion in select single joints • Clinical understanding, application, and basis synthesis of multiple national scientific/medical guidelines and position stands	

CEP

B.   Perform a preparticipation health screening including review the participant's medical history and knowledge, their needs and goals, the program's potential benefits, and additional required testing and data. (cont.)

Knowledge or Skill Statement	Explanation/Examples	Resources
Skill in effective interview techniques **Skill** in medication recognition **Skill** in auscultation methods for common cardiopulmonary abnormalities **Skill** in data collection during baseline intake assessment **Skill** in assessment and interpretation of information collected during the baseline intake assessment **Skill** in formulating an exercise program based on the information collected during the baseline intake assessment **Skill** in selection, application, and monitoring of exercise testing for healthy and patient populations **Skill** in muscle strength, endurance, and flexibility assessments for healthy and patient populations **Skill** in patient preparation and ECG electrode application for resting and exercise ECG	• Evaluate arteries for adequate pulses and bruits, lungs for emphysema, the heart for heart failure, murmurs, etc. • Techniques to appropriately acquire individual patient information that may influence patient participation status • Interpretation of graded exercise tests, blood pressure and heart rate response, ECG interpretation, oxygen saturation, and gas exchange and ventilatory responses • Practice the frequency, intensity, time, type, volume, and progression (FITT-VP) principle for aerobic, muscle strength and endurance, and flexibility exercise based on the goals, limitations, and ability of the patient. • Determine testing protocols that are safe and effective for the individual; know the procedure and be able to effectively explain it to the individual; know testing termination criteria. • Practice one repetition maximum bench press and leg press, push-up test, curl up (crunch test), YMCA bench press test, sit and reach (trunk flexion), range of motion in select single joints • Practice finding the anatomical landmarks for ECG lead placement; dry the skin, alcohol prep the landmarks, and shave body hair (if necessary).	*ACSM's Guidelines for Exercise Testing and Prescription* (GETP), 10th edition (6) • Chapter 5 *ACSM's Guidelines for Exercise Testing and Prescription* (GETP), 10th edition (6) • Chapter 5 *ACSM's Guidelines for Exercise Testing and Prescription* (GETP), 10th edition (6) • Chapters 4 and 5 *ACSM's Guidelines for Exercise Testing and Prescription* (GETP), 10th edition (6) • Chapter 4

C.   Evaluate the participant's risk to ensure safe participation and determine level of monitoring/supervision in a preventive or rehabilitative exercise program.

Knowledge or Skill Statement	Explanation/Examples	Resources
Knowledge of applied exercise physiology principles **Knowledge** of cardiovascular, pulmonary, and metabolic pathologies; their clinical progression; diagnostic testing; and medical regimens/procedures to treat **Knowledge** of pre-exercise readiness assessment as delineated in the current edition of *ACSM's Guidelines for Exercise Testing and Prescription*	• Understand the acute and chronic responses and adaptations exercise has on the body. These include the cardiorespiratory responses, metabolic responses, neuromuscular responses, and muscular fatigue. • Understanding of clinical information necessary to assess disease status, indications of clinical progression, and possible methods of treatment • Understanding of self-guided screening for physical activity and exercise testing recommendations based on risk factors	*ACSM's Guidelines for Exercise Testing and Prescription* (GETP), 10th edition (6) • Chapter 2 *ACSM's Guidelines for Exercise Testing and Prescription* (GETP), 10th edition (6) • Chapter 2 *ACSM's Guidelines for Exercise Testing and Prescription* (GETP), 10th edition (6)

CEP

C. Evaluate the participant's risk to ensure safe participation and determine level of monitoring/supervision in a preventive or rehabilitative exercise program. (cont.)

Knowledge or Skill Statement	Explanation/Examples	Resources
Knowledge of the participant's risk factor profile (*i.e.*, cardiovascular, pulmonary, and metabolic) to determine level of exercise supervision using ACSM, American Heart Association (AHA), and American Association of Cardiovascular and Pulmonary Rehabilitation (AACVPR) risk stratification criteria **Knowledge** of indications and contraindications to exercise testing **Knowledge** of functional and diagnostic exercise testing methods, including symptom-limited maximal and submaximal aerobic testing **Knowledge** of interpretation of electrocardiograms (ECGs) for abnormalities (*e.g.*, arrhythmias, blocks, ischemia, infarction) **Knowledge** of normal and abnormal (*i.e.*, signs/symptoms) endpoints for termination of exercise testing **Knowledge** of testing and interpretation of muscle strength/endurance and flexibility **Knowledge** of commonly used medication for cardiovascular, pulmonary, and metabolic diseases **Knowledge** of current published guidelines for treatment of cardiovascular, pulmonary, and metabolic pathologies (*e.g.*, American College of Cardiology [ACC]/AHA Joint Guidelines, Global Initiative for Chronic Obstructive Lung Disease [GOLD], American Diabetes Association [ADA] guidelines)	• Understanding of self-guided screening for physical activity, risk factors, exercise testing recommendations • Understanding of cardiovascular, pulmonary, and metabolic disorder variables that affect the decisions regarding administration of and exercise test • Knowledge of parameters of exercise test modalities, test protocols, disease diagnosis, severity and prognosis, functional testing, and return-to-work testing • Be able to identify resting and exercise abnormalities including, but not limited to, bundle-branch blocks, sinus bradycardia and tachycardia, sinus arrest, atrial fibrillation and flutter, ventricular tachycardia and fibrillation, ST depression and elevation, and premature ventricular and atrial contractions. • Clinical understanding of absolute and relative indications for terminating exercise testing • Knowledge of one repetition maximum bench press and leg press, push-up test, bench press test, sit and reach (trunk flexion), and range of motion in select single joints to evaluate muscle strength/endurance and flexibility • Understanding medications' normal and abnormal effects on resting and exercise cardiovascular, pulmonary, and metabolic diseases • Clinical understanding, application, and basis of multiple national scientific/medical guidelines and position stands	• Chapters 2, 3, and 5 *ACSM's Guidelines for Exercise Testing and Prescription* (GETP), 10th edition (6) • Chapter 5 *ACSM's Guidelines for Exercise Testing and Prescription* (GETP), 10th edition (6) • Chapter 5 *ACSM's Guidelines for Exercise Testing and Prescription* (GETP), 10th edition (6) • Chapter 4 *ACSM's Guidelines for Exercise Testing and Prescription* (GETP), 10th edition (6) • Appendix A
Skill in the determination of participant risk and level of monitoring using participant health history, medical history, medical records and additional diagnostic assessments **Skill** in risk stratification using established guidelines (ACSM, AHA vs. informal) **Skill** in selection, application, and monitoring of exercise tests for apparently healthy participants and those with chronic disease **Skill** in ECG interpretation and interpreting exercise test results	• Determine readiness for exercise and evaluate who requires physician clearance for exercise and physician supervision during exercise testing. • Understanding of and management of testing protocols that are safe and effective for the individual; know the procedure and be able to effectively explain it to the individual; know testing termination criteria and data collection during test stages. • Understand clinical significance in identifying normal resting ECGs, normal changes with ECGs during exercise, abnormal ECG changes during exercise, know dangerous arrhythmias, and exercise termination criteria.	*ACSM's Guidelines for Exercise Testing and Prescription* (GETP), 10th edition (6) • Chapter 2 *ACSM's Guidelines for Exercise Testing and Prescription* (GETP), 10th edition (6) • Chapters 4 and 5

D. Review available participant information and determine outstanding information and testing required before program entry.

Knowledge or Skill Statement	Explanation/Examples	Resources
Knowledge of the epidemiology, pathophysiology, progression, risk factors, key clinical findings, and treatments of chronic diseases **Knowledge** of the techniques (*e.g.*, lab results, diagnostic tests) used to diagnose chronic diseases, their indications, limitations, risks, and normal and abnormal results **Knowledge** of commonly used medications in patients with chronic diseases, their mechanisms of action, and side effects	• Understanding of chronic diseases related to health, the physical changes that accompany a particular disease or syndrome, risk factors as related to the individual, and treatments and particular clinical findings of the diseases. • Understanding of diagnostic techniques and lab results to determine if a participant with a chronic disease has limitations before program implementation. • Know the mechanisms, effects, and interactions of commonly prescribed medications for patients with chronic diseases.	*ACSM's Exercise Management for Persons with Chronic Diseases and Disabilities*, 4th edition (2)
Skill in the understanding and application of medical terminology **Skill** in the interpretation of medical records	• Review and be familiar with medical terminology to understand doctor's notes and medical records.	*ACSM's Exercise Management for Persons with Chronic Diseases and Disabilities*, 4th edition (2)

E. Assess resting physical measures to determine baseline status (*e.g.*, height, weight, vital signs, body composition).

Knowledge or Skill Statement	Explanation/Examples	Resources
Knowledge of techniques for assessing signs and symptoms associated with pathological conditions (*e.g.*, peripheral pulses, blood pressure, edema, pain) **Knowledge** of medical therapies for chronic diseases and their effect on resting vital signs and symptoms **Knowledge** of abnormal signs and symptoms in apparently healthy individuals and those with chronic disease	• Understanding of signs and symptoms of pathological conditions such as vital signs (pulses, blood pressure, respiration, body temperature), edema, and pain • Know how resting vital signs and symptoms are affected by various medical therapies. • Know signs and symptoms of those with chronic diseases as well as those who are apparently healthy.	*ACSM's Exercise Management for Persons with Chronic Diseases and Disabilities*, 4th edition (2)
Skill in assessing resting physical measures to determine baseline status (*e.g.*, height, weight, vital signs, body composition)	• Understanding and ability to use the various methods for determining baseline physical measurements, height, weight, vital signs, and body composition in all clients.	*ACSM's Guidelines for Exercise Testing and Prescription* (GETP), 10th edition (6)

CEP

F. Determine baseline exercise status using a variety of procedures as needed (*e.g.*, graded exercise testing, strength, flexibility, balance, exercise history).

Knowledge or Skill Statement	Explanation/Examples	Resources
Knowledge of testing protocols used to assess aerobic capacity, graded exercise testing, strength, flexibility and balance **Knowledge** of contraindications to symptom-limited, maximal exercise testing and factors associated with complications (*e.g.*, probability of coronary heart disease, abnormal blood pressure) **Knowledge** of medical therapies for chronic diseases and their effect on the physiologic response to exercise **Knowledge** of current practice guidelines and recommendations (*e.g.*, American Heart Association, American Diabetes Association) for the prevention, evaluation, treatment, and management of chronic diseases **Knowledge** of the timing of daily activities (*e.g.*, medications, dialysis, meals, glucose monitoring) and their effect on exercise in patients with chronic diseases	• Understanding of and ability to perform aerobic capacity, graded exercise testing, and strength, flexibility, and balance tests. • Check for contraindications to symptom-limited exercise testing and factors associated with complications, not limited to heart disease and abnormal blood pressure. • Understanding of how medical therapies affect the physiological response to exercise for those with chronic diseases. • Awareness of the ongoing guidelines and recommendations from organizations such as the American College of Sports Medicine, American Heart Association, American Diabetes Association, and others for the prevention, evaluation, treatment, and management of chronic diseases • Understand how the timing of daily activities affects patients with chronic diseases and their monitoring/medication schedule; ability to work with patients to gather this information and apply it in context of exercise	*ACSM's Guidelines for Exercise Testing and Prescription* (GETP), 10th edition (6)
Skill in matching the appropriate exercise test to the participant's individual needs and functional abilities	• Know how to select and match the appropriate exercise test to the individual needs and functional abilities of the participant.	*ACSM's Guidelines for Exercise Testing and Prescription* (GETP), 10th edition (6)

DOMAIN II: EXERCISE PRESCRIPTION

A. Develop a clinically appropriate exercise prescription using all available information (*e.g.*, clinical and physiological status, goals, and behavioral assessment).

Knowledge or Skill Statement	Explanation/Examples	Resources
Knowledge of applied exercise physiology principles **Knowledge** of the frequency, intensity, time, and type (FITT) principle for cardiovascular, muscular fitness/resistance training, and flexibility exercise prescription **Knowledge** of cardiovascular, pulmonary, and metabolic pathologies; their clinical progression; diagnostic testing; and medical regimens/procedures to treat **Knowledge** of the effects of physical inactivity, including bed rest, and methods to counteract these changes **Knowledge** of normal physiologic responses to exercise **Knowledge** of abnormal responses/signs and symptoms to exercise associated with different pathologies (*e.g.*, cardiovascular, pulmonary, metabolic) **Knowledge** of validated tools of measurement of psychosocial health status **Knowledge** of functional and diagnostic exercise testing methods, including symptom-limited maximal and submaximal aerobic testing **Knowledge** of normal and abnormal (*i.e.*, signs/symptoms) endpoints for termination of exercise testing **Knowledge** of tests to assess and interpret muscle strength/endurance and flexibility **Knowledge** of commonly used medication for cardiovascular, pulmonary, and metabolic diseases and their effect on exercise prescription **Knowledge** of exercise principles (prescription, progression/maintenance, and supervision) for apparently healthy participants and participants with cardiovascular, pulmonary, and/or metabolic diseases	• Understand the acute and chronic responses and adaptations exercise has on the body. These include the cardiorespiratory responses, metabolic, and neuromuscular responses and muscular fatigue. • Understanding of the frequency, intensity, time, type, total volume and progression (FITT-VP) principles and how to manipulate each principle to achieve desired exercise volume and response • Understanding of how diagnostic testing and medical regimens/procedures can assess clinical progression of disease and/or exercise effects • Understanding of deconditioning effects of bed rest and inactivity on the various body systems (*e.g.*, cardiovascular, pulmonary, muscular) • Metabolic equivalent (MET) requirements for various physical activities; arm vs. leg exercise differences in hemodynamics; volume of oxygen consumed per unit of time ($\dot{V}O_2$); myocardial oxygen consumption; neuromuscular, vascular, and metabolic adaptations; muscle hypertrophy • Knowledge of absolute and relative contraindications to exercise and abnormal responses/signs and symptoms for cardiovascular, pulmonary, and metabolic disease stated • Five-factor model of personality, transtheoretical model, *Diagnostic and Statistical Manual of Mental Disorders* (*DSM*), classes of mood disorders, subtypes of anxiety disorders • Knowledge of parameters of exercise test modalities, test protocols, disease diagnosis, severity and prognosis, functional testing, and return-to-work testing • Clinical understanding of absolute and relative indications for terminating exercise testing	*ACSM's Guidelines for Exercise Testing and Prescription* (GETP), 10th edition (6) • Chapter 6 *ACSM's Guidelines for Exercise Testing and Prescription* (GETP), 10th edition (6) • Chapter 2 *ACSM's Guidelines for Exercise Testing and Prescription* (GETP), 10th edition (6) • Chapter 5 *ACSM's Guidelines for Exercise Testing and Prescription* (GETP), 10th edition (6) • Chapter 5 *ACSM's Guidelines for Exercise Testing and Prescription* (GETP), 10th edition (6) • Chapter 4 *ACSM's Guidelines for Exercise Testing and Prescription* (GETP), 10th edition (6) • Appendix A *ACSM's Guidelines for Exercise Testing and Prescription* (GETP), 10th edition (6) • Chapters 6–11 *ACSM's Guidelines for Exercise Testing and Prescription* (GETP), 10th edition (6) • Chapters 6–11 *ACSM's Metabolic Calculations Handbook* (3)

A. Develop a clinically appropriate exercise prescription using all available information (*e.g.*, clinical and physiological status, goals, and behavioral assessment). (cont.)		
Knowledge or Skill Statement	**Explanation/Examples**	**Resources**
Knowledge of appropriate mode, volume, and intensity of exercise to produce desired outcomes for apparently healthy participants and those with cardiovascular, pulmonary, and metabolic diseases **Knowledge** of the application of metabolic calculations **Knowledge** of goal development strategies **Knowledge** of behavioral assessment tools (*e.g.*, SF-36, health-related quality of life, Chronic Respiratory Disease Questionnaire) and strategies for use **Knowledge** of psychological issues associated with acute and chronic illness (*e.g.*, anxiety, depression, social isolation, suicidal ideation)	• One repetition maximum bench press and leg press, push-up test, curl up (crunch test), Young Men's Christian Association (YMCA) bench press test, sit and reach (trunk flexion), range of motion in select single joints • Understanding medications' normal and abnormal effects on resting and exercise cardiovascular, pulmonary, and metabolic diseases • Knowledge of the FITT-VP principle and the components of a single exercise session: warm-up, stretching, conditioning phase (or sports-related exercise) and cool-down • Exercise program design specific to the individual (novice vs. advanced exerciser) and their goals; exercise program design to help manage chronic disease (hypertension, diabetes, dyslipidemia, obesity, asthma, chronic obstructive pulmonary disease [COPD], etc.) • Understanding how to calculate and apply $\dot{V}O_2$ equations for walking, running, leg cycling, arm cranking, and stepping • Set goals that are specific, measurable, and challenging but realistic (*e.g.*, specific, measurable, attainable, realistic, and time-bound [SMART] goals). • Application of health-related quality of life, their target populations, strategies for their use, and how results may affect exercise prescription • Know how these conditions may affect exercise program adherence and motivation; social support groups; referral to other health care professionals.	
Skill in interpretation of functional and diagnostic exercise testing with applications to exercise prescription **Skill** in interpretation of muscular strength/endurance testing with applications to exercise prescription **Skill** in developing an exercise prescription based on a participant's clinical status	• Design and implement an exercise program that is safe and effective for the individual based on his or her functional ability and known risk factors/disease(s). • Design and implement a resistance training program that is safe and effective for the individual based on his or her functional ability and known risk factors/disease(s). • Develop an exercise program that is safe for the individual based on their clinical status yet effective to manage/treat his or her risk factors/disease(s).	*ACSM's Guidelines for Exercise Testing and Prescription* (GETP), 10th edition (6) • Chapters 4 and 6–11 *ACSM's Guidelines for Exercise Testing and Prescription* (GETP), 10th edition (6) • Chapters 9–11

CEP

B. Review the exercise prescription and exercise program with the participant, including home exercise, compliance, and participant's expectations and goals.

Knowledge or Skill Statement	Explanation/Examples	Resources
Knowledge of applied exercise physiology principles **Knowledge** of normal physiologic responses to exercise **Knowledge** of abnormal responses/signs and symptoms to exercise associated with different pathologies (*e.g.*, cardiovascular, pulmonary, metabolic) **Knowledge** of anthropometric measurements and their interpretation **Knowledge** of participant-centered goal setting **Knowledge** of exercise principles (prescription, progression/maintenance, and supervision) for apparently healthy participants and participants with cardiovascular, pulmonary, and/or metabolic diseases **Knowledge** of the frequency, intensity, time, and type (FITT) principle for cardiovascular, muscular fitness/resistance training, and flexibility exercise prescription **Knowledge** of appropriate mode, volume, and intensity of exercise to produce desired outcomes for apparently healthy participants and those with cardiovascular, pulmonary, and metabolic diseases **Knowledge** of the application of metabolic calculations **Knowledge** of goal development strategies **Knowledge** of terminology appropriate to provide the client with education regarding his or her exercise prescription **Knowledge** of instructional techniques for safe and effective prescription implementation and understanding by participant **Knowledge** of the timing of daily activities with exercise (*e.g.*, medications, meals, insulin/glucose monitoring) **Knowledge** of disease-specific strategies and tools to improve tolerance of exercise (*e.g.*, breathing techniques, insulin pump use and adjustments, prophylactic nitroglycerin)	• Understand the acute and chronic responses and adaptations exercise has on the body. These include the cardiorespiratory responses, neuromuscular responses, and muscular fatigue. • Metabolic equivalent (MET) requirements for various physical activities; arm vs. leg exercise differences in hemodynamics; volume of oxygen consumed per unit of time ($\dot{V}O_2$); myocardial oxygen consumption; neuromuscular adaptations; muscle hypertrophy • Knowledge of absolute and relative contraindications to exercise and abnormal responses/signs and symptoms for cardiovascular, pulmonary, and metabolic disease stated • Body mass index (BMI), circumferences, skinfold measurements, hydrodensitometry, dual-energy x-ray absorptiometry, bioimpedance and their clinical significance • Set goals that are specific, measurable, and challenging but realistic (*e.g.*, specific, measurable, attainable, realistic, and time-bound [SMART] goals) • Knowledge of the frequency, intensity, time, type, total volume and progression (FITT-VP) principle and the components of a single exercise session: warm-up, stretching, conditioning phase (or sports-related exercise), and cool-down • Understanding of FITT-VP principles and how manipulation of each affects the exercise prescription for cardiovascular strength/endurance, muscular fitness/resistance training, and flexibility • Exercise program design specific to the individual (novice vs. advanced exerciser) and their goals; exercise program design to help manage chronic disease (hypertension, diabetes, dyslipidemia, obesity, asthma, chronic obstructive pulmonary disorder [COPD], etc.) • Knowledge of calculating $\dot{V}O_2$/MET equations for walking, running, leg cycling, arm cranking, and stepping to design the exercise program based on the patient's ability (*e.g.*, MET level)	*ACSM's Guidelines for Exercise Testing and Prescription* (GETP), 10th edition (6) • Chapter 2 *ACSM's Guidelines for Exercise Testing and Prescription* (GETP), 10th edition (6) • Chapter 4 *ACSM's Guidelines for Exercise Testing and Prescription* (GETP), 10th edition (6) • Chapters 6–11 "Pulmonary Rehabilitation: Joint ACCP/AACVPR Evidence-Based Guidelines" (8) *ACSM's Guidelines for Exercise Testing and Prescription* (GETP), 10th edition (6) • Chapters 6–11 *ACSM's Metabolic Calculations Handbook* (3) *ACSM's Guidelines for Exercise Testing and Prescription* (GETP), 10th edition (6) • Appendix A

B. Review the exercise prescription and exercise program with the participant, including home exercise, compliance, and participant's expectations and goals. (cont.)		
Knowledge or Skill Statement	**Explanation/Examples**	**Resources**
Knowledge of instructional strategies for improving exercise adoption and maintenance **Knowledge** of common barriers to exercise compliance and strategies to address these (*e.g.*, physical, psychological, environmental, demographic) **Knowledge** of instructional techniques to assess participant's expectations and goals **Knowledge** of risk factor reduction programs and alternative community resources (*e.g.*, dietary counseling, weight management/Weight Watchers, smoking cessation, stress management, physical therapy/back care)	• Set goals that are specific, measurable, and challenging but realistic (*e.g.*, SMART goals). • Ability to educate individuals on a practical level. Avoid "technical" terms and choose basic terms (*e.g.*, chest instead of pectoralis major). • Communicating to participant via various methods (*e.g.*, verbal, visual, written), proper technique, theory, and rational for implementation of an effective exercise prescription • Optimal times to exercise with relation to eating and blood sugar (energy levels), medication peak times and their effects on exercise performance, insulin use/injection site recommendations, evening exercise, and hypoglycemia risk • Be able to respond/recommend the appropriate strategy to maximize exercise safety and the conditioning effect and minimize any adverse reactions. • Develop patient-centered strategies to overcome exercise barriers. • Set goals that are specific, measurable, and challenging but realistic (*e.g.*, SMART goals). • Be familiar with various programs and services that assist with improving cardiac, pulmonary, and metabolic health.	
Skill in communicating with participants from a wide variety of educational backgrounds **Skill** in effectively communicating exercise prescription and exercise techniques **Skill** in applying various models to optimize patient compliance and adherence in order to achieve patient goals	• Practice communicating in a way that the patient will understand and will not be intimidated. • Describe/explain the exercise program so the patient will understand what they are doing and why. • Consider personal factors, behavioral factors, enjoyment, incentives, social support, environmental factors, conveniences, etc.	

C. Instruct the participant in the safe and effective use of exercise modalities, exercise plan, reporting symptoms, and class organization.

Knowledge or Skill Statement	Explanation/Examples	Resources
Knowledge of applied exercise physiology principles **Knowledge** of normal physiologic responses to exercise **Knowledge** of abnormal responses/signs and symptoms to exercise associated with different pathologies (*e.g.*, cardiovascular, pulmonary, metabolic) **Knowledge** of the timing of daily activities with exercise (*e.g.*, medications, meals, insulin/glucose monitoring) **Knowledge** of commonly used medication for cardiovascular, pulmonary, and metabolic diseases **Knowledge** of lay terminology for explanation of exercise prescription **Knowledge** of the operation of various exercise equipment/modalities **Knowledge** of proper biomechanical technique for exercise (*e.g.*, gait assessment, proper weightlifting form) **Knowledge** of muscle strength/endurance and flexibility modalities and their safe application and instruction **Knowledge** of tools to measure exercise tolerance (heart rate/pulse, blood pressure, glucometry, oximetry, rating of perceived exertion, dyspnea scale, pain scale) **Knowledge** of principles and application of exercise session organization	• Understand the acute and chronic responses and adaptations exercise has on the body. These include the cardiorespiratory responses, neuromuscular responses, and muscular fatigue. • Metabolic equivalent (MET) requirements for various physical activities; arm vs. leg exercise differences in hemodynamics; volume of oxygen consumed per unit of time ($\dot{V}O_2$); myocardial oxygen consumption; neuromuscular adaptations; muscle hypertrophy • Knowledge of absolute and relative contraindications to exercise and abnormal responses/signs and symptoms for cardiovascular, pulmonary, and metabolic disease states • Optimal times to exercise with relation to eating and blood sugar (energy levels), medication peak times and their effects on exercise performance, insulin use/injection site recommendations, evening exercise, and hypoglycemia risk • Understanding medications' normal and abnormal effects on resting and exercise cardiovascular, pulmonary, and metabolic diseases • Ability to educate individuals on a practical level. Avoid "technical" terms and choose basic terms (*e.g.*, chest instead of pectoralis major). • Be familiar with equipment settings and adjustments; demonstrate proper technique; know common errors when using various exercise modalities. • Knowledge of proper anatomical positioning to aerobic and resistance training modalities • Be familiar with numerous resistance training exercises and stretches, their proper applications, and common mistakes. • Understand how to use and interpret these tools; know how the measurements relate to exercise tolerance (*e.g.*, blood glucose readings that are too low or too high for exercise). • Warm-up, stretching, conditioning exercise, cool-down	*ACSM's Guidelines for Exercise Testing and Prescription* (GETP), 10th edition (6) • Chapter 2 *ACSM's Guidelines for Exercise Testing and Prescription* (GETP), 10th edition (6) • Chapter 11 • Appendix A *ACSM's Guidelines for Exercise Testing and Prescription* (GETP), 10th edition (6) • Appendix A *Essentials of Strength Training and Conditioning*, 3rd edition (12) • Chapters 13 and 14 *ACSM's Guidelines for Exercise Testing and Prescription* (GETP), 10th edition (6) • Chapters 4, 5, and 11 *ACSM's Guidelines for Exercise Testing and Prescription* (GETP), 10th edition (6) • Chapter 6

C. Instruct the participant in the safe and effective use of exercise modalities, exercise plan, reporting symptoms, and class organization. (cont.)

Knowledge or Skill Statement	Explanation/Examples	Resources
Skill in the observational assessment of participants **Skill** in communicating with participants from a wide variety of educational backgrounds **Skill** in communicating with participants regarding the proper organization of exercise sessions	• Ability to assess a patient's exercise technique, posture, movements, balance, etc. • Communicate in a way that the patient will understand and will not be intimidated. • Describe/explain the exercise program so the patient will understand what they are doing and why.	

D. Reassess and update the exercise prescription based on the participant's progress and feedback.

Knowledge or Skill Statement	Explanation/Examples	Resources
Knowledge of systems for tracking participant progress in both preventive and rehabilitative exercise programs **Knowledge** of typical participant progress in a preventive and rehabilitative exercise program given gender, age, clinical status, specifics of the exercise program (*e.g.*, walking only vs. comprehensive monitored program), and rate of program participation	• Use various systems for tracking participant's progress in both preventive and rehabilitative programs. • Know progress of a typical participant in a rehabilitative and preventive program given specifics of the program. Know how gender, age, and clinical status affect the participant's progress and rate of program participation.	*ACSM's Exercise Management for Persons with Chronic Diseases and Disabilities*, 4th edition (2)
Skill in assessing adequacy of participant progress in a preventive or rehabilitative exercise program given gender, age, clinical status, specifics of the exercise program (*e.g.*, walking only vs. comprehensive monitored program), and rate of program participation	• Assess how the participant progresses in a rehabilitative or preventive exercise program. Make adjustments as needed based on participation.	*ACSM's Exercise Management for Persons with Chronic Diseases and Disabilities*, 4th edition (2)

DOMAIN III: PROGRAM IMPLEMENTATION AND ONGOING SUPPORT

A. Implement the program (*e.g.*, exercise prescription, education, counseling, and goals).

Knowledge or Skill Statement	Explanation/Examples	Resources
Knowledge of abnormal responses/signs and symptoms to exercise associated with different pathologies (*i.e.*, cardiovascular, pulmonary, metabolic) **Knowledge** of normal and abnormal 12-lead and telemetry electrocardiogram (ECG) interpretation	• Knowledge of absolute and relative contraindications to exercise and abnormal responses/signs and symptoms for cardiovascular, pulmonary, and metabolic disease stated • Determine and identify normal resting ECG, normal changes with ECG during exercise, abnormal ECG changes during exercise, and various arrhythmias.	*ACSM's Guidelines for Exercise Testing and Prescription* (GETP), 10th edition (6) • Chapter 2 "Position Stand: Exercise and Hypertension" (4) *ACSM's Guidelines for Exercise Testing and Prescription* (GETP), 10th edition (6)

CEP

A.   Implement the program (*e.g.*, exercise prescription, education, counseling, and goals). (cont.)

Knowledge or Skill Statement	Explanation/Examples	Resources
Knowledge of the frequency, intensity, time, and type (FITT) principle for cardiovascular, muscular fitness/resistance training, and flexibility exercise prescription **Knowledge** of exercise progression/maintenance and supervision for apparently healthy participants and participants with cardiovascular, pulmonary, and/or metabolic diseases **Knowledge** of disease-specific strategies and tools to improve tolerance of exercise (*e.g.*, breathing techniques, insulin pump use and adjustments, prophylactic nitroglycerin) **Knowledge** of instructional strategies for improving exercise adoption and maintenance **Knowledge** of strategies to maximize exercise compliance (*e.g.*, overcoming barriers, values clarification, goals setting) **Knowledge** of the operation of various exercise equipment/modalities **Knowledge** of proper biomechanical technique for exercise (*e.g.*, gait, weightlifting form) **Knowledge** of tools to measure clinical exercise tolerance (*e.g.*, heart rate, glucometry, oximetry, subjective assessments) **Knowledge** of the principles and application of exercise session organization **Knowledge** of commonly used medications for cardiovascular, pulmonary, and metabolic diseases **Knowledge** of exercise program monitoring (*e.g.*, telemetry, oximetry, glucometry) **Knowledge** of principles and application of muscular strength/endurance and flexibility training **Knowledge** of methods to assess participant's educational goals **Knowledge** of counseling techniques to optimize participant's disease management, risk reduction, and goal attainment	• Clinical understanding of the frequency, intensity, time, and type, volume and progression (FITT-VP) principle and how to manipulate it based on changes in participants' disease status, progression/regression, maintenance, and supervision • Knowledge and clinical understanding of the effect of participants disease status (cardiovascular, pulmonary, and/or metabolic) on exercise progression/maintenance and supervision • Be able to respond/recommend the appropriate strategy to maximize exercise safety and the conditioning effect and minimize any adverse reactions. • Patient education on the benefits of exercise specific to the patient; developing exercise programs that meet the needs of the patient; patient-centered approaches that consider the patient's priorities, risk factors, and psychosocial status • Develop patient-centered strategies to overcome exercise barriers; develop specific, measurable, attainable, realistic, and time-bound (SMART) goals with the patient; consider what is most important to the patient. • Be familiar with equipment settings and adjustments; demonstrate proper technique; know common errors when using various exercise modalities. • Knowledge of proper anatomical positioning to aerobic and resistance training modalities • Understand how to use and interpret these tools; know how the measurements relate to exercise tolerance (*e.g.*, blood glucose readings that are too low or too high for exercise). • Warm-up, stretching, conditioning exercise, cool-down • Understanding medications' normal and abnormal effects on resting and exercise cardiovascular, pulmonary, and metabolic diseases	• Chapter 6 *ACSM's Guidelines for Exercise Testing and Prescription* (GETP), 10th edition (6) *ACSM's Guidelines for Exercise Testing and Prescription*, 10th edition (6) • Chapter 2 *ACSM's Guidelines for Exercise Testing and Prescription* (GETP), 10th edition (6) • Chapters 4, 5, and 11 *ACSM's Guidelines for Exercise Testing and Prescription* (GETP), 10th edition (6) • Chapter 6 *ACSM's Guidelines for Exercise Testing and Prescription* (GETP), 10th edition (6) • Appendix A *ACSM's Guidelines for Exercise Testing and Prescription* (GETP), 10th edition (6) • Chapters 9–11 *ACSM's Guidelines for Exercise Testing and Prescription* (GETP), 10th edition (6) • Chapter 6 *Essentials of Strength Training and Conditioning*, 3rd edition (12) • Chapters 13 and 14

A. Implement the program (*e.g.*, exercise prescription, education, counseling, and goals). (cont.)		
Knowledge or Skill Statement	**Explanation/Examples**	**Resources**
	• Knowledge and clinical understanding of various exercise monitoring tools/techniques with specific attention to individual patient safety parameters • Understanding of various resistance exercises and stretches: Understand proper technique, body alignment and posture, muscles/joints involved, and common mistakes. • Knowledge and understanding of various methods (*e.g.*, questionnaires, surveys, tests) to assess participants educational goals/needs • Establish rapport, show interest and empathy, listen actively, then provide information and advice.	
Skill in educating participants on the use and effects of medications **Skill** in the application of metabolic calculations **Skill** in communicating the exercise prescription and related exercise programming techniques **Skill** in observation of clients for problems associated with comprehension and performance of their exercise program **Skill** in muscular strength/endurance and flexibility training	• Provide patients with an understanding of how their medications work, what the benefits are, and the importance of medication compliance; speak to the patient in lay terms. • Knowledge of calculating ($\dot{V}O_2$)/ metabolic equivalent (MET) equations for walking, running, leg cycling, arm cranking, and stepping to design the exercise program based on the patient's ability (*e.g.*, MET level) • Describe/explain the exercise program so the patient will understand what they are doing and why. • Ask for patient feedback to ensure the patient understands what he or she is doing and how to do it; follow up with observation; reeducate when necessary. • Understanding of various resistance exercises and stretches: Practice proper technique, body alignment, and posture; be familiar with muscles/joints involved and common mistakes.	*ACSM's Guidelines for Exercise Testing and Prescription* (GETP), 10th edition (6) • Appendix A *ACSM's Metabolic Calculations Handbook* (3) *ACSM's Guidelines for Exercise Testing and Prescription* (GETP), 10th edition (6) • Chapter 6 *Essentials of Strength Training and Conditioning*, 3rd edition (12) • Chapters 13 and 14

CEP

B. Continually assess participant feedback, clinical signs and symptoms, and exercise tolerance, and provide feedback to the participant about their exercise, general program participation, and clinical progress.

Knowledge or Skill Statement	Explanation/Examples	Resources
Knowledge of cardiovascular, pulmonary, and metabolic pathologies; their clinical progression; diagnostic testing; and medical regimens/procedures to treat **Knowledge** of normal and abnormal exercise responses and signs and symptoms associated with different pathologies (*i.e.*, cardiovascular, pulmonary, metabolic) **Knowledge** of normal and abnormal 12-lead and telemetry electrocardiogram (ECG) interpretation **Knowledge** of normal and abnormal heart and lung sounds **Knowledge** of the components of a participant's medical history necessary to screen during program participation **Knowledge** of appropriate mode, volume, and intensity of exercise to produce desired outcomes for apparently healthy participants and those with cardiovascular, pulmonary, and metabolic diseases **Knowledge** of psychological issues associated with acute and chronic illness (*e.g.*, depression, social isolation, suicidal ideation) **Knowledge** of the timing of daily activities with exercise (*e.g.*, medications, meals, insulin/glucose monitoring) **Knowledge** of how medications or missed dose(s) of medications impact exercise and its progression **Knowledge** of methods to provide participant feedback relative to their exercise, general program participation, and clinical progress	• Understanding of how diagnostic testing and medical regimens/procedures can assess clinical progression of disease and/or effects of exercise • Knowledge of absolute and relative contraindications to exercise and abnormal responses/signs and symptoms for cardiovascular, pulmonary, and metabolic disease stated • Know the anatomical landmarks for ECG lead placement and skill to identify/minimize artifact, identify normal resting ECG and exercise ECG changes, and know/identify dangerous arrhythmias. • Understand the clinical descriptions and auscultation sounds for normal and abnormal heart and lung sounds. • Knowledge of and interpretation of established exercise screening tools (*e.g.*, Physical Activity Readiness Questionnaire [PAR-Q], American Heart Association [AHA]/American College of Sports Medicine [ACSM] Health/Fitness Facility Participation Screening Questionnaire) and individual medical history for program participation • Exercise program design specific to the individual (novice vs. advanced exerciser) and their goals; exercise program design to help manage chronic disease (hypertension, diabetes, dyslipidemia, obesity, asthma, chronic obstructive pulmonary disease [COPD], etc.) • Know how these conditions may affect exercise adherence and motivation; social support groups; referral to other health care professionals. • Optimal times to exercise in relation to eating and blood sugar (energy levels), medication peak times and their effects on exercise performance, insulin use/injection site recommendations, evening exercise, and hypoglycemia risk • Understand the dangers of missed doses of medication and the possible effects on exercise participation. • Make necessary adjustments to the patients exercise program based on feedback (*e.g.*, increase exercise variety) for optimal outcomes.	*Guidelines for Cardiac Rehabilitation and Secondary Prevention Programs*, 5th edition (7) • Chapter 9 *ACSM's Guidelines for Exercise Testing and Prescription* (GETP), 10th edition (6) • Chapter 2 *ACSM's Guidelines for Exercise Testing and Prescription* (GETP), 10th edition (6) • Chapter 2 *ACSM's Guidelines for Exercise Testing and Prescription* (GETP), 10th edition (6) • Chapters 6–11 *ACSM's Guidelines for Exercise Testing and Prescription* (GETP), 10th edition (6) • Chapter 10 • Appendix A

CEP

B. Continually assess participant feedback, clinical signs and symptoms, and exercise tolerance, and provide feedback to the participant about their exercise, general program participation, and clinical progress. (cont.)

Knowledge or Skill Statement	Explanation/Examples	Resources
Skill in auscultation methods for common cardiovascular and pulmonary abnormalities **Skill** in the assessment of normal and abnormal response to exercise **Skill** in adjusting the exercise program based on participant's signs and symptoms, feedback, and exercise response **Skill** in communicating exercise techniques, program goals, and clinical monitoring and progress **Skill** in applying and interpreting tools for clinical assessment (*e.g.,* telemetry, oximetry and glucometry, perceived rating scales)	• Evaluate arteries for adequate pulses and bruits, lungs for emphysema, the heart for heart failure, murmurs, etc. • Identify any of the nine major symptoms of cardiovascular, pulmonary, or metabolic disease; identify normal responses to exercise (*e.g.,* heart rate, blood pressure, respirations, peripheral fatigue). • Make necessary adjustments to the patients' exercise program based on feedback for optimal outcomes and safety (*e.g.,* reduce or increase exercise intensity or duration). • Educate the patients in lay terminology on proper exercise technique, setting realistic goals, and how you assess their progress. • Understand the practice and use of these tools for measurements related to exercise tolerance (*e.g.,* blood glucose readings that are too low or too high for exercise, exercise intensity based on rating of perceived exertion [RPE] scales).	*ACSM's Guidelines for Exercise Testing and Prescription* (GETP), 10th edition (6) • Chapter 2 *ACSM's Guidelines for Exercise Testing and Prescription* (GETP), 10th edition (6) • Chapters 9–11

C. Reassess and update the program (*e.g.*, exercise, education, and client goals) based on the participant's progress and feedback.

Knowledge or Skill Statement	Explanation/Examples	Resources
Knowledge of techniques to determine participant's medical history through available documentation **Knowledge** of normal physiologic responses to exercise **Knowledge** of abnormal responses/signs and symptoms to exercise associated with different pathologies (*e.g.*, cardiovascular, pulmonary, metabolic) **Knowledge** of participant's educational and behavioral goals and methods to obtain them **Knowledge** of counseling techniques focusing on participant goal attainment **Knowledge** of exercise progression/maintenance and supervision for apparently healthy participants and participants with cardiovascular, pulmonary, and/or metabolic diseases **Knowledge** of appropriate mode, volume, and intensity of exercise to produce desired outcomes for apparently healthy participants and those with cardiovascular, pulmonary, and metabolic diseases **Knowledge** of strategies to maximize exercise compliance (*e.g.*, overcoming barriers, values clarification, goals setting) **Knowledge** of risk factor reduction programs and alternative community resources (*e.g.*, dietary counseling/Weight Watchers, smoking cessation, physical therapy/back care) **Knowledge** of proper biomechanical technique for exercise (*e.g.*, gait, weightlifting form) **Knowledge** of clinical monitoring of the exercise program (*e.g.*, telemetry, oximetry and glucometry, adjusting exercise intensity) **Knowledge** of commonly used medication for cardiovascular, pulmonary, and metabolic diseases **Knowledge** of the application and instruction of muscle strength/endurance and flexibility modalities **Knowledge** of modification of the exercise prescription for clinical changes and attainment of participant's goals	• Self-guided, professionally guided screenings for physical activity • Know the normal responses to exercise (*e.g.*, heart rate, blood pressure, respirations, peripheral fatigue). • Knowledge of absolute and relative contraindications to exercise and abnormal responses/signs and symptoms for cardiovascular, pulmonary, and metabolic disease states • Active listening, ask open-ended questions, clarify and summarize their statements. • Establish rapport, show interest and empathy, listen actively, provide information and advice; help set specific, measurable, attainable, realistic, and time-bound (SMART) goals. • Appropriate rate of progression based on health status, exercise tolerance, and exercise goals; monitor for adverse effects once when exercises are progressed; know recommendations to enhance exercise adherence. • Exercise program design specific to the individual (novice vs. advanced exerciser) and their goals and desired physiological outcome; exercise program design to help manage chronic disease (hypertension, diabetes, dyslipidemia, obesity, asthma, chronic obstructive pulmonary disease [COPD], etc.) • Develop patient-centered strategies to overcome exercise barriers; develop SMART goals with the patient; consider what is most important to the patient. • Be familiar with various methods of improving cardiac, pulmonary, and metabolic health. • Knowledge of proper anatomical positioning to aerobic and resistance training modalities • Knowledge and clinical understanding of various exercise monitoring tools/techniques to establish exercise programming with attention to individual patient safety parameters	*ACSM's Guidelines for Exercise Testing and Prescription* (GETP), 10th edition (6) • Chapter 2 *ACSM's Guidelines for Exercise Testing and Prescription* (GETP), 10th edition (6) • Chapter 2 *ACSM's Guidelines for Exercise Testing and Prescription* (GETP), 10th edition (6) • Chapters 6–11 *ACSM's Guidelines for Exercise Testing and Prescription* (GETP), 10th edition (6) • Chapters 6 and 11 *ACSM's Guidelines for Exercise Testing and Prescription* (GETP), 10th edition (6) • Chapters 9–11 "Resistance Exercise Update in Individuals With and Without Cardiovascular Disease: 2007 Update: A Scientific Statement from the American Heart Association" (14) *ACSM's Guidelines for Exercise Testing and Prescription* (GETP), 10th edition (6) • Appendix A *ACSM's Guidelines for Exercise Testing and Prescription* (GETP), 10th edition (6) • Chapter 6 *Essentials of Strength Training and Conditioning*, 3rd edition (12) • Chapters 13 and 14

C. Reassess and update the program (*e.g.*, exercise, education, and client goals) based on the participant's progress and feedback. (cont.)		
Knowledge or Skill Statement	**Explanation/Examples**	**Resources**
Knowledge of community resources available to the participant following discharge from the program	• Understanding medications' normal and abnormal effects on resting and exercise cardiovascular, pulmonary, and metabolic diseases • For various resistance exercises and stretches: Understand proper technique, body alignment and posture, muscles/joints involved, and common mistakes. • Make necessary adjustments to the patients' exercise program based on feedback and exercise responses for optimal outcomes and safety (*e.g.*, reduce or increase exercise intensity or duration). • Help facilitate a smooth transition from rehabilitation to continuing health behavior changes (*e.g.*, joining a fitness club, social support groups).	
Skill in modifying the exercise program based on participant's signs and symptoms, feedback, and exercise responses **Skill** in using metabolic calculations and clinical data to adjust the exercise prescription **Skill** in observation of participant for problems associated with comprehension and performance of their exercise program **Skill** in communicating exercise techniques, program goals, and clinical monitoring and progress **Skill** in applying and interpreting tools for clinical assessment (*e.g.*, telemetry, oximetry and glucometry, perceived rating scales)	• Exercise program modifications based on the patient's exercise tolerance, their likes/dislikes with the program, and their adaptations/responses to the program • Practice adjusting exercise prescriptions to meet the physical abilities and desired energy expenditure (*e.g.*, current metabolic equivalent [MET] level) of the patient (*e.g.*, appropriate exercise mode, intensity level). • Practice talking with the patient/obtaining patient feedback to ensure they understand the program, know proper exercise technique and understand progression; educate the patient in a manner that they understand, the principles of exercise (*e.g.*, frequency, intensity, time, and type, volume and progression [FITT-VP]), proper exercise technique, and the goals of the exercise program, and practice monitoring applicable clinical data (*e.g.*, electrocardiogram [ECG], blood pressure). • Educate the patients in lay terminology on proper exercise technique, setting realistic goals, and how you assess their progress. • Understand the practice and use of these tools for measurements related to exercise tolerance (*e.g.*, blood glucose readings that are too low or too high for exercise, exercise intensity based on rating of perceived exertion [RPE] scales).	*ACSM's Guidelines for Exercise Testing and Prescription* (GETP), 10th edition (6) • Chapters 6 and 11 "Compendium of Physical Activities: An Update of Activity Codes and MET intensities" (1) *ACSM's Guidelines for Exercise Testing and Prescription* (GETP), 10th edition (6) • Chapters 9–11

D. Maintain participant records to document progress and clinical status.

Knowledge or Skill Statement	Explanation/Examples	Resources
Knowledge of participant's medical history through available documentation **Knowledge** of cardiovascular, pulmonary, and metabolic pathologies; diagnostic testing; and medical management regimens and procedures **Knowledge** of commonly used medication for cardiovascular, pulmonary, and metabolic diseases **Knowledge** of Health Insurance Portability and Accountability Act (HIPAA) regulations relative to documentation **Knowledge** of medical documentation (*e.g.*, progress notes, SOAP notes—subjective, objective, assessment, and plan)	• Self-guided, professionally guided screenings for physical activity • Understanding of how diagnostic testing and medical regimens/procedures can assess clinical status progression of disease • Understanding medication effects on resting and exercise vitals; cardiovascular, pulmonary, and metabolic diseases as well as side effects • Promotion of access for consumers to health insurance, privacy protection of health care data, standardize billing, and insurance claims processing in the health care industry • Know how to document all data collected during assessments, testing and training, and goal setting; SOAP notes.	*ACSM's Guidelines for Exercise Testing and Prescription* (GETP), 10th edition (6) • Chapter 2 *ACSM's Guidelines for Exercise Testing and Prescription* (GETP), 10th edition (6) • Appendix A *Drugs for the Heart*, 6th edition (13)
Skill in applying knowledge of medical documentation and regulations **Skill** in summarizing participants' exercise sessions, outcomes, and clinical issues into an appropriate medical record	• Contract law, informed consent, Tort law, negligence, malpractice, standards of practice (*e.g.*, practice peer-developed guidelines, report incidents, communicate critical information in a timely manner) • Practice documenting the details (mode, intensity, duration) of the exercises performed, any issues, abnormal responses, or significant findings during the session.	*Drugs for the Heart*, 6th edition (13)

DOMAIN IV: LEADERSHIP AND COUNSELING

A. Educate the participant about performance and progression of aerobic, strength, and flexibility exercise programs.

Knowledge or Skill Statement	Explanation/Examples	Resources
Knowledge of physiological responses and signs and symptoms to exercise associated with different pathologies (*i.e.*, cardiovascular, pulmonary, metabolic) **Knowledge** of exercise (as written previously) principles (prescription, progression/maintenance, and supervision) for apparently healthy participants and participants with cardiovascular, pulmonary, and/or metabolic diseases	• Help the patient understand abnormal responses/signs and symptoms for cardiovascular, pulmonary, and metabolic disease. • Explain the frequency, intensity, time, and type, volume and progression (FITT-VP) principle and the components of a single exercise session: warm-up, stretching, conditioning phase (or sports-related exercise), and cool-down; special exercise considerations for various clinical populations.	*ACSM's Guidelines for Exercise Testing and Prescription* (GETP), 10th edition (6) • Chapter 2 *ACSM's Guidelines for Exercise Testing and Prescription* (GETP), 10th edition (6) • Chapters 6–11 *ACSM's Guidelines for Exercise Testing and Prescription* (GETP), 10th edition (6) • Chapters 4, 5, and 11

CEP

A. Educate the participant about performance and progression of aerobic, strength, and flexibility exercise programs. (cont.)

Knowledge or Skill Statement	Explanation/Examples	Resources
Knowledge of exercise progression, maintenance, and supervision for apparently healthy participants and participants with cardiovascular, pulmonary, and/or metabolic diseases **Knowledge** of tools for measuring clinical exercise tolerance (*e.g.*, heart rate, glucometry, subjective rating scales) **Knowledge** of the application and instruction of muscle strength/endurance and flexibility modalities **Knowledge** of exercise modalities and the operation of associated equipment **Knowledge** of proper biomechanical techniques (*e.g.*, gait assessment, resistance training form) **Knowledge** of methods to educate participant in proper exercise programming and progression **Knowledge** of the timing of daily activities with exercise (*e.g.*, medications, meals, insulin/glucose monitoring) **Knowledge** of disease-specific strategies and tools to improve exercise tolerance (*e.g.*, breathing techniques, insulin pump use, prophylactic nitroglycerin) **Knowledge** of behavioral strategies for improving exercise adoption and maintenance **Knowledge** of barriers to exercise compliance and associated strategies (*e.g.*, physical, psychological, environmental)	• Knowledge and use of the FITT-VP principle and components for exercise progression of various patient population • Understand how to use and interpret these tools; know how the measurements relate to exercise tolerance (*e.g.*, blood glucose readings that are too low or too high for exercise). • Demonstrate numerous resistance training exercises and stretches, their proper applications, and common mistakes. • Demonstrate various exercise machines/modalities, proper setup, adjustments, proper technique, and common errors. • Explain proper anatomical positioning for aerobic and resistance training modalities. • Knowledge of techniques to educate patients on the benefits of exercise specific to the patient; discuss how the exercise program meet the needs of the patient; patient-centered approaches that consider the patient's priorities, risk factors and psychosocial status; use terminology that they will understand. • Optimal times to exercise with relation to eating and blood sugar (energy levels), medication peak times and their effects on exercise performance, insulin use/injection site recommendations, evening exercise, and hypoglycemia risk • Explain how disease-specific adjunct therapies and techniques can improve exercise tolerance (*e.g.*, breathing retraining, insulin pump use and adjustment, prophylactic nitroglycerin). • Knowledge and implementation of behavioral strategies (*e.g.*, counseling, education, scheduling) to improve adoption of exercise and maintenance • Knowledge of and skill in developing patient-centered strategies to overcome exercise barriers	*ACSM's Guidelines for Exercise Testing and Prescription* (GETP), 10th edition (6) • Chapters 9–11 *Essentials of Strength Training and Conditioning*, 3rd edition (12) • Chapters 13 and 14 *Essentials of Strength Training and Conditioning*, 3rd edition (12) • Chapter 14 *ACSM's Guidelines for Exercise Testing and Prescription* (GETP), 10th edition (6) • Chapter 10 • Appendix A *Pollock's Textbook of Cardiovascular Disease and Rehabilitation* (9)

CEP

A. Educate the participant about performance and progression of aerobic, strength, and flexibility exercise programs. (cont.)

Knowledge or Skill Statement	Explanation/Examples	Resources
Skill in communication of exercise techniques, prescription, and progression **Skill** in the assessment of participant symptoms, biomechanics, and exercise effort	• Describe/explain the exercise program so the patient will understand what they are doing and why (*e.g.*, proper technique, FITT-VP principle, how and when to progress); use a terminology that the patient will understand. • Practice in recognizing adverse symptoms from exercise, proper movement and gait patterns, and subjective/objective exercise monitoring (*e.g.*, rating of perceived exertion [RPE], heart rate).	*ACSM's Guidelines for Exercise Testing and Prescription* (GETP), 10th edition (6) • Chapter 4

B. Provide disease management and risk factor reduction education based on the participant's medical history, needs, and goals.

Knowledge or Skill Statement	Explanation/Examples	Resources
Knowledge of education program development based on participant's medical history, needs, and goals **Knowledge** of methods to educate participant in risk factor reduction **Knowledge** of published national standards on risk factors for cardiovascular, pulmonary, and metabolic disease **Knowledge** of risk factor reduction programs and alternative community resources (*e.g.*, dietary counseling/Weight Watchers, smoking cessation, physical therapy/back care) **Knowledge** of strategies to improve participant compliance to risk factor reduction **Knowledge** of goal development strategies **Knowledge** of counseling techniques **Knowledge** of validated tools for measurement of psychosocial health status (*e.g.*, SF-36, strait-trait anxiety, Beck depression) **Knowledge** of psychological issues associated with acute and chronic illness (*e.g.*, anxiety, depression, social isolation, suicidal ideation)	• Patient-centered approach to counseling and educating patients; establish rapport, listen actively, show interest, recognize their stage of readiness to change, provide education that is applicable and timely for the patient. • Knowledge and implementation of various methods of patient education (*e.g.*, videos, handouts, consultations) methods to assess and educate participant on risk factor reduction • Knowledge and attainment of national standards of risk factor reduction for cardiovascular, pulmonary, and metabolic diseases; their target populations; strategies for their use; and how results may effect program participation • Be familiar with various methods of improving cardiac, pulmonary, and metabolic health. • Skill and knowledge to recognize possible "high-risk" situations that may cause a relapse in healthy behavior change (*e.g.*, vacations, bad weather); suggest alternatives, refer to other health care professional when appropriate	*ACSM's Guidelines for Exercise Testing and Prescription* (GETP), 10th edition (6) • Chapters 3 and 11

CEP

B. Provide disease management and risk factor reduction education based on the participant's medical history, needs, and goals. (cont.)		
Knowledge or Skill Statement	**Explanation/Examples**	**Resources**
Knowledge of outcome evaluation methods (*e.g.*, American Association of Cardiovascular and Pulmonary Rehabilitation [AACVPR] outcomes model)	• Set goals that are specific, measurable, and challenging but realistic (*e.g.*, specific, measurable, attainable, realistic, and time-bound [SMART] goals). • Understand the key components of counseling for health behavior: listen actively, show empathy, ask open-ended questions, establish rapport, know stages of change, etc. • Knowledge of health-related quality of life, their target populations, strategies for their use, and how results may affect program participation • Understanding of how these conditions may affect exercise adherence and motivation; social support groups; and referral to other health care professionals • Understand the core components of rehabilitation and assessment/outcomes for each component.	
Skill in communicating with participants from a wide variety of backgrounds **Skill** in selection of participant outcome parameters	• Understanding how to communicate in a way that the patient will understand and will not be intimidated • Knowledge and understanding the selection of appropriate participant outcome parameters. Select outcomes that are relevant to the patient and measurable (*e.g.*, achieve a resting blood pressure of <120/80 mm Hg).	

C. Create a positive environment for participant adherence and outcomes by incorporating effective motivational skills, communication techniques, and behavioral strategies.		
Knowledge or Skill Statement	**Explanation/Examples**	**Resources**
Knowledge of current behavior facilitation theories (*e.g.*, health belief model, transtheoretical model) **Knowledge** of behavioral strategies and coaching methods for improving exercise adoption and maintenance **Knowledge** of communication strategies that foster a positive environment	• Understand stages of change, processes of change, motivational readiness for change. • Knowledge and skill in choosing appropriate behavioral strategies (*e.g.*, patient education on the benefits of exercise specific to the patient; developing exercise programs that meet the needs of the patient; patient-centered approaches that consider the patient's priorities, risk factors, and psychosocial status)	*Behavior Modification: What It Is and How To Do It,* 9th edition (11) • xvii, p. 462

C. Create a positive environment for participant adherence and outcomes by incorporating effective motivational skills, communication techniques, and behavioral strategies. (cont.)

Knowledge or Skill Statement	Explanation/Examples	Resources
Knowledge of methods to educate participant in motivational skills and behavioral strategies **Knowledge** of barriers to exercise compliance (*e.g.*, physical, psychological, environmental) **Knowledge** of community resources available for participant use following discharge from the program	• Knowledge and use of communication strategies that provide the patient with social support, rewards/incentives; find activities or an environment that will be enjoyable for the patient (*e.g.*, exercise in groups) • Knowledge of educational methods for participant motivation and implementation of behavioral strategies (*e.g.*, counseling, education, scheduling) • Identify potential barriers to consistent exercise and apply strategies to overcome them; develop patient-centered strategies to overcome exercise barriers. • Help facilitate a smooth transition from rehabilitation to continuing health behavior changes (*e.g.*, joining a fitness club, social support groups).	

D. Collaborate and consult with health care professionals to address clinical issues and provide referrals to optimize participant outcomes.

Knowledge or Skill Statement	Explanation/Examples	Resources
Knowledge of cardiovascular, pulmonary, and metabolic pathologies; clinical progression; diagnostic testing; medical regimens; and treatment procedures **Knowledge** of techniques to determine participant's medical history through available documentation **Knowledge** of commonly used medication for cardiovascular, pulmonary, and metabolic diseases **Knowledge** of tools for measuring clinical exercise tolerance (*e.g.*, heart rate, glucometry, subjective rating scales) **Knowledge** of risk factor reduction programs and alternative community resources (*e.g.*, dietary counseling/Weight Watchers, smoking cessation, physical therapy/back care) **Knowledge** of psychological issues associated with acute and chronic illness (*e.g.*, anxiety, depression, suicidal ideation)	• Understand how exercise affects cardiovascular, pulmonary, and metabolic pathologies. Understand how diagnostic testing and medical regimens/procedures can assess clinical progression of disease and/or exercise effects. • Self-guided, professionally guided screenings for physical activity • Understanding medication effects on resting and exercise vitals; cardiovascular, pulmonary, and metabolic diseases as well as side effects • Understand how to use and interpret these tools; know how the measurements relate to exercise tolerance (*e.g.*, blood glucose readings that are too low or too high for exercise). • Be familiar with various methods of improving cardiac, pulmonary, and metabolic health.	*ACSM's Guidelines for Exercise Testing and Prescription* (GETP), 10th edition (6) • Chapter 2 *ACSM's Guidelines for Exercise Testing and Prescription* (GETP), 10th edition (6) • Appendix A *ACSM's Guidelines for Exercise Testing and Prescription* (GETP), 10th edition (6) • Chapter 12

D. Collaborate and consult with health care professionals to address clinical issues and provide referrals to optimize participant outcomes. (cont.)		
Knowledge or Skill Statement	**Explanation/Examples**	**Resources**
Knowledge of assessment tools to measure psychosocial health status **Knowledge** of accepted methods of referral **Knowledge** of community resources available for participant use following program discharge	• How these conditions may affect exercise adherence and motivation; social support groups; referral to other health care professionals • Five-factor model of personality, transtheoretical model, *Diagnostic and Statistical Manual of Mental Disorders (DSM)*, classes of mood disorders, subtypes of anxiety disorders • Recognize signs and symptoms of various issues (*e.g.*, eating disorders, mental health states) that may require referral to another health care professional; know who to refer to and suggest appropriate professional; understand the appropriate protocol for referral including documentation and staff involved. • Help facilitate a smooth transition from rehabilitation to continuing health behavior changes (*e.g.*, joining a fitness club, social support groups).	
Skill in collaborative decision making **Skill** in interpretation of psychosocial assessment tools	• Practice making decisions with the patient; decision-making theory, decisional balance. • Practice determining and understanding a patient's psychosocial status based on the results of assessments tools (*e.g.*, *Diagnostic and Statistical Manual of Mental Disorders IV [DSM-IV]*); make appropriate referral when necessary.	

DOMAIN V: LEGAL AND PROFESSIONAL CONSIDERATIONS

A. Evaluate the exercise environment to minimize risk and optimize safety by following routine inspection procedures based on established facility and industry standards and guidelines.		
Knowledge or Skill Statement	**Explanation/Examples**	**Resources**
Knowledge of government and industry standards and guidelines (*e.g.*, American Association of Cardiovascular and Pulmonary Rehabilitation [AACVPR], Health Insurance Portability and Accountability Act [HIPAA], Occupational Health and Safety Administration [OHSA]) **Knowledge** of the operation, calibration, and maintenance of exercise equipment	• Make sure you and your facility are following proper protocols, minimizing risk, and maximizing safety. • Understand how to maintain the equipment, be able to recognize problems with the equipment (*e.g.*, a treadmill that needs to be calibrated), and know to fix the problem or contact the appropriate personnel.	*ACSM's Guidelines for Exercise Testing and Prescription* (GETP), 10th edition (6) • Appendix B

CEP

B. Perform regular inspections of emergency equipment and practice emergency procedures (*e.g.*, crash cart, advanced cardiac life support procedures, activation of emergency medical system).

Knowledge or Skill Statement	Explanation/Examples	Resources
Knowledge of standards of practice during emergency situations (*e.g.*, American Heart Association [AHA]) **Knowledge** of local and institutional procedures for activation of the emergency medical system **Knowledge** of standards for inspection of emergency medical equipment	• Cardiopulmonary resuscitation (CPR), automated external defibrillator (AED), advanced cardiac life support (ACLS), activating emergency medical service (EMS), assisting the code team, basic first aid, proper documentation • Knowledge of institutional policy and procedures for activation of emergency response (*i.e.*, Code Team, EMS, etc.) • Knowledge of and skill to be able to perform periodic reviews of the emergency equipment to ensure it is operational	*ACSM's Guidelines for Exercise Testing and Prescription* (GETP), 10th edition (6) • Appendix B
Skill in the application of basic life support procedures and external defibrillator use	• Obtain and maintain CPR/AED certification; participate in announced and unannounced emergency drills.	*ACSM's Guidelines for Exercise Testing and Prescription* (GETP), 10th edition (6) • Appendix B

C. Promote awareness and accountability and minimize risk by informing participants of safety procedures, self-monitoring of exercise, and related symptoms.

Knowledge or Skill Statement	Explanation/Examples	Resources
Knowledge of signs and symptoms of exercise intolerance **Knowledge** of the timing of daily activities with exercise (*e.g.*, medications, meals, insulin/glucose monitoring) **Knowledge** of commonly used medications for cardiovascular, pulmonary, and metabolic diseases **Knowledge** of communication techniques to ensure safety in participant's self-monitoring and symptom management **Knowledge** of contraindicated and higher risk exercises and proper exercise form to minimize risk	• Knowledge of absolute and relative contraindications to exercise and abnormal responses/signs and symptoms for cardiovascular, pulmonary, and metabolic disease states • Optimal times to exercise with relation to eating and blood sugar (energy levels), medication peak times and their effects on exercise performance, insulin use/injection site recommendations, evening exercise, and hypoglycemia risk. • Understanding medication effects on resting and exercise vitals; cardiovascular, pulmonary, and metabolic diseases as well as side effects • Educate patients in a way that they understand you (*e.g.*, lay terminology); ask for feedback to confirm that they understand how to self-monitor themselves. • Know common exercise errors and how to correct them; identify high risk exercises and offer alternative, safer ones.	*ACSM's Guidelines for Exercise Testing and Prescription* (GETP), 10th edition (6) • Chapter 5 *ACSM's Guidelines for Exercise Testing and Prescription* (GETP), 10th edition (6) • Chapter 11 • Appendix A *ACSM's Guidelines for Exercise Testing and Prescription* (GETP), 10th edition (6) • Chapter 11 • Appendix A *Essentials of Strength Training and Conditioning*, 3rd edition (12) • Chapter 14

C.	Promote awareness and accountability and minimize risk by informing participants of safety procedures, self-monitoring of exercise, and related symptoms. (cont.)	

Knowledge or Skill Statement	Explanation/Examples	Resources
Skill in the instruction and modification of exercises to minimize risk of injury	• Educate participant in proper exercise technique, body alignment, and overall form for safe and effective exercise training; demonstrate alternative exercises when needed for safe participation.	*Essentials of Strength Training and Conditioning*, 3rd edition (12) • Chapters 13 and 14

D.	Comply with Health Insurance Portability and Accountability Act (HIPAA) laws and industry-accepted professional, ethical, and business standards in order to maintain confidentiality, optimize safety, and reduce liability.	

Knowledge or Skill Statement	Explanation/Examples	Resources
Knowledge of HIPAA regulations relative to documentation and protecting patient privacy (*e.g.*, written and electronic medical records) **Knowledge** of the use and limitations of informed consent **Knowledge** of advanced directives and implications for rehabilitation programs **Knowledge** of professional responsibilities and their implications related to liability and negligence	• Educate and knowledge of institutional and federal regulations regarding HIPAA and protecting patient privacy. • Conveys an understanding of the tests/exercises, risks, option to choose to participate • Living will, personal directive • Follow peer-reviewed guidelines, maintain professional credentials, understand your scope of practice, instruct patients, document your services, report incidents, and maintain equipment.	

E.	Promote a positive image of the program by engaging in healthy lifestyle practices.	

Knowledge or Skill Statement	Explanation/Examples	Resources
Knowledge of common sources of health information, education, and promotion techniques	• Be familiar with various, credible sources of information and professional organizations that will educate patients on health and well-being (*e.g.*, American Heart Association [AHA]).	
Skill in the practice and demonstration of a healthy lifestyle	• Practice what you "preach"; exercise and be active regularly; eat a healthy diet; set a good example.	

CEP

F.	Select and participate in continuing education programs that enhance knowledge and skills on a continuing basis, maximize effectiveness, and increase professionalism in the field.	
Knowledge or Skill Statement	**Explanation/Examples**	**Resources**
Knowledge of continuing education opportunities as required for maintenance of professional credentials **Knowledge** of total quality management (TQM) and continuous quality improvement (CQI) concepts and application to personal professional growth	• Know what is required (*e.g.*, how many Continuing Education Credits [CECs]) to maintain professional certification(s); focus on areas for professional growth/areas of current practice. • Continuously improve the quality of your knowledge and skills through continuing education.	ACSM's Web site (5) • Especially see "Certification" section *ACSM's Guidelines for Exercise Testing and Prescription* (GETP), 10th edition (6) • Appendix D

REFERENCES

ACSM REFERENCES:

1. Ainsworth BE, Haskell WL, Whitt MC, et al. Compendium of physical activities: an update of activity codes and MET intensities. *Med Sci Sports Exerc*. 2000;32:S498–S504.
2. American College of Sports Medicine. *ACSM's Exercise Management for Persons with Chronic Diseases and Disabilities*. 4th ed. Champaign (IL): Human Kinetics; 2016. 416 p.
3. American College of Sports Medicine. *ACSM's Metabolic Calculations Handbook*. Baltimore (MD): Lippincott Williams & Wilkins; 2006. 111 p.
4. American College of Sports Medicine. Position stand: exercise and hypertension. *Med Sci Sports Exerc*. 2004;36:533–553.
5. American College of Sports and Medicine Web site [Internet]. Indianapolis (IN): American College of Sports Medicine; [cited 2017 April]. Available from: http://www.acsm.org
6. Riebe D, senior editor. *ACSM's Guidelines for Exercise Testing and Prescription*. 10th ed. Philadelphia (PA): Wolters Kluwer; 2018.

NON-ACSM REFERENCES:

7. American Association of Cardiovascular and Pulmonary Rehabilitation. *Guidelines for Cardiac Rehabilitation and Secondary Prevention Programs*. 5th ed. Champaign (IL): Human Kinetics; 2013. 336 p.
8. American College of Chest Physicians/American Association of Cardiovascular and Pulmonary Rehabilitation Guidelines Panel. Pulmonary rehabilitation: joint ACCP/AACVPR evidence-based guidelines. *Chest*. 1997;112:1363–96.
9. Durstine JL, Moore GE, LaMonte MJ, Franklin BA, eds. *Pollock's Textbook of Cardiovascular Disease and Rehabilitation*. Champaign (IL): Human Kinetics; 2008. 411 p.
10. Fletcher GF, Balady GJ, Amsterdam EA, et al. Exercise standards for testing and training: a statement for healthcare professionals from the American Heart Association. *Circulation*. 2001;104(14): 1694–740.
11. Martin G, Pear J. *Behavior Modification: What It Is and How To Do It*. 9th ed. Boston (MA): Pearson Education/Allyn & Bacon; 2011. xvii, 462 p.
12. National Strength and Conditioning Association. *Essentials of Strength Training and Conditioning*. 3rd ed. Champaign (IL): Human Kinetics; 2008.
13. Opie LH. *Drugs for the Heart*. 6th ed. Philadelphia (PA): Saunders; 2004. 437 p.
14. Williams MA, Haskell WL, Ades PA, et al. Resistance exercise update in individuals with and without cardiovascular disease: 2007 update: a scientific statement from the American Heart Association. *Circulation*. 2007;116: 572–84.

Note: CEP certification candidates may also review the practice examinations found in Part 1, ACSM Certified Personal Trainer (CPT) and Part 2, ACSM Certified Exercise Physiologist (EP-C).

DIRECTIONS: Each of the numbered items or incomplete statements in this section is followed by answers or by completions of the statement. Select the ONE lettered answer or completion that is BEST in each case.

1. During a medical emergency, which of the following medications is an endogenous catecholamine that can be used to increase blood flow to the heart and brain?
   A) Lidocaine
   B) Oxygen
   C) Atropine
   D) Epinephrine

2. If a healthy young man who weighs 80 kg exercises at an intensity of 45 mL $\cdot$ kg^{-1} $\cdot$ min^{-1} for 30 min, five times per week, how long (assuming an isocaloric diet) would it take him to lose 10 lb?
   A) 9 wk
   B) 11 wk
   C) 13 wk
   D) 15 wk

3. Which of the following techniques can be used to diagnose coronary artery disease and assess heart wall motion abnormalities, ejection fraction, and cardiac output?
   A) Electrocardiography
   B) Radionuclide imaging
   C) Echocardiography
   D) Cardiac spirometry

4. Which of the following would be an adequate initial exercise prescription for a patient who has had a heart transplant?
   A) High intensity, short duration, small muscle groups, and high frequency
   B) High intensity, long duration, small muscle groups, and high frequency
   C) Moderate intensity, 6 d $\cdot$ wk^{-1}, large muscle groups, and moderate duration
   D) Low intensity, 3 d $\cdot$ wk^{-1}, large muscle groups, and moderate duration

5. Individuals with diabetes should follow exercise guidelines to avoid unnecessary risks. The following list of recommendations should include all of the following *except* _____.
   A) Avoiding injection of insulin into an exercising muscle
   B) Exercising with a partner
   C) Exercising only when temperature and humidity are moderate
   D) Avoiding exercise during peak insulin activity

6. Which of the following is a reversible pulmonary condition caused by some type of irritant (*e.g.*, dust, pollen) and characterized by bronchial airway narrowing, dyspnea, coughing, and, possibly, hypoxia and hypercapnia?
   A) Emphysema
   B) Bronchitis
   C) Asthma
   D) Pulmonary vascular disease

7. A supraventricular ectopic rhythm that results from a focus of automaticity located in the bundle of His is an example of _____.
   A) Ventricular arrhythmia
   B) Junctional arrhythmia
   C) Atrioventricular (AV) block
   D) Premature ventricular contraction

8. Which of the following statements regarding contraindications to graded exercise testing is accurate?
   A) Some individuals have risk factors that outweigh the potential benefits from exercise testing and the information that may be obtained.
   B) Absolute contraindications refer to individuals for whom exercise testing should not be performed until the situation or condition has stabilized.
   C) Relative contraindications include patients who might be tested if the potential benefit from exercise testing outweighs the relative risk.
   D) All of the above statements are true.

9. Cardiac impulses originating in the sinoatrial node and then spreading to both atria, causing atrial depolarization, are represented on the electrocardiogram (ECG) as a _____.
   A) P wave
   B) QRS complex
   C) ST segment
   D) T wave

10. For previously sedentary individuals, a 20%–30% reduction in all-cause mortality can be obtained from physical activity (PA) with a daily energy expenditure of _____.
    A) 50–80 kcal $\cdot$ d^{-1}
    B) 80–100 kcal $\cdot$ d^{-1}
    C) 150–200 kcal $\cdot$ d^{-1}
    D) >400 kcal $\cdot$ d^{-1}

11. Exercise has been shown to reduce mortality in people with coronary artery disease. Which of the following mechanisms is *not* responsible?
    A) The effect of exercise on other risk factors
    B) Reduced myocardial oxygen demand at rest and at submaximal workloads
    C) Reduced platelet aggregation
    D) Decreased endothelial-mediated vasomotor tone

12. Which behavioral change model is often used in cardiac rehabilitation and diabetes management programs because it suggests that individuals who perceive they are susceptible to serious disease are more likely to engage in behaviors to prevent the health problem from occurring?
    A) Motivational interviewing
    B) Social cognitive theory
    C) Disease observation model
    D) Health Belief Model

13. Which of the following treatment strategies is most commonly used in patients with multiple vessel disease that is not responding to other treatments?
    A) Percutaneous transluminal coronary angioplasty (PTCA)
    B) Coronary artery stent
    C) Coronary artery bypass graft (CABG) surgery
    D) Pharmacologic therapy

14. Which of the following statements *best* describes the exercise precautions for patients with an automatic implantable cardioverter defibrillator (AICD)?
    A) Persons with AICD must be monitored closely during exercise, keeping the heart rate (HR) 10 beats or more below the activation rate for a shock.
    B) Persons with AICD are not at risk for an inappropriate shock because most AICDs are set to an HR of 300 bpm.
    C) Persons with AICD can inactivate the AICD before high-intensity exercise to avoid the risk of shock.
    D) Persons with AICD can exercise at or above the cutoff HR but only if monitored by instantaneous ECG telemetry.

15. Healthy, untrained individuals have an anaerobic threshold at approximately what percentage of their maximal volume of oxygen consumed per unit of time ($\dot{V}O_{2max}$)?
    A) 25%
    B) 55%
    C) 75%
    D) 95%

16. Which of the following medications reduces myocardial ischemia by lowering myocardial oxygen demand, is used to treat typical and variant angina, but has *not* been shown to reduce post-myocardial infarction (MI) mortality?
    A) β-Adrenergic blockers
    B) Niacin
    C) Aspirin
    D) Nitrates

17. A 35-yr-old female client asks the exercise physiologist to estimate her energy expenditure. She weighs 110 lb and pedals the cycle ergometer at 50 rpm with a resistance of 2.5 kp for 60 min. The physiologist should report which of the following caloric values?
    A) 250 cal
    B) 510 cal
    C) 770 cal
    D) 1,700 cal

18. The cardiac rehabilitation's medical director orders a prerehabilitation ECG on a 50-yr-old man. The exercise physiologist performing the ECG notes the machine error message reads artifact in the precordial lead V_4. To correct the artifact, an exercise physiologist would check which of the following lead positions for adhesive contact?
    A) Fourth intercostal space, left sternal border
    B) Fourth intercostal space, right sternal border
    C) Midaxillary line, fifth intercostal space
    D) Midclavicular line, fifth intercostal space

19. Which of the following cardiac indices increases curvilinearly with the work rate until it reaches near maximum at a level equivalent to approximately 50% of aerobic capacity, increasing only slightly thereafter?
    A) Stroke volume
    B) HR
    C) Cardiac output
    D) Systolic blood pressure (BP)

20. A 55-yr-old cardiac rehabilitation patient returned from vacation with the following complaints: elevation in BP, slight chest pain, shortness of breath with chest wheezing, and dryness and burning of the mouth and throat. Based on this information, the exercise physiologist would suspect that the patient was exposed to which of the following environments?
    A) Extreme cold
    B) Extreme heat
    C) High altitude
    D) High humidity

21. Which of the following is an absolute indication to terminate a symptom-limited maximal exercise test?
    A) Achievement of ≥85% of the age-predicted maximal heart rate (HR_{max})
    B) Signs of poor perfusion (cyanosis or pallor)
    C) Systolic BP ≥250 mm Hg
    D) Development of bundle-branch block

22. An individual's maximal exercise test is terminated secondary to symptoms of myocardial ischemia. Which of the following variables monitored during the test would be the most reliable estimate of ischemic threshold when prescribing exercise for this individual?
    A) Rating of perceived exertion (RPE)
    B) HR_{max}
    C) Rate-pressure product (RPP)
    D) Maximal metabolic equivalent (MET) level achieved

23. An exercise physiologist monitoring the ECG of a cardiac rehabilitation patient observes QT-interval shortening and ST-segment scooping during exercise. Based on this observation, the physiologist can suspect that the patient is treated with which of the following medications?
    A) β-Blockers
    B) Calcium channel blockers
    C) Potassium
    D) Digitalis

24. The exercise physiologist is orienting a 60-yr-old patient entering cardiac rehabilitation after having CABG 3 wk ago. All of the following statements are correct except _____.
    A) The patient should avoid upper body resistance training because of sternal and leg wounds for 4–6 mo.
    B) The clinician should observe for infection or discomfort along the incision.
    C) The patient should be monitored for chest pain, dizziness, and dysrhythmias.
    D) The patient should avoid high-intensity exercise early in the rehabilitation period.

25. Which of the following tests would give the best confirmation of diabetes?
    A) Fasting blood glucose test
    B) Oral glucose tolerance test
    C) Glycolated hemoglobin (HbA1C)
    D) Total blood count

26. Moderate aerobic exercise is recommended for most adults when prescribing exercise. What is considered to be moderate intensity in regard to aerobic training?
    A) 40%–59% heart rate reserve (HRR)/$\dot{V}O_{2max}$
    B) 39%–60% HRR/$\dot{V}O_{2max}$
    C) 45%–75% HRR/$\dot{V}O_{2max}$
    D) 55%–80% HRR/$\dot{V}O_{2max}$

27. During which times should the most caution be taken when beginning an exercise program with an individual with diabetes?
    A) Early morning and late evening
    B) Late morning
    C) Afternoon
    D) Evening

28. While monitoring the ECG of a cardiac rehabilitation patient, a progressive lengthening of the PR interval until a dropped QRS complex is observed. Based on this observation, what kind of AV block are you observing?
    A) First degree
    B) Mobitz type I
    C) Mobitz type II
    D) Third degree

29. You are asked to review an ECG strip for evidence of myocardial ischemia and/or injury. On what areas of the ECG should you focus?
    A) Q wave
    B) PR interval
    C) ST segment
    D) T wave

30. Which of the following cold-weather activities has been shown to increase HR up to 97% HR_{max} and systolic BP up to 200 mm Hg, resulting in a potentially dangerous increase in risk of morbidity and mortality for individuals with cardiovascular disease (CVD)?
    A) Ice skating
    B) Shoveling snow
    C) Building snowman
    D) Walking on ice

31. In an ECG recording, the presence of certain combinations of ST-segment abnormalities (i.e., elevation and/or depression) and significant Q waves may be suggestive of what condition?
    A) Acute MI
    B) Left ventricular hypertrophy
    C) Right bundle-branch block
    D) Ventricular aneurysm

32. What is the relative oxygen consumption rate for walking on a treadmill at 3.5 mph with a 10% grade?
    A) $18.17 \text{ mL} \cdot \text{kg}^{-1} \cdot \text{min}^{-1}$
    B) $27.96 \text{ mL} \cdot \text{kg}^{-1} \cdot \text{min}^{-1}$
    C) $29.76 \text{ mL} \cdot \text{kg}^{-1} \cdot \text{min}^{-1}$
    D) $31.28 \text{ mL} \cdot \text{kg}^{-1} \cdot \text{min}^{-1}$

33. All of the following statements regarding the clinical exercise physiologist administering clinical exercise tests are true *except* _____.
    A) The clinical exercise physiologist will review and interpret the results of the test and report them to the supervising physician.
    B) The clinical exercise physiologist must have the knowledge to recognize and treat complications of exercise testing.
    C) The clinical exercise physiologist must have knowledge of cardiac arrhythmias and the ability to recognize and treat serious arrhythmias.
    D) The clinical exercise physiologist may administer clinical exercise tests without the personal supervision of a physician, but a qualified physician must be in the immediate vicinity and available for all emergencies.

34. Why is it important to choose the appropriate BP cuff size?
    A) A cuff too small will give a lower reading for both the systolic and diastolic pressures.
    B) If cuff size encircles <80% of the upper arm, measurement will be inaccurate.
    C) When deflating the cuff, you will not be able to maintain a deflation rate of 2–3 mm Hg $\cdot$ s^{-1}.
    D) Both B and C

35. What percentage of the peak work rate from the incremental exercise test should be used to evaluate the intensities an individual with chronic obstructive pulmonary disease (COPD) is likely to experience during everyday life?
    A) 75%–90%
    B) 80%–90%
    C) 75%–85%
    D) 70%–90%

36. Which of the following is most likely to represent nonischemic or atypical chest pain?
    A) Pain in one or both arms or shoulders
    B) Pain provoked by cold weather or excitement
    C) Pain that is substernal across the mid thorax area
    D) Pain in the left submammary or hemithorax area

37. According to *ACSM's Guidelines for Exercise Testing and Prescription*, 10th ed., moderate intensity exercise is defined as _____.
    A) 30%–<40% HRR or oxygen consumption reserve ($\dot{V}O_2R$), 2–<3 METs, RPE 9–11, an intensity that causes slight increases in HR and breathing
    B) ≥60% HRR or $\dot{V}O_2R$, ≥6 METs, RPE ≥14, an intensity that causes substantial increases in HR and breathing
    C) 40%–<60% HRR or $\dot{V}O_2R$, 3–<6 METs, RPE 12–13, an intensity that causes noticeable increases in HR and breathing
    D) 35%–<50% HRR or $\dot{V}O_2R$, 2–<4 METs, RPE 10–12, an intensity that causes moderate increases in HR and breathing

38. Which of the following is the proper emergency response for a patient who has experienced a cardiac arrest but now is breathing and has a palpable pulse?
    A) Continue the exercise test to determine why the patient had this response.
    B) Place the patient in the recovery position with the head to the side to prevent airway obstruction.
    C) Place the patient in a comfortable seated position.
    D) Start phase I cardiac rehabilitation.

39. A patient weighing 200 lb sets the treadmill at 4.0 mph with a 5% grade. At peak exercise, his BP is 150/90 mm Hg, HR is 150 bpm, and respiratory quotient is 1.0. What is his estimated absolute energy expenditure?
    A) 1.07 L $\cdot$ min^{-1}
    B) 2.17 L $\cdot$ min^{-1}
    C) 4.28 L $\cdot$ min^{-1}
    D) 8.56 L $\cdot$ min^{-1}

40. Which of the following procedures provides the *least* sensitivity and specificity in the diagnosis of coronary artery disease?
    A) Coronary angiography
    B) Echocardiography
    C) Electrocardiography
    D) Radionuclide imaging

41. What does flow-resistive training (a type of breathing retraining) teach patients with pulmonary disease?
    A) To effectively breathe through a progressively smaller airway
    B) Coordinate breathing with activities of daily living
    C) Increase respiratory muscle endurance and strength
    D) Increase ventilatory threshold

42. Patients enrolled in an outpatient cardiac rehabilitation program can begin upper body resistance training at ≥5–10 lb (or <50% of maximal voluntary contraction [MVC]) approximately how soon after their coronary artery bypass surgery?
    A) 4–6 wk
    B) 6–8 wk
    C) 10–12 wk
    D) Only after they have been cleared by their surgeon

43. In patients with a new implantable cardioverter defibrillator (ICD), mild upper body extremity range of motion (ROM) activities can be initiated how soon after device implantation?
    A) After the first 72 h
    B) After the first 24 h
    C) Within the first 24 h
    D) As soon as the patent's pain tolerance permits

44. Which of the following is the thickest, middle layer of the artery wall that is composed predominantly of smooth muscle cells and is responsible for vasoconstriction and vasodilation?
    A) Endothelium
    B) Intima
    C) Media
    D) Adventitia

45. Data obtained from a clinical exercise test can be useful for all of the following *except* _____.
    A) Determining a return to work date prior to a patient undergoing CABG surgery
    B) Predicting prognosis in patients with known heart disease
    C) Developing an exercise prescription for a patient in cardiac rehabilitation
    D) Evaluating preoperative risk

46. What is the total energy expenditure for a 70-kg man doing an exercise session composed of 5 min of warm-up at 2.0 METs, 20 min of treadmill running at 9 METs, 20 min of leg cycling at 8 METs, and 5 min of cool-down at 2.5 METs?
    A) 162 kcal
    B) 868 kcal
    C) 444 kcal
    D) 1,256 kcal

47. Both the American College of Sports Medicine (ACSM)/American Heart Association (AHA) Primary Physical Activity Recommendation and the Primary Physical Activity Recommendations from the *2008 Physical Activity Guidelines Committee Report* suggest that healthy adults should participate in which of the following exercise prescriptions for aerobic activity?
    A) 20 min · d^{-1}, five times a week or 75 min · wk^{-1} of low intensity PA
    B) 30 min · d^{-1}, five times a week or 150 min · wk^{-1} of moderate intensity exercise
    C) 20 min · d^{-1}, three times a week or 75 min · wk^{-1} of moderate intensity exercise
    D) 30 min · d^{-1}, five times a week or 150 min · wk^{-1} of vigorous intensity exercise

48. Which of the following statements regarding an emergency plan is *true*?
    A) The emergency plan does not need to be written down as long as everyone understands it.
    B) As long as everyone knows his or her individual responsibilities during an emergency, a list of each staff member's responsibilities is not needed.
    C) All emergency situations must be documented with dates, times, actions, people involved, and outcomes.
    D) There is no need to practice emergencies as long as the staff members fully understand their responsibilities.

49. Orthopnea is _____.
    A) Dyspnea caused by physical exertion
    B) Dyspnea at rest in a recumbent position that is relieved by sitting upright or standing
    C) The same as orthostatic hypotension
    D) Dyspnea that occurs going from a recumbent position to a standing position

50. Which of the following is characterized by an inflammation and edema of the trachea and bronchial tubes, hypertrophy of the mucous glands that narrows the airway, arterial hypoxemia that leads to vasoconstriction of smooth muscle in the pulmonary arterioles and venules, and in the presence of continued vasoconstriction results in pulmonary hypertension?
    A) Emphysema
    B) Bronchitis
    C) Pulmonary hypertension
    D) Asthma

51. The progressive overload principle is defined as _____.
    A) Employing controlled movements during a specific ROM
    B) Performing less sets per muscle group and increasing the number of days per week muscle groups are trained
    C) Performing more sets per muscle group and increasing the number of days per week muscle groups are trained
    D) Performing a one repetition maximum (1-RM) test every 6 wk

52. Which of the following is *not* a characteristic of ventricular tachycardia?
    A) Wide QRS complex ($\geq$120 ms)
    B) AV dissociation (P waves and QRS complexes have no relationship)
    C) Flutter waves at a rate of 250–350 atrial depolarizations per minute
    D) Three or more consecutive ventricular beats at 100 bpm

53. Which of the following is the minimum that will improve muscular strength, particularly among novice participants?
    A) One set of a resistance training exercise
    B) Two sets of a resistance training exercise
    C) Three sets of a resistance training exercise
    D) Four sets of a resistance training exercise

54. Which type of AV block occurs with a PR interval that progressively lengthens beyond 0.20 s until a P wave fails to conduct?
    A) First degree
    B) Second degree, Mobitz type I
    C) Second degree, Mobitz type II
    D) Third degree

55. The best measurement of exercise capacity (METs) is obtained by which of the following?
    A) Using exercise time on a standard protocol to estimate peak METs
    B) Using standard ACSM equations to calculate METs from peak workload
    C) Using the Borg RPE scale
    D) Using open-circuit indirect spirometry to determine maximal oxygen uptake ($\dot{V}O_{2\,max}$)

56. The progressive accent to higher altitudes will result in which two physiological responses?
    A) Increased arterial oxygen levels and increased cardiac output
    B) Increased arterial oxygen levels and decreased cardiac output
    C) Decreased arterial oxygen levels and decreased cardiac output
    D) Decreased arterial oxygen levels and increased cardiac output

57. Which exertional heat illness occurs when the body cannot sustain the level of $\dot{Q}$ needed to support skin blood flow for thermoregulation and blood flow for metabolic requirements of exercise?
    A) Heat cramps
    B) Syncope
    C) Heat exhaustion
    D) Heat stroke

58. For patients with congestive heart failure, which of the following statements is *true*?
    A) Patients may not exceed a workload of 5 METs.
    B) Warm-up and cool-down periods should be limited to 5 min.
    C) Patients should expect no significant improvement in exercise capacity.
    D) Peripheral adaptations are largely responsible for an increase in exercise tolerance.

59. Which of the following populations would benefit *most* from regular muscular strength and endurance training?
    A) Postmenopausal women
    B) Athletes <14 yr of age
    C) Stroke survivors
    D) Hypertensive adults

60. Which of the following ECG interpretations involves a QRS complex duration that exceeds 0.11 s and a P wave precedes the QRS complex if it is present?
    A) AV conduction delay
    B) Normal cardiac function
    C) Supraventricular aberrant conduction
    D) Acute MI

61. Bilateral ankle edema that is most evident at night is a characteristic sign of _____.
    A) Congestive heart failure
    B) Pulmonary hypertension
    C) Metabolic syndrome
    D) Coronary artery disease

62. In the "readiness to change model," which stage is it recommended to use multiple resources to stress the importance of a desired change?
    A) Precontemplation
    B) Contemplation
    C) Preparation
    D) Instruction

63. Which should be lowered as an effective strategy in limiting the progression and promoting regression of atherosclerosis?
    A) Low-density lipoprotein (LDL) cholesterol
    B) High-density lipoprotein (HDL) cholesterol
    C) Triglycerides (TGs)
    D) Blood platelets

64. Which of the following medications does *not* affect exercise HR response?
    A) Angiotensin-converting enzyme (ACE) inhibitors and angiotensin II blockers
    B) Calcium channel blockers
    C) Thyroid medications
    D) β-Blockers

65. Which of the following treadmill protocols would be appropriate for an individual with intermittent claudication?
    A) Bruce
    B) Modified Åstrand
    C) Naughton
    D) Balke and Ware

66. Medications may directly alter the ECG response during exercise and result in false-positive tests. The drug *most* likely to have this effect is _____.
    A) Lidocaine (Xylocaine)
    B) Propranolol (Inderal)
    C) Digitalis (Lanoxin)
    D) Reserpine (Serpasil)

67. Compared with data obtained during a previous graded exercise test when no medications were taken, a patient now taking propranolol (Inderal) would have which response to the same submaximal exercise intensity during a second test?
    A) A higher RPP
    B) A larger QRS duration
    C) A lower HR
    D) Greater ST-segment depression

CEP

68. Jane, a 47-yr-old female with no prior history of regular exercise recently completed a 12-wk exercise training program. Her routine consisted of walking and/or bike riding three times per week, for 30 min. Originally, Jane found that going up the stairs was rather difficult, often leaving her short of breath. Jane is now able to walk up multiple flights of stairs with ease. Her increase in aerobic endurance is an example of what type of relationship?
    A) Linear relationship
    B) Dose-response relationship
    C) Principle of adaptation relationship
    D) Inverse–linear relationship

69. False-negative test results limit the diagnostic value of an exercise test. The incidence of false negatives is related to all but one of the following. Which is *not* related to false-negative results?
    A) Insufficient level of stress
    B) Single vessel coronary artery disease
    C) Monitoring an insufficient number of ECG leads
    D) Lack of metabolic determination (*i.e.*, $\dot{V}O_{2max}$)

70. Sounds heard during measurement of BP are produced by _____.
    A) The closing of the mitral valve
    B) The closing of the aortic valve and pulmonary valves
    C) The contraction of the ventricle
    D) Turbulent blood flow

71. For individuals with heart failure, what intensity and duration should be used for their exercise program?
    A) RPE 9–13; 30–60 min · d^{-1}
    B) RPE 11–14; 15–30 min · d^{-1}
    C) RPE 9–13; 15–30 min · d^{-1}
    D) RPE 11–14; 30–60 min · d^{-1}

72. Which muscular endurance test controls for repetition duration and posture alignment, which increases the test's reliability?
    A) Curl-up test
    B) Young Men's Christian Association (YMCA) bench press test
    C) 1-RM test
    D) Push-up test

73. At a set workload (*e.g.*, 4 METs), myocardial oxygen consumption of a patient with coronary artery disease is reduced following endurance training as evidenced by a decrease in _____.
    A) Systolic ejection period
    B) RPE
    C) HR
    D) Whole-body oxygen consumption

74. When prescribing exercise for patients with atherosclerosis, which of the following is *true*?
    A) Training HR among patients who are status post-MI are altered by α-blocking agents.
    B) Patients with peripheral arterial disease should exercise to leg pain level 3 (on 4-point scale), with intermittent rest periods.
    C) Most patients with stable angina who are cleared to participate in outpatient exercise programs (*i.e.*, YMCA) can exercise safely with moderate angina levels (2+).
    D) During the initial phase (1–3 d after the event) of inpatient programs, activities should be restricted to moderate intensity (3–5 METs).

75. Studies show the least physically active populations to include all of the following *except* _____.
    A) Obese
    B) Elderly
    C) Less educated
    D) Upper middle class

76. ST-segment elevation may occur in all of the following *except* _____.
    A) Coronary artery spasm
    B) A ventricular aneurysm
    C) An acute MI
    D) Subendocardial ischemia

77. Which of the following statements are *false* concerning stroke volume in healthy adults?
    A) A greater preload will increase stroke volume.
    B) Increased arterial BP and greater ventricular outflow resistance will reduce stroke volume.
    C) During exercise, stroke volume increases to 50%–60% of maximal capacity, after which increases in cardiac output are largely caused by further increases in HR.
    D) Stroke volume is equal to the ratio of end-diastolic volume to end-systolic volume.

78. Long-term conditioning results in adaptations of the cardiovascular system. When measured at the same submaximal exercise intensity, these adaptations result in a decrease in _____.
    A) Stroke volume
    B) HR
    C) Cardiac output
    D) Arteriovenous oxygen difference

79. An increase in maximal attainable RPP following successful CABG surgery for severe angina suggests _____.
    A) Decreased myocardial oxygen demand
    B) Increased cardiac output during submaximal exercise
    C) Increased maximum coronary blood flow
    D) Increased extraction of oxygen by the myocardium

80. Greater oxygen delivery is provided to the myocardium in all of the following situations *except* _____.
    A) Severe coronary artery disease
    B) Increase HR
    C) Increase coronary blood flow
    D) Increase cardiac output

81. Which of the following would you not expect to occur with increased workload?
    A) Increased O_2
    B) Increased peripheral resistance
    C) Increased cardiac output
    D) Increased mean arterial pressure

82. Which of the following is *not* associated with exercise-induced myocardial ischemia?
    A) Angina pectoris
    B) ST-segment depression
    C) Impaired left ventricular function
    D) Decreased RPP

83. While at rest, physically inactive men compared to physically active men of the same weight and age typically have a _____.
    A) Higher BP
    B) Higher metabolic rate
    C) Higher cardiac output
    D) Lower stroke volume

84. Myocardial oxygen consumption is highly correlated with RPP. Which variables are used to determine RPP?
    A) Systolic BP and stroke volume
    B) Mean arterial pressure and HR
    C) Systolic pressure and HR
    D) Pulse pressure and HR

85. Which of the following would be the *best* marker of ischemic threshold?
    A) HR
    B) BP
    C) Oxygen uptake
    D) RPP

86. Long-term participation by healthy persons in activities such as running, cycling, and swimming results in the following adaptations during maximum exercise *except* _____.
    A) Increased oxidative capacity of a given mass of muscle
    B) Increased venous return
    C) Increased HR
    D) Increased blood flow through active muscles

87. When conducting a symptom-limited maximal exercise test, relative indications for terminating the test include _____.
    A) Moderate to severe angina
    B) Subject's request to stop
    C) Drop in systolic BP >10 mm Hg (persistently below baseline) despite an increase in workload, *in the absence* of other evidence of ischemia
    D) Signs of poor perfusion (*i.e.*, cyanosis or pallor)

88. Which method of determining exercise intensity is mostly recommended for individuals with autonomic neuropathy?
    A) HRR
    B) BP
    C) $\dot{V}O_2R$
    D) RPE

89. A reversible or transient perfusion defect on a myocardial perfusion imaging test is diagnostic for which of the following?
    A) MI
    B) Transient ischemic attack (TIA), or "mini-stroke"
    C) Exertional myocardial ischemia
    D) Angina pectoris

90. Which of the following statements regarding BP and resistance exercise (weightlifting) is correct?
    A) People with even mild CVD should never perform resistance exercise.
    B) BP elevations are highest during isometric muscular actions.
    C) BP elevations during resistance exercise are independent of the muscle mass involved.
    D) Typically, BP elevations seen during maximal resistance exercise are less than those observed during maximal aerobic exercise.

91. Which of the following is generally true of the hemodynamic exercise response in a patient who has received a cardiac transplant when compared to age-matched healthy individuals?
    A) Exercising HR is usually elevated.
    B) BP is attenuated at rest and during exercise.
    C) HR returns to rest faster.
    D) HR returns to rest slower.

92. The primary effects of chronic exercise training on blood lipids include _____.
    A) Decreased TG and increased HDL
    B) Decreased total cholesterol and LDL
    C) Decreased HDL and increased LDL
    D) Decreased total cholesterol and increased HDL

93. Which of the following statements concerning the surgical treatment of coronary artery disease is *true*?
    A) A coronary artery stent carries a lower rate of revascularization than does PTCA.
    B) Atherectomy is a prerequisite requirement for PTCA.
    C) Venous grafts are significantly superior to arterial grafts in terms of patency.
    D) Long-term outcome of laser angioplasty is unknown and thus rarely used.

94. A cardiac patient is taking a β-blocker medication. During an exercise test, you would expect _____.
    A) An ST-segment depression because β-blockers depress the ST segment on the resting ECG
    B) An increase in the anginal threshold compared with a test without the medication
    C) No change in HR or BP compared with a test without the medication
    D) A slight decrease or no effect on BP compared with a test without the medication

95. If an individual is in the action stage of the "stages of motivational readiness," he or she _____.
    A) Has been physically active on a regular basis for <6 mo
    B) Participates in some exercise but does so irregularly
    C) Intends to start exercising in the next 6 mo
    D) Has been physically active on a regular basis for >6 mo

96. Following termination of a graded exercise (stress) test, a 12-lead ECG is _____.
    A) Monitored immediately and then every 1–2 min for 5 min of recovery or until exercise-induced changes are at baseline
    B) Monitored immediately and then at 2 and 5 min after the test
    C) Monitored immediately only
    D) Monitored and recorded only if any signs or symptoms arise during recovery

97. What is the best test to help determine ejection fraction at rest and during exercise?
    A) Angiogram
    B) Thallium stress test
    C) Single-photon emission computed tomography test
    D) Multiple-gated acquisition (MUGA) (blood pool imagery) study

98. Which of the following is *not* part of an emergency plan?
    A) The plan should list the schedule of each staff member so that they can all be accounted for during an emergency.
    B) The plan must be written.
    C) The plan should outline each specific action.
    D) The staff should be prepared and trained in the plan.

99. Which of the following is not true for an individual who suffered a cerebral vascular accident and wishes to return to work?
    A) Patients should be educated on avoidance and precautions.
    B) Assessment of muscular strength and endurance are needed.
    C) They should not be encouraged to return to work.
    D) Exercise programs should be specific to occupational requirements.

100. Which of the following statements about confidentiality is *not* correct?
    A) All records must be kept by the program director/manager under lock and key.
    B) Data must be available to all individuals who need to see it.
    C) Data should be kept on file for at least 1 yr before being discarded.
    D) Sensitive information (*e.g.*, participant's name) needs to be protected.

CEP

CEP EXAMINATION ANSWERS AND EXPLANATIONS

1—D. Epinephrine

Epinephrine is an endogenous catecholamine that optimizes blood flow to the heart and brain by increasing aortic diastolic pressure and preferentially shunting blood to the internal carotid artery. Lidocaine is an antiarrhythmic agent that can decrease automaticity in the ventricular myocardium as well as raise the fibrillation threshold. Supplemental oxygen ensures adequate arterial oxygen content and greatly enhances tissue oxygenation. Atropine is a parasympathetic blocking agent used to treat bradyarrhythmias.

2—C. 13 wk

The steps are as follows:

a. Convert relative $\dot{V}O_2$ to absolute $\dot{V}O_2$ by multiplying relative $\dot{V}O_2$ ($mL \cdot kg^{-1} \cdot min^{-1}$) by his body weight.

b. The young man weights 80 kg. Therefore,

$$Absolute\ \dot{V}O_2 = relative\ \dot{V}O_2 \times body\ weight$$
$$= 45\ mL \cdot kg^{-1} \cdot min^{-1} \times 80\ kg$$
$$= 3{,}600\ mL \cdot min^{-1}$$

c. To get $L \cdot min^{-1}$, divide $mL \cdot min^{-1}$ by 1,000

$$3{,}600\ mL \cdot min^{-1}/1{,}000 = 3.60\ L \cdot min^{-1}$$

d. Multiply $3.60\ L \cdot min^{-1}$ by the constant 5.0 to get $kcal \cdot min^{-1}$

$$3.60\ L \cdot min^{-1} \times 5.0 = 18.0\ kcal \cdot min^{-1}$$

e. Multiply $18.0\ kcal \cdot min^{-1}$ by the total number of minutes that he exercises ($\sim$30 min 5 times per week = 150 total minutes) to get the total caloric expenditure

$$18.0\ kcal \cdot min^{-1} \times 150\ min = 2{,}700\ kcal \cdot wk^{-1}$$

f. Divide by 3,500 to get pounds of fat

$2{,}700\ kcal \cdot wk^{-1}/3{,}500\ kcal \cdot lb^{-1}$ of fat = 0.7714 lb of fat $\cdot wk^{-1}$

g. Divide 10 lb by 0.7714 to get how many weeks it will take him to lose 10 lb of fat

10 lb of fat/0.7714 = 12.96 wk or approximately 13.0 wk

3—C. Echocardiography

In the diagnosis of coronary artery disease, electrocardiography, radionuclide imaging, and echocardiography are commonly used by themselves or with other tests. However, echocardiography uses sound waves to assess heart wall motion, abnormalities, ejection fraction, systolic and diastolic function, and cardiac output. Other important diagnostic studies for coronary artery disease include coronary angiography.

4—C. Moderate intensity, 6 d $\cdot$ wk^{-1}, large muscle groups, and moderate duration

Patients who have had heart transplant should exercise at an RPE of between 11 and 16 (moderate) and not use a target HR prescription. Duration should include a prolonged warm-up and cooldown. In addition, resistance training can be used in moderation after 8–12 wk (follow sternotomy special considerations).

5—C. Exercising only when temperature and humidity are moderate

Recommended precautions for the exercising patient with diabetes include wearing proper footwear, maintaining adequate hydration, monitoring blood glucose level regularly, always wearing a medical identification bracelet or other form of identification, avoiding injecting insulin into exercising muscles, always exercising with a partner, and avoiding exercise during peak insulin activity. There is no reason why a patient with diabetes cannot exercise at any time if proper precautions are followed.

6—C. Asthma

Bronchitis is inflammation of the main air passages to the lungs. Bronchitis can be acute or chronic. Acute bronchitis is characterized by a cough, with or without the production of sputum, and can last several days or weeks. Chronic bronchitis, a type of chronic obstructive pulmonary disease, is characterized by the presence of a productive cough that lasts for 3 mo or more per year for at least 2 yr. Emphysema usually refers to a long-term, progressive disease of the lungs that causes shortness of breath. Emphysema is called an obstructive lung disease because the destruction of lung tissue around the alveoli makes these air sacs unable to hold their functional shape upon exhalation. Pulmonary vascular disease is a category of disorders that affect the blood circulation in the lungs. Examples include pulmonary arterial hypertension and pulmonary edema.

7—B. Junctional arrhythmia

A junctional arrhythmia is a supraventricular ectopic rhythm that results from a focus of automaticity located in the bundle of His. A ventricular arrhythmia could be a premature ventricular complex (PVC) in which one of the ventricles depolarizes first and then spreads to the other ventricle or ventricular fibrillation, which is often triggered by the simultaneous conduction of ischemic ventricular cells within multiple locations of the ventricles. An AV block result when supraventricular impulses are delayed in the AV node. A premature ventricular contraction occurs when the ventricles are prematurely depolarized.

8—D.   All of the above statements are true.

All of these statements are true regarding contraindications to exercise testing.

9—A.   P wave

The cardiac impulse originating in the sinoatrial node that spreads to both atria causing atrial depolarization is indicated on the ECG as a P wave. Atrial repolarization usually is not seen on the ECG because it is obscured by the ventricular electrical potentials. Ventricular depolarization is represented on the ECG by the QRS complex. Ventricular repolarization is represented on the ECG by the ST segment, the T wave, and, at times, the U wave.

10—C. $150–200 \text{ kcal} \cdot \text{d}^{-1}$

A minimal caloric threshold of 150–200 kcal of PA per day is associated with a significant 20%–30% reduction in risk of all-cause mortality, and this should be the initial goal for previously sedentary individuals.

11—D.   Decreased endothelial-mediated vasomotor tone

The mechanisms responsible for a reduction in deaths from coronary artery disease include its effect on other risk factors, reduced myocardial oxygen demand both at rest and at submaximal workloads (resulting in an increased ischemic and anginal threshold), reduced platelet aggregation, and improved endothelial-mediated vasomotor tone.

12—D.   Health Belief Model

The Health Belief Model (HBM) is centered on the idea that an individual will be more likely to engage in corrective behaviors if he or she meets the following criteria: (a) believe he or she is susceptible to disease, (b) believe the disease has serious consequences, (c) believe taking action reduces their susceptibility to the condition or its severity, (d) believe benefits of taking action outweigh the costs, (e) believe they can successfully perform actions, and (f) are exposed to factors that prompt action.

13—C.   Coronary artery bypass graft (CABG) surgery

CABG surgery usually is reserved for patients who have a poor prognosis for survival or are unresponsive to pharmacologic treatment, stents, or PTCA. Such patients include those with angina, left main coronary artery stenosis, multiple vessel disease, and left ventricular dysfunction.

14—A.   Persons with AICD must be monitored closely during exercise, keeping the heart rate (HR) 10 beats or more below the activation rate for a shock.

There are many benefits of chronic exercise for a patient with an AICD. Several precautions need to be taken, however, including monitoring the HR and knowing the rate at which the AICD is set to shock the patient. The rate for activation is preset and varies for each patient.

15—B.   55%

The anaerobic threshold is normally expressed as a percentage of an individual's $\dot{V}O_{2max}$. For example, if $\dot{V}O_{2max}$ occurs at 6 mph on a treadmill test and a sharp rise in blood lactate concentration above resting levels is seen at 3 mph, then the anaerobic threshold is said to be 50% $\dot{V}O_{2max}$. In well-trained athletes, anaerobic threshold typically occurs at 70%–80% $\dot{V}O_{2max}$. In untrained individuals, it occurs much sooner at 50%–60% $\dot{V}O_{2max}$. This is because the adaptations from regular aerobic exercise have not occurred (*e.g.*, increased mitochondria and capillary density).

16—D.   Nitrates

Nitrates relax peripheral venous vessels, which decrease preload, attenuate myocardial oxygen demand, and alleviate ischemia. Nitrates do not reduce the risk of post-MI mortality. β-Adrenergic blockers reduce myocardial ischemia by lowering myocardial oxygen demand. These agents lower BP, control ventricular arrhythmias, and significantly reduce first-year mortality rates in patients after MI by 20%–35%. Niacin lowers low-density lipids by inhibiting secretion of lipoproteins from the liver. Aspirin is a platelet inhibitor.

17—B.   510 cal

The steps are as follows:

a. Choose the ACSM's leg cycling formula.

b. Write down your knowns and convert the values to the appropriate units.

110 lb/2.2 = 50 kg
50 rpm × 6 m = 300 m · min^{-1}
2.5 kp = 2.5 kg
60 min of cycling

c. Write down the ACSM leg cycling formula.

Leg cycling $(mL \cdot kg^{-1} \cdot min^{-1}) =$
$(1.8 \times$ work rate/body weight$) +$
$3.5 + 3.5$ $(mL \cdot kg^{-1} \cdot min^{-1})$

d. Calculate the work rate.

Work rate $= kg \cdot m \cdot min^{-1}$
$= 2.5 \, kg \cdot 300 \, m \cdot min^{-1}$
$= 750 \, kg \cdot m \cdot min^{-1}$

e. Substitute the known values for the variable name.

$mL \cdot kg^{-1} \cdot min^{-1} = (1.8 \times 750/50) + 3.5 + 3.5$

f. Solve for the unknown.

$mL \cdot kg^{-1} \cdot min^{-1} = 27 + 3.5 + 3.5$
Gross leg cycling $\dot{V}O_2 = 34 \, mL \cdot kg^{-1} \cdot min^{-1}$

g. To find out how many calories she expends, we must first convert her oxygen consumption to absolute terms.

Absolute $\dot{V}O_2$ = relative $\dot{V}O_2 \times$ body weight
$= 34 \, mL \cdot kg^{-1} \cdot min^{-1}$
$= 1,700 \, mL \cdot min^{-1}$

h. Convert $mL \cdot min^{-1}$ to $L \cdot min^{-1}$ by dividing by 1,000.

$1,700 \, mL \cdot min^{-1}/1,000 = 1.7 \, L \cdot min^{-1}$

i. Next, we must see how many calories she expends in 1 min by multiplying her absolute $\dot{V}O_2$ (in $L \cdot min^{-1}$) by the constant 5.0.

$1.7 \, L \cdot min^{-1} \times 5.0 = 8.5 \, kcal \cdot min^{-1}$

j. Finally, multiply the number of calories she expends in 1 min by the number of minutes that she cycles.

$8.5 \, kcal \cdot min^{-1} \times 60 \, min = 510$ total calories

18—D. Midclavicular line, fifth intercostal space

The proper anatomic location of V_4 is the midclavicular line, fifth intercostal space. Precordial leads V_1 and V_2 are located at the fourth intercostal space, right and left sternal borders. There is no precordial lead site at the midaxillary line, fifth intercostal space.

19—A. Stroke volume

During exercise, stroke volume increases curvilinearly with work rate until it reaches near maximum at a level equivalent to approximately 50% of aerobic capacity, increasing only slightly thereafter. The left ventricle is able to contract with greater force during exercise because of a greater end-diastolic volume and enhanced mechanical ability of muscle fibers to produce force.

20—A. Extreme cold

Exposure to cold causes vasoconstriction (higher BP response); lowers the anginal threshold in patients with angina; can provoke angina at rest (variant or Prinzmetal angina); and can induce asthma, general dehydration, and dryness or burning of the mouth and throat.

21—B. Signs of poor perfusion (cyanosis or pallor)

The development of a bundle-branch block and a systolic BP of $\geq 250 \, mm \, Hg$ are relative indications to terminate a symptom-limited maximal exercise test. The achievement of $\geq 85\%$ age-predicted HR_{max} would indicate the termination of an exercise test with a predetermined intensity goal, which diminishes the sensitivity of the test. Signs of poor perfusion are an absolute indication to terminate the test.

22—C. Rate-pressure product (RPP)

The RPP should be used to prescribe exercise for this individual because it is a repeatable estimate of the ischemic threshold. RPP is also a more reliable estimate of ischemic threshold than external workload, which is why it is the best choice.

23—D. Digitalis

Digitalis is used to treat heart failure and certain arrhythmias. Shortening of the QT interval and a "scooping" of the ST–T complex characterize the effects of digitalis on the ECG.

24—A. The patient should avoid upper body resistance training because of sternal and leg wounds for 4–6 mo.

Avoiding tension on the upper body typically is recommended for 8–12 wk, not for 2–4 mo. All of the other precautions are appropriate.

25—C. Glycolated hemoglobin (HbA1C)

HbA1C is a blood chemistry test that reflects glucose levels in the blood over a 2–3 mo period. Levels greater than or equal to 6.5% are diagnostic for diabetes.

26—A. 40%–59% heart rate reserve (HRR)/$\dot{V}O_{2max}$

Moderate intensity for aerobic training would be 40%–59% of a person's HRR and/or $\dot{V}O_{2max}$. Vigorous intensities would be 60%–89% HRR/$\dot{V}O_{2max}$, and light/low intensities would range from 30% to 39% HRR/$\dot{V}O_{2max}$.

27—A. Early morning and late evening

Exercising early in the morning may result in elevated blood glucose levels after exercise. Avoid exercise prior to bed to avoid hypoglycemia when sleeping. This is due to the release of the counterregulatory hormones epinephrine and glucagon.

28—B. Mobitz type I

Second-degree AV block is subdivided into two types: Mobitz type I and Mobitz type II. Mobitz type I also is known as the Wenckebach phenomenon. In this condition, the conduction of the impulse through the AV junction becomes increasingly more difficult, resulting in a progressively longer PR interval, until a QRS complex is dropped following a P wave. This indicates that the AV junction failed to conduct the impulse from the atria to the ventricles. This pause allows the AV node to recover, and the following P wave is conducted with a normal or slightly shorter PR interval.

29—C. ST segment

ST segments are considered to be sensitive indicators of myocardial ischemia or injury. A Q wave is a negative deflection of a QRS complex preceding an R wave. A "pathologic" Q wave is an indication of an old transmural MI. The PR interval is the time that it takes from the initiation of an electrical impulse in the sinoatrial node to the initiation of electrical activity in the ventricles. The T wave indicates ventricular repolarization.

30—B. Shoveling snow

Shoveling snow can quickly create a potential crisis for an individual with CVD due to a triad of common physiological responses. Snow shoveling raises the HR up to 97% HR_{max} and systolic BP up to 200 mm Hg. Also, cold outdoor temperatures cause whole body and facial cooling which can lower the threshold for the onset of angina during exercise. Additionally, activities in cold temperatures that involve the upper body and increase metabolism further increase the risk for individuals with CVD.

31—A. Acute MI

An ECG is an excellent tool for detecting cardiac rhythm and conduction abnormalities, chamber enlargements, ischemia, and infarction. In an ECG recording, ST-segment elevation with an absence of R waves that are replaced by Q waves is a sign of acute MI.

32—C. $29.76 \text{ mL} \cdot \text{kg}^{-1} \cdot \text{min}^{-1}$

The steps are as follows:

a. Choose the ACSM's walking formula.

b. Write down your knowns and convert the values to the appropriate units.

$3.5 \text{ mph} \times 26.8 = 93.8 \cdot \text{min}^{-1}$
$10\% \text{ grade} = 0.10$

c. Write down the ACSM's walking formula.

walking $(\text{kg}^{-1} \cdot \text{min}^{-1}) = (0.1 \times \text{speed}) + (1.8 \times \text{speed} \times \text{fractional grade}) + 3.5 \text{ (mL} \cdot \text{kg}^{-1} \cdot \text{min}^{-1})$

d. Substitute the known values for the variable name.

$\text{mL} \cdot \text{kg}^{-1} \cdot \text{min}^{-1} = (0.1 \times 93.8) + (1.8 \times 93.8 \times 0.1) + 3.5 \text{ mL} \cdot \text{kg}^{-1} \cdot \text{min}^{-1} = 9.8 + 16.884 + 3.5$

e. Solve for the unknown.

$\text{mL} \cdot \text{kg}^{-1} \cdot \text{min}^{-1} = 9.38 + 16.884 + 3.5$
gross walking $\dot{V}O = 29.76 \text{ mL} \cdot \text{kg}^{-1} \cdot \text{min}^{-1}$

33—A. The clinical exercise physiologist will review and interpret the results of the test and report them to the supervising physician.

The clinical exercise physiologist will not review and interpret the results of the test; this is done by the physician. The physician does not have to be directly present in the exercise testing room but must be available for emergencies. The clinical exercise physiologist must possess the cognitive skills to recognize and treat exercise testing complications and/or serious arrhythmias.

34—B. If cuff size encircles <80% of the upper arm, measurement will be inaccurate.

While choosing too small of a cuff will lead to an inaccurate reading, it will tend to overestimate systolic and diastolic pressures. The deflation rate is not dependent on cuff size but technique by technician.

35—B. 80%–90%

To evaluate the work-related activity levels that are likely to be incorporated into everyday life, a constant work rate test using 80%–90% of the peak work achieved during the incremental exercise test is ideal, especially when the test is performed on a treadmill.

CEP

36—D. Pain in the left submammary or hemithorax area

Chest pain in the left submammary or hemithorax area is generally not ischemic in origin. Atypical or nonischemic chest pain may be caused by many conditions other than angina pectoris including musculoskeletal conditions, costochondritis, abdominal gas, or infection.

37—C. 40%–<60% HRR or $\dot{V}O_2R$, 3–<6 METs, RPE 12–13, an intensity that causes noticeable increases in HR and breathing

ACSM defines moderate intensity exercise as an exercise workload of 40%–<60% HRR or $\dot{V}O_2R$, 3–<6 METs, RPE 12–13, at an intensity that causes noticeable increases in HR and breathing. This level of exercise may be suitable for a cardiac rehabilitation patient who has completed many of the prescribed exercise sessions with an estimated or actual peak oxygen consumption ($\dot{V}O_{2peak}$) of ≥8 METs.

38—B. Place the patient in the recovery position with the head to the side to prevent airway obstruction.

The proper response to a patient who has experienced a cardiac arrest yet is breathing and has a pulse is to call to the emergency medical system immediately; place the patient in the recovery position, with the head to the side to avoid an airway obstruction; and then stay with the patient and continue to monitor his or her vital signs.

39—B. $2.17 \text{ L} \cdot \text{min}^{-1}$

The steps are as follows:

a. Choose the ACSM's walking formula.

b. Write down your knowns and convert the values to the appropriate units.

5% grade = 0.05
4.0 mph = $107.2 \text{ m} \cdot \text{min}^{-1}$
200 lb = 90.91 kg

c. Write down the ACSM's walking formula:

walking $(\text{kg}^{-1} \cdot \text{min}^{-1})$ = $(0.1 \times \text{speed})$ + $(1.8 \times \text{speed} \times \text{fractional grade})$ + $3.5 \ (\text{mL} \cdot \text{kg}^{-1} \cdot \text{min}^{-1})$

d. Substitute knowns:

$\dot{V}O_2 = (0.1 \times 107.2) + (1.8 \times 107.2 \times 0.05) + 3.5$

e. Solve:

$\dot{V}O_2 = 23.87 \text{ mL} \cdot \text{kg}^{-1} \cdot \text{min}^{-1}$
$\dot{V}O_2 = 23.83 \times 90.01 \text{ kg}/1,000$
$\dot{V}O_2 = 2.17 \text{ L} \cdot \text{min}^{-1}$

40—C. Electrocardiography

Electrocardiography is the least sensitive and specific of all these tests. Directly visualizing the coronary arteries using coronary angiography provides the highest sensitivity and specificity. Radionuclide imaging and echocardiography have about the same sensitivity and specificity.

41—A. To effectively breathe through a progressively smaller airway

Flow-resistive training involves breathing through a progressively smaller airway or opening. Paced breathing helps to coordinate breathing with activities of daily living. Respiratory muscle training increases respiratory muscle endurance and strength. Ventilatory threshold is the breakpoint in ventilation during exercise and likely reflects a balance between lactate production and removal.

42—C. 10–12 wk

Because of the median sternotomy used to provide access for cardiovascular surgery, it is common to provide ROM and weight load restrictions for upper limb movement. These instructions are conveyed at discharge and may vary somewhat. However, they are usually set at 5–10 lb or <50% MVC for 10–12 wk postoperatively.

43—B. After the first 24 h

Mobilization of the upper extremities may be useful in preventing joint complications after ICD implantation. Guidelines suggest that gentle ROM activities begin after the first 24 h to reduce the risk of lead displacement.

44—C. Media

The media contains most of the smooth muscle cells, which maintain arterial tone. The endothelium comprises a single layer of cells that forms a tight barrier between blood and the arterial wall to resist thrombosis, promote vasodilation, and inhibit smooth muscle cells from migration and proliferation into the intima. The intima is the very thin, innermost layer of the artery wall and is composed mainly of connective tissue with some smooth muscle cells. The adventitia is the outermost layer of the arterial wall and consists of connective tissue, fibroblasts, and a few smooth muscle cells. Adventitia is highly vascularized and provides the media and intima with oxygen and other nutrients.

45—A. Determining a return to work date prior to a patient undergoing CABG surgery

Data from a clinical exercise test performed after a cardiac event or procedure is useful in developing return to work guidelines for patients. Due to the somewhat unpredictable nature of post-CABG recovery (*i.e.*, possible postoperative complications, individual variability in recovery, etc.), it is not appropriate to use data from a clinical exercise test performed prior to surgery to predict a return to work date.

46—C.   444 kcal

First, determine the MET level for each activity.

Warm-up is 2.0 METs × 5 min = 10 METs
Treadmill is 9.0 METs × 20 min = 180 METs
Cycle is 8.0 METs × 20 min = 160 METs
Cool-down is 2.50 METs × 5 min = 12.5 METs

Then, determine the total number of MET for all activities. 10 + 180 + 160 + 12.5 = 362.5. Multiply 362.5 METs by 3.5 (because 1 MET = $3.5 \cdot mL \cdot kg^{-1} \cdot min^{-1}$), which is equal to $1{,}268.75$ mL $\cdot$ kg^{-1}.

Multiply 1,268.75 mL $\cdot$ kg^{-1} by body weight (70 kg), which is equal to 88,812.5 mL. Divide that number by 1,000 (because 1,000 mL = 1 L), which is equal to 88.81 L. Multiply 88.81 L by 5 (because 5 kcal = 1 L of oxygen consumed), which is equal to 444 kcal.

47—B.   30 min $\cdot$ d^{-1}, five times a week or 150 min $\cdot$ wk^{-1} of moderate intensity exercise

The ACSM/AHA Primary Physical Activity Recommendations suggest that all healthy individuals aged 18–65 yr should participate in moderate intensity, aerobic PA for a minimum of 30 min on 5 d of the week or vigorous intensity, aerobic activity for a minimum of 20 min on 3 d of the week. The Primary Physical Activity Recommendations from the *2008 Physical Activity Guidelines Committee Report* suggests that all Americans should participate in an amount of energy expenditure equivalent to 150 min $\cdot$ wk^{-1} of moderate intensity, aerobic activity or 75 min $\cdot$ wk^{-1} of vigorous intensity, aerobic activity.

48—C.   All emergency situations must be documented with dates, times, actions, people involved, and outcomes.

The emergency plan must be written down and available in all testing and exercise areas. The plan should list the specific responsibilities of each staff member, required equipment, and predetermined contacts for an emergency response. All emergencies must be documented with dates, times, actions, people involved, and results. The plan should be practiced with both announced and unannounced drills periodically. All staff members,

including nonclinical staff members, should be trained in the emergency plan.

49—B.   Dyspnea at rest in a recumbent position that is relieved by sitting upright or standing

Orthopnea refers to dyspnea occurring at rest in the recumbent position that is relieved promptly by sitting upright or standing. Paroxysmal nocturnal dyspnea refers to dyspnea that begins usually 2–5 h after the onset of sleep, which may be relieved by sitting on the side of the bed or standing to get out of bed. Both conditions are symptoms of left ventricular dysfunction.

50—B.   Bronchitis

Signs and symptoms of bronchitis include chronic cough, mucus production, and mucous gland enlargement that involves the large airways. The body attempts to heal by depositing collagen in the airway walls. The effects include further airway narrowing, an increase in airway resistance decreasing ventilation to the lung, increased perfusion resulting in ventilation–perfusion mismatch, arterial hypoxemia, and pulmonary arterial hypertension. Common clinical symptoms of emphysema are shortness of breath or coughing, sputum production notable in the morning, hypoxemia, and eventual cor pulmonale. Emphysema primarily involves abnormalities of the lung parenchyma and smaller airways. Asthma is an episodic reversible condition that is characterized by increased airway reactivity to various stimuli resulting in widespread reversible narrowing of the airways. Pulmonary hypertension is a mean pulmonary artery pressure at rest >25 mm Hg or >30 mm Hg with exercise.

51—C.   Performing more sets per muscle group and increasing the number of days per week muscle groups are trained

The progressive overload principle incorporates more repetitions per muscle group while increasing the number of days per week muscle groups are trained.

52—C.   Flutter waves at a rate of 250–350 atrial depolarizations per minute

Ventricular tachycardia is characterized by three or more consecutive ventricular beats per minute or faster, a wide QRS complex (≥120 ms), AV dissociation (the P waves and QRS complexes have no relationship) and a QRS complex that does not have the morphology of bundle-branch block. Atrial flutter is characterized by flutter waves at a rate of 250–350 atrial depolarizations per minute.

CEP

53—A.   One set of a resistance training exercise

A single set of a resistance exercise will improve muscular strength, particularly among novice participants. The first set of a resistance exercise is responsible for the majority of the benefits derived even from multiple-set routines. Although two to four set prescriptions provide superior results with a multitude of other benefits, 10 to 12 single-set exercises working various muscle groups may prove to be beneficial for the person just beginning resistance training.

54—B.   Second degree, Mobitz type I

Second degree: Mobitz type I (Wenckebach). PR interval lengthens until a P wave fails to conduct.

55—D.   Using open-circuit indirect spirometry to determine maximal oxygen uptake ($\dot{V}O_{2\,max}$)

Exercise time on a standard protocol and the ACSM equations are both useful for estimating the attained MET level during clinical exercise testing. However, the analysis of expired gases obtained during indirect spirometry is the best method for accurately measuring exercise capacity.

56—D.   Decreased arterial oxygen levels and increased cardiac output

Higher altitudes (2,400–4,000 m or 7,874–13,123 ft) have a decreased atmospheric pressure which reduces the partial pressure of oxygen in the inspired air. This change will result in a physiological decrease in arterial oxygen levels and the immediate compensatory response includes increased ventilation and cardiac output ($\dot{Q}$).

57—C.   Heat exhaustion

Heat exhaustion is often associated with fatigue and peripheral vascular dilation resulting in hypotension, blood pooling, and cardiovascular insufficiency. This blood pooling reduces intravascular heat transport from the core to the skin and diminishes thermoregulation. Heat cramps are muscle spasms that may occur in association with strenuous activity, syncope is a temporary loss of consciousness, and heat stroke is caused by hyperthermia of >40° C or 104° F.

58—D.   Peripheral adaptations are largely responsible for an increase in exercise tolerance.

Physical conditioning in patients with heart failure and moderate to severe left ventricular dysfunction results in improved functional capacity and quality of life and reduced symptoms. Peripheral adaptation (increased skeletal muscle oxidative enzymes and improved mitochondrial size and density) are responsible for the increase in exercise tolerance.

59—A.   Postmenopausal women

A reduction in the risk of osteoporosis, low back pain, hypertension, and diabetes are associated with resistance training. In addition, the benefits of increased muscular strength, bone density, enhanced strength of connective tissue, and the increase or maintenance of lean body mass may also occur. These adaptations are beneficial for all ages, including middle-aged and older adults, and, in particular, postmenopausal women who may experience a more rapid loss of bone mineral density.

60—C.   Supraventricular aberrant conduction

Supraventricular aberrant conduction — QRS complex is ≥0.11 s; widened QRS usually with unchanged initial vector; P present or absent but with relationship to QRS.

61—A.   Congestive heart failure

Bilateral ankle edema that is most evident at night is a characteristic sign of congestive heart failure (or bilateral chronic venous insufficiency). Unilateral edema of a limb often results from venous thrombosis or lymphatic blockage in the limb. Generalized edema (known as anasarca) occurs in those with the nephrotic syndrome, severe heart failure, or hepatic cirrhosis.

62—A.   Precontemplation

Patients express lack of interest in making change. Moving patients through this stage involves the use of multiple resources to stress the importance of the desired change. This can be achieved through written materials, educational classes, physician and family persuasion, and other means.

63—A.   Low-density lipoprotein (LDL) cholesterol

Lowering total cholesterol and LDL cholesterol has proved to be effective in reducing and even reversing atherosclerosis. The goal is to reduce the availability of lipids to the injured endothelium. In primary prevention trials, lowering total cholesterol and LDL cholesterol has been shown to reduce the incidence and mortality of coronary artery disease.

64—A.   Angiotensin-converting enzyme (ACE) inhibitors and angiotensin II blockers

ACE inhibitor and angiotensin II receptor blockers: $\leftrightarrow$ HR (R and E)
Calcium channel blockers: $\uparrow$ or $\uparrow$ or $\leftrightarrow$ HR (R and E)
β-Blockers: $\downarrow$ HR (R and E)
Thyroid medications: $\uparrow$ HR (R and E)

65—C. Naughton

The Naughton protocol is appropriate for diseased populations. It is more gradual with increases in intensity and it uses a lower speed than other common protocols (*e.g.*, Bruce protocol). The speed remains constant (2 mph) throughout the test. The grade starts at 0% and increases every 2 min. Small increments in grade allow claudication times to be stratified according to peripheral arterial disease severity.

66—C. Digitalis (Lanoxin)

Digitalis can modify the ST–T contour and slow AV conduction. Digitalis may produce characteristic scooping of the ST–T complex. The ST segment and T wave are fused together, and it can be impossible to tell where one ends and the other begins. This may occur when digitalis is in the therapeutic range. With digitalis toxicity, digitalis can cause virtually any arrhythmia and all degrees of AV.

67—C. A lower HR

Inderal is a β-blocker that diminishes the effect of norepinephrine and epinephrine and lowers HR.

68—B. Dose-response relationship

The dose-response relationship shows that an increase in the volume of exercise results in an increase in health and fitness benefits.

69—D. Lack of metabolic determination (*i.e.*, $\dot{V}O_{2max}$)

Sufficient physiological stress is needed to reach an ischemic threshold. There can be compensation by collateral circulation with single vessel disease. Sufficient ECG leads (*e.g.*, 12-lead) are required to monitor a complete view of the heart. However, not determining $\dot{V}O_{2max}$ is not a cause for a false negative.

70—D. Turbulent blood flow

When measuring BP, blood flows in spurts as the pressure in the artery rises above the pressure in the cuff and then drops back down beyond the cuffed region of the arm. This results in turbulence that produces the audible sounds (Korotkoff sounds).

71—D. RPE 11–14; 30–60 min · d^{-1}

Individuals with heart failure should exercise 3–5 d · wk^{-1} at an intensity of 11–14 on a 6–20 RPE scale. They should increase up to 30 min · d^{-1} and then to 60 min · d^{-1} by free or treadmill walking or the use of a cycle ergometer.

72—B. Young Men's Christian Association (YMCA) bench press test

The YMCA bench press test, mentioned in the *ACSM's Guidelines for Exercise Testing and Prescription*, 10th ed., Chapter 4, has a standardized repetition rate of 30 lifts per minute, which controls for repetition duration. The test is also done while in a supine position, against a flat surface, which accounts for posture alignment.

73—C. HR

Myocardial oxygen consumption is increased by a number of variables, including increased HR. A decreased HR at a given intensity (4 METs) would reduce myocardial oxygen consumption. The other three choices do not directly affect myocardial oxygen demand.

74—B. Patients with peripheral arterial disease should exercise to leg pain level 3 (on 4-point scale), with intermittent rest periods.

The guidelines recommend patients with peripheral arterial disease achieve 3 (intense pain) on the 4-point claudication scale during exercise. Rest periods should then be allowed until the pain fully resolves before continuing exercise.

75—D. Upper middle class

Obese and elderly persons are often less physically active because of various physical or medical limitations (*e.g.*, osteoarthritis, frailty). The less educated are often not aware of the important health and fitness benefits of being physically active on a regular basis.

76—D. Subendocardial ischemia

The most common ECG change with subendocardial ischemia is ST-segment depression, *not* ST-segment elevation. ST-segment depression indicates insufficient blood flow (*i.e.*, ischemia) to the heart muscle.

77—D. Stroke volume is equal to the ratio of end-diastolic volume to end-systolic volume.

For healthy adults, stroke volume is calculated by subtracting end-systolic volume from end-diastolic volume.

78—B. HR

Adaptations to long-term aerobic activity include an increased oxidative capacity of the exercised muscles, increased blood flow through active muscles, and increased venous blood flow return to the heart. These adaptations (*i.e.*, increased aerobic fitness) result in a decreased HR at the same level of submaximal exercise intensity.

79—C. Increased maximum coronary blood flow

RPP is an indicator of myocardial oxygen demand. An increase in maximal RPP indicates that there is improved/increased blood flow to the coronary arteries.

CEP

80—A. Severe coronary artery disease

Severe coronary artery disease will result in less oxygen delivery to the myocardium because of blockage(s), which will reduce or limit oxygenated blood flow to the myocardium.

81—B. Increased peripheral resistance

During increasing aerobic activity, there is a volume load on the heart and cardiovascular system, which causes a *decrease* in peripheral vascular resistance. This volume load results in a rise in systolic BP and no change or a slight decrease in diastolic BP. An increase in O_2, cardiac output, and mean arterial pressure is typically seen with an increased workload.

82—D. Decreased RPP

RPP is a measure of the stress put on the cardiac muscle (myocardial oxygen demand) based on the number of times it needs to beat per minute and the arterial BP that it is pumping against (HR × systolic BP). A decreased RPP indicates less myocardial oxygen demand. An *increased* RPP can be associated with exercise-induced myocardial ischemia.

83—D. Lower stroke volume

Regular aerobic activity typically increases stroke volume at rest. Increased aerobic fitness usually results in a lower resting HR (HR_{rest}). The lower HR prolongs diastole (ventricular filling), increasing end-diastolic volume and enables more blood to be ejected with each beat. So, physically inactive men will typically have a lower stroke volume compared to physically active men of the same age and weight.

84—C. Systolic pressure and HR

For example, HR is 80 bpm, systolic pressure is 140.

85—D. RPP

RPP (HR × systolic BP) is a measure or indicator of the stress put on the cardiac muscle (myocardial oxygen demand), making it a better indicator of the ischemic threshold compared to HR or BP alone. Oxygen uptake is not a direct measure of ischemia.

86—C. Increased HR

HR during maximal exercise will not increase with adaptations from long-term PA. HR during maximal exercise is related to age.

87—D. Signs of poor perfusion (*i.e.*, cyanosis or pallor)

Although all of the options are potential reasons for terminating a symptom limited maximal exercise test, only "D" is a relative contraindication for termination. If benefits of exercise testing outweigh the risks, this contraindication may be superseded.

88—D. RPE

RPE, because individuals with autonomic neuropathy may show blunted HR and BP responses to exercise.

89—C. Exertional myocardial ischemia

A reversible perfusion defect is caused by decreased uptake of the radionuclide isotope by the myocardium due to the relative reduction of blood flow to the ischemic tissue during exercise. This may or may not be accompanied by symptoms of angina pectoris. This abnormality is not seen when myocardial perfusion is evaluated at rest.

90—B. BP elevations are highest during isometric muscular actions.

During isometric contractions, constant — rather than rhythmic — force is generated by the skeletal muscle fibers. This constant force exerts pressure on the blood vessels, which results in occlusion (or blocking) of blood flow through the vessels. Because of this vascular resistance and the heart's efforts to overcome it, BP is highest during isometric contractions. Because of the associated cardiovascular challenges, isometric contractions should be avoided, particularly among those with known CVD.

91—D. HR returns to rest slower.

Because a transplanted heart is denervated, it lacks direct autonomic control of HR. Without parasympathetic innervation, HR is slower to return to preexercise levels.

92—A. Decreased TG and increased HDL

Chronic exercise training has its greatest benefit on lowering TG and increasing HDL. Changes in total cholesterol or LDL cholesterol are influenced more by dietary habits and body weight than by exercise training.

93—A. A coronary artery stent carries a lower rate of revascularization than does PTCA.

Restenosis occurs within 6 mo in approximately 30%–50% of patients who have had a PTCA, whereas a stent has about a 25% failure rate and the drug-eluting stent having a restenosis rate in the low single digits. Atherectomy can be used along with PTCA and is useful when the PTCA catheter cannot pass through the artery, but atherectomy is not a prerequisite for PTCA. Internal mammary artery grafts are preferred over saphenous venous grafts because of superior patency (90% vs. <50% at 10 yr). About 25%–50% of patients will experience a restenosis within 6 mo of laser angioplasty.

94—B. An increase in the anginal threshold compared with a test without the medication

β-Blockers increase the anginal threshold by reducing myocardial oxygen demand at rest and during exercise. This occurs through a reduction in chronotropic (HR) and inotropic (strength of contraction) responses. BP is also reduced at rest and during exercise by a reduction in cardiac output (reduced chronotropic and inotropic response) and a reduction in total peripheral resistance. β-Blockers do not produce ST-segment changes on the resting ECG.

95—A. Has been physically active on a regular basis for <6 mo

Stages of motivational readiness describe five categories of readiness to change or maintain behavior. As applied to PA or exercise, they are precontemplation (stage 1), contemplation (stage 2), preparation (stage 3), action (stage 4), and maintenance (stage 5). The action stage is when the person is engaged in PA or exercise that meets the current ACSM's recommendations for PA but has not maintained this program for 6 mo or more.

96—A. Monitored immediately and then every 1–2 min for 5 min of recovery or until exercise-induced changes are at baseline

The 12-lead ECG should be recorded immediately after exercise and then every 1–2 min for 5 min or until exercise-induced ECG changes are at baseline.

97—D. Multiple-gated acquisition (MUGA) (blood pool imagery) study

MUGA study may be performed to assess resting and exercise cardiac function related to cardiac output, ejection fraction, and wall motion. In this test, technetium-99m is injected into the bloodstream, where it attaches to red blood cells. Areas where the blood pools, such as the ventricles, are visualized by the technetium emissions.

98—A. The plan should list the schedule of each staff member so that they can all be accounted for during an emergency.

Accounting for staff in an emergency is not essential. Writing down the plan is essential so that the staff can read it as part of their training as well as have a document to refer to during an emergency. Delineating specific actions by each staff member in an emergency situation and training the staff in these actions obviously are integral parts of any emergency plan.

99—C. They should not be encouraged to return to work.

Exercise programs consisting of aerobic and resistance training specific to provide muscular strength and endurance appropriate for their previous occupation, and improve their ability to work, self-efficacy, and comfort with working after their illness, as long as adjustments are appropriately made.

100—C. Data should be kept on file for at least 1 yr before being discarded.

There is no accepted minimal or maximal amount of time that data should be stored. Clearly, however, data must be stored in a confidential (lock-and-key) manner, and discretion must be used when sharing data.

CEP EXAMINATION QUESTIONS BY DOMAIN

Use the following table as a guide to assist you in your studying process. It is important to note that some questions can be classified as testing multiple domains by the knowledge and skills (KSs).

Domain Number	I	II	III	IV	V
Domain Name	Patient/Client Assessment	Exercise Prescription	Program Implementation and Ongoing Support	Leadership and Counseling	Legal and Professional Considerations
Percentage of Questions from Domain	30%	30%	20%	15%	5%
Question Numbers	3, 7, 8, 9, 16, 18, 19, 20, 21, 22, 25, 27, 28, 29, 30, 31, 33, 36, 37, 40, 44, 52, 54, 60, 65, 66, 67, 69, 70, 88	2, 4, 5, 6, 10, 11, 17, 23, 24, 26, 32, 39, 41, 46, 47, 53, 58, 59, 63, 64, 73, 74, 75, 76, 77, 89, 90, 94, 96, 97	15, 34, 35, 42, 43, 45, 51, 55, 68, 71, 72, 78, 79, 80, 81, 87, 91, 92, 93, 99	12, 13, 14, 49, 50, 56, 57, 61, 62, 82, 83, 84, 85, 86, 95	1, 38, 48, 98, 100

A Editors for the Previous Two Editions

EDITORS FOR THE 4TH EDITION

SENIOR EDITOR

Gregory B. Dwyer, PhD, FACSM, ACSM-ETT, ACSM-CES, ACSM-RCEP, ACSM-PD
East Stroudsburg University
East Stroudsburg, Pennsylvania

ASSOCIATE EDITORS

Nancy J. Belli, MA, ACSM-HFS
Asphalt Green
New York, New York

Meir Magal, PhD, FACSM, ACSM-CES
North Carolina Wesleyan College
Rocky Mount, North Carolina

Paul Sorace, MS, ACSM-RCEP
Hackensack University Medical Center
Hackensack, New Jersey

EDITORS FOR THE 3RD EDITION

SENIOR EDITORS

Khalid W. Bibi, PhD
Professor and Chair, Department of Sports Medicine,
Health & Human Performance
Professor, Graduate School of Education
Canisius College
Buffalo, New York

Michael G. Niederpruem, MS
Vice President of Certification
American Health Information Management Association
Chicago, Illinois

Contributors to the Previous Two Editions

CONTRIBUTING AUTHORS TO THE FOURTH EDITION

Nancy J. Belli, MA, ACSM-HFS
Asphalt Green
New York, New York
Cases: Domain of Legal, Professional, Business, and Marketing for CPT

Clinton Brawner, MS, FACSM, ACSM-RCEP, ACSM-CES
Henry Ford Hospital
Detroit, Michigan
Cases: Domain of Patient/Client Assessment for CES (Electrocardiograms)

Nikki Carosone Russo, MS, ACSM-CPT
Long Island University
Brooklyn, New York
Cases: Domain of Exercise Programming and Implementation for CPT

Brian Coyne, MEd, ACSM-RCEP, ACSM/NCPAD-CIFT
Duke University Health System
Durham, North Carolina
Cases: Domain of Exercise Counseling and Behavioral Strategies for HFS

Donald M. Cummings, PhD, ACSM-CES
East Stroudsburg University
East Stroudsburg, Pennsylvania
Cases: Domain of Exercise Prescription for CES

Shala E. Davis, PhD, FACSM, ACSM-ETT, ACSM-CES, ACSM-PD
East Stroudsburg University
East Stroudsburg, Pennsylvania
Cases: Domain of Leadership and Counseling for CES

Kimberly DeLeo, BS, PTA, ACSM-CPT
Health and Exercise Connections, LLC
Middleboro, Massachusetts
Cases: Domain of Legal, Professional, Business, and Marketing for CPT

Julie J. Downing, PhD, FACSM, ACSM-CPT, ACSM-HFS
Central Oregon Community College
Bend, Oregon
Cases: Domain of Health and Fitness Assessment for HFS

Shawn Drake, PT, PhD, ACSM-RCEP, ACSM-PD
Arkansas State University
Jonesboro, Arkansas
Cases: Domain of Exercise Prescription and Implementation for EP-C

Trent A. Hargens, PhD, ACSM-CES
James Madison University
Harrisonburg, Virginia
Cases: Domain of Patient/Client Assessment for CES

Dennis Kerrigan, PhD, ACSM-CES
Henry Ford Hospital
Detroit, Michigan
Cases: Domain of Patient/Client Assessment for CES (Electrocardiograms)

Frederick Klinge, MBA, ACSM-HFS
Ochsner Health System/Varsity Sports
New Orleans, Louisiana
Cases: Domain of Management for HFS

Timothy S. Maynard, MS, ACSM-PD
Providence Hospital
Mobile, Alabama
Cases: Domain of Legal and Professional Considerations for CES

Matthew W. Parrott, PhD, ACSM-HFS
H-P Fitness, LLC
Kansas City, Missouri
Cases: Domain of Legal/Professional for HFS

James H. Ross, MS, ACSM-RCEP, ACSM-CES
Wake Forest University
Winston-Salem, North Carolina
Cases: Domain of Exercise Prescription for CES

Tom Spring, MS, FAACVPR, ACSM-CPT, ACSM-HFS, ACSM-CES
WebMD Health Services
Detroit, Michigan
Cases: Domain of Initial Client Consultation and Assessment for CPT

David E. Verrill, MS, FAACVPR, ACSM-RCEP, ACSM-CES
University of North Carolina at Charlotte
Charlotte, North Carolina
Cases: Domain of Program Implementation and Ongoing Support for CES

Janet P. Wallace, PhD, FACSM, ACSM-CES, ACSM-PD
Indiana University
Bloomington, Indiana
Cases: Domain of Exercise Prescription for CES

Michael J. Webster, PhD, FACSM, ACSM-CES
University of Southern Mississippi
Hattiesburg, Mississippi
Cases: Domain of Exercise Leadership and Client Education for CPT

CONTRIBUTORS TO THE 3RD EDITION

CHAPTER AUTHORS

Chapter 1

Jeffrey J. Betts, PhD
Health Sciences Department
Central Michigan University
Mt. Pleasant, Michigan

Elaine Filusch Betts, PhD, PT, FACSM
Physical Therapy
Central Michigan University
Mt. Pleasant, Michigan

Chad Harris, PhD
Department of Kinesiology
Boise State University
Boise, Idaho

Chapter 2

Michael Deschenes, PhD, FACSM
Kinesiology Department
College of William & Mary
Williamsburg, Virginia

Chapter 3

Deborah Riebe, PhD, FACSM
Department of Kinesiology
University of Rhode Island
Kingston, Rhode Island

Robert S. Mazzeo, PhD, FACSM
Department of Integrative Physiology
University of Colorado
Boulder, Colorado

David S. Criswell, PhD
Department of Applied Physiology and Kinesiology
University of Florida
Gainesville, Florida

Chapter 4

Carol Ewing Garber, PhD, FFAHA, ACSM
Department of Biobehavioral Sciences
Teachers College
Columbia University
New York, New York

Chapter 5

Andrea Dunn, PhD, FACSM
Klein Buendel Inc.
Golden, Colorado

Bess H. Marcus, PhD
Community Health and Psychiatry and Human Behavior
Brown University
Providence, Rhode Island

David E. Verrill, MS, FAACVPR
Presbyterian Hospital
Presbyterian Center for Preventive Cardiology
Charlotte, North Carolina

Chapter 6

Stephen C. Glass, PhD, FACSM
Department of Movement Science
Grand Valley State University
Allendale, Michigan

Chapter 7

Frederick S. Daniels, MS, MBA
CPTE Health Group
Nashua, New Hampshire

Nancy J. Belli, MA
Physical Activity Department
Plus One Holdings, Inc.
New York, New York

Kathy Donofrio
Swedish Covenant Hospital
Chicago, Illinois

Chapter 8

Kathleen M. Cahill, MS, ATC
Sugar Land, Texas

John W. Wygand, MA
Adelphi University
Human Performance Laboratory
Garden City, New York

Julie J. Downing, PhD, FACSM
Central Oregon Community College
Health and Human Performance
Bend, Oregon

Chapter 9

Janet R. Wojcik, PhD
Department of Health and Physical Education
Winthrop University
Rock Hill, South Carolina

R. Carlton Bessinger, PhD, RD
Department of Human Nutrition
Winthrop University
Rock Hill, South Carolina

Chapter 10

Frederick S. Daniels, MS
CPTE Health Group
Nashua, New Hampshire

Gregory B. Dwyer, PhD, FACSM
Department of Exercise Science
East Stroudsburg University
East Stroudsburg, Pennsylvania

Chapter 11

Khalid W. Bibi, PhD
Sports Medicine, Health and Human Performance
Canisius College
Buffalo, New York

Dennis W. Koch, PhD
Human Performance Center
Canisius College
Buffalo, New York

Chapter 12

Theodore J. Angelopoulos, PhD, MPH
Center for Lifestyle Medicine
University of Central Florida
Orlando, Florida

Joshua Lowndes, MA
Center for Lifestyle Medicine
University of Central Florida
Orlando, Florida

CHAPTER CONTRIBUTORS

Chapter 1

John Mayer, PhD, DC
Spine and Sport Foundation
San Diego, California

Brian Undermann, PhD, ATC, FACSM
Department of Exercise and Sports Science
University of Wisconsin-La Crosse
La Crosse, Wisconsin

Chapter 10

Neal I. Pire, MA
Plus One Fitness
New York, New York

Kathy Donofrio
Swedish Covenant Hospital
Chicago, Illinois

Chapter 11

Stephen C. Glass, PhD, FACSM
Department of Movement Science
Grand Valley State University
Allendale, Michigan

ACSM Certified Clinical Exercise Physiologist. *See* CEP

ACSM Certified Exercise Physiologist. *See* EP-C

ACSM Certified Personal Trainer. *See* CPT

CEP
  case studies, 157–184
    answers and explanations, 185–206
  domains
    Domain I (patient/client assessment)
      case study related to, 157–158
      job task analysis information and
        resources, 207–213
    Domain II (exercise prescription)
      case studies related to, 158–169
      job task analysis information and
        resources, 214–219
    Domain III (program implementation
      and ongoing support)
      case study related to, 169–172
      job task analysis information and
        resources, 219–226
    Domain IV (leadership and
      counseling)
      case study related to, 172–173
      job task analysis information and
        resources, 226–231
    Domain V (legal and professional
      considerations)
      case studies related to, 173–175
      job task analysis information and
        resources, 231–234
  ECG case studies, 175–184
    answers and explanations, 202–206
  examination, 235–243
    answers and explanations, 244–253
    questions by domain, 253
  job task analysis, 207–234
    exercise prescription (Domain II)
      clinically appropriate prescription
        development, 214–215
      instruction in safe and effective
        use of exercise modalities,
        218–219
      prescription and program review
        with participant, 216–217
    leadership and counseling (Domain IV)
      collaboration with health care
        professionals, 230–231
      creation of positive environment,
        229–230
      education about disease
        management and risk factor
        reduction, 228–229
      education about performance and
        progress, 226–228

    legal and professional considerations
      (Domain V)
      continuing education, 234
      emergency equipment and
        procedures, 232
      environment evaluation and facility
        inspection, 231
      Health Insurance Portability
        and Accountability Act
        (HIPAA), 233
      healthy lifestyle practices, 233
      safety procedures and self-
        monitoring, 232–233
    patient/client assessment (Domain I)
      participant risk evaluation,
        monitoring, and supervision,
        210–211
      physician referral and medical
        records, 207
      preparticipation screening,
        208–210
    program implementation and ongoing
      support (Domain III)
      participant feedback assessment,
        222–223
      participant records, progress, and
        clinical status, 226
      program implementation,
        219–221
      program reassessment and updating,
        224–225
CPT
  case studies, 3–12
    answers and explanations, 12–19
  domains
    Domain I (initial client consultation and
      assessment)
      case study related to, 3–4
      job task analysis information and
        resources, 21–28
    Domain II (exercise programming and
      implementation)
      case studies related to, 4–8
      job task analysis information and
        resources, 29–41
    Domain III (exercise leadership and
      client education)
      case studies related to, 8–11
      job task analysis information and
        resources, 41–46
    Domain IV (legal, professional,
      business, and marketing)
      case study related to, 11–12
      job task analysis information and
        resources, 46–56

  examination, 59–66
    answers and explanations, 67–77
    questions by domain, 77
  job task analysis, 21–56
    exercise leadership and client education
      (Domain III)
      client education, knowledge base,
        and fitness-related information,
        43–46
      creating positive exercise experience,
        41–43
    exercise programming and
      implementation (Domain II)
      client feedback, satisfaction, and
        enjoyment, 41
      exercise modality selection, 30–32
      frequency, intensity, time, and
        type (FITT) determination,
        32–34
      modify frequency, intensity, time,
        and type (FITT), 40
      monitoring client technique and
        exercise response, 38–39
      program review with client, 35–38
      training program determination,
        29–30
    initial client consultation and
      assessment (Domain I)
      behavioral readiness evaluation for
        exercise adherence, 23
      client data, risk stratification, action
        plan, and physical assessment,
        22–23
      client instructions and initial
        documents, 21
      client interview, 22
      fitness assessments, goal setting,
        and baseline for program
        development, 24–28
      reassessment plan/timeline
        development, 28
    legal, professional, business, and
      marketing (Domain IV)
      ACSM Code of Ethics, 51–52
      business plan development, 52–53
      collaboration with health care
        professionals and organizations,
        47–48
      confidentiality and privacy, 56
      continuing education program
        participation, 51
      copyrights and intellectual property,
        55–56
      insurance and industry-accepted
        practices, 54

CPT (continued)
marketing, networking, and promotion, 53–54
medical clearance, 46–47
modeling healthy lifestyle practices, 55
risk management program, 48–51
EP-C
case studies, 81–89
answers and explanations, 90–95
domains
Domain I (health and fitness assessment)
case study related to, 81–83
job task analysis information and resources, 97–105
Domain II (exercise prescription, implementation, and ongoing support)
case study related to, 83–84
job task analysis information and resources, 106–121
Domain III (exercise counseling and behavioral strategies)
case study related to, 84–85
job task analysis information and resources, 121–126
Domain IV (legal and professional)
case study related to, 85–87
job task analysis information and resources, 126–130
Domain V (management)
case study related to, 87–89
job task analysis information and resources, 130–133

examination, 135–142
answers and explanations, 143–153
questions by domain, 153
job task analysis, 97–133
exercise counseling and behavioral strategies (Domain III)
behavioral and motivational strategies, 122–124
communication techniques, 121–122
educational resources, 124–125
support within scope of practice and referral, 126
exercise prescription, implementation, and ongoing support (Domain II)
cardiorespiratory exercise prescription, FITT principle, 108–110
determining program to achieve desired outcomes and goals, 106–108
environmental conditions and prescription modification, 120–121
flexibility, muscular strength, muscular endurance, FITT principle, 111–114
healthy special populations, 118–120
participants with controlled cardiovascular, pulmonary, and metabolic diseases and other clinical populations, 117–118
progression guidelines for resistance, aerobic, and flexibility activities, 114

screening, health appraisal, exercise history, and fitness assessment review, 106
weight management program, 115–117
health and fitness assessment (Domain I)
anthropometric and body composition assessments, 105
assessment protocols and preparticipation health screening, 97
cardiorespiratory fitness assessments, 101–103
muscular strength, muscular endurance, and flexibility, 103–104
participant's readiness, 98–100
selection and preparation for healthy participants and those with controlled disease, 100–101
legal and professional (Domain IV)
injury prevention program, emergency policies and procedures, 129–130
risk management guidelines, 126–128
management (Domain V)
communication techniques and professional relationships, 133
fiscal resources, 131
human resources, 130
marketing plan, 132–133
policies and procedures for health/fitness facilities, 131–132